Pathogenesis, Diagnosis and Management of Colorectal Cancer

Pathogenesis, Diagnosis and Management of Colorectal Cancer

Editor: Lancel Herring

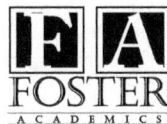

FA
FOSTER
ACADEMICS

www.fosteracademics.com

www.fosteracademics.com

FA
FOSTER
A C A D E M I C S

Cataloging-in-Publication Data

Pathogenesis, diagnosis and management of colorectal cancer / edited by Lancel Herring.
     p. cm.
Includes bibliographical references and index.
ISBN 978-1-63242-748-9
1. Colon (Anatomy)--Cancer--Pathogenesis. 2. Rectum--Cancer--Pathogenesis.
3. Colon (Anatomy)--Cancer--Diagnosis. 4. Rectum--Cancer--Diagnosis.
5. Colon (Anatomy)--Cancer--Treatment. 6. Rectum--Cancer--Treatment. I. Herring, Lancel.
RC280.C6 P38 2019
616.994 347--dc23

Foster Academics,
118-35 Queens Blvd., Suite 400,
Forest Hills, NY 11375, USA

ISBN 978-1-63242-748-9 (Hardback)

Contents

Preface

The purpose of the book is to provide a glimpse into the dynamics and to present opinions and studies of some of the scientists engaged in the development of new ideas in the field from very different standpoints. This book will prove useful to students and researchers owing to its high content quality.

Colorectal cancer refers to the cancer of the rectum or colon. Its symptoms are a change in bowel movement, weight loss, blood in the stool and a persistent state of exhaustion. Consumption of processed meat, red meat and alcohol, lack of physical activity, obesity and smoking are considered risk factors that contribute to the occurrence of this cancer. It can be diagnosed by performing a colonoscopy or sigmoidoscopy, or by a microscopical examination of a tissue sample. A referral medical imaging determines the spread or localization of the disease. Colorectal cancer can be treated through a combination of chemotherapy, radiation therapy, surgery and targeted therapy. Depending on the stage of the tumor and patient's health, treatment can be palliative or done with the intent to cure. The topics covered in this extensive book deal with the core aspects of colorectal cancer. Its aim is to present researches pertaining to the pathogenesis, diagnosis and management of colorectal cancer. It will prove to be immensely beneficial to students and researchers in this field.

At the end, I would like to appreciate all the efforts made by the authors in completing their chapters professionally. I express my deepest gratitude to all of them for contributing to this book by sharing their valuable works. A special thanks to my family and friends for their constant support in this journey.

Editor

Robot-Assisted Colonic Resections for Cancer

Monica Ortenzi, Giovanni Lezoche,
Roberto Ghiselli and Mario Guerrieri

Abstract

Minimally invasive surgery for colon cancer, if compared with open surgery, has shown similar oncologic outcomes, and it has become the standard management for malignant colonic disease. Its benefits appear yet in early post-operative period such as less postoperative pain, earlier recovery of gastrointestinal functions and shorter hospital stay. Robotic surgery was born in the attempt to overcome the intrinsic limitations of laparoscopic technique. It offers the possibility to have a tridimensional magnified view of surgical field and to use wristed instrument to perform an accurate dissection and lymphadenectomy. It provides the possibility to rotate at 360 degrees the instruments, facilitating considerably the performance of intracorporeal ileo-colic anastomosis in right colectomy. We want to illustrate the feasibility and technique to carry out right and left colectomy in a robotic-assisted way and its advantages with respect to laparoscopic surgery.

Keywords: robot-assisted, surgery, laparoscopy, colon, cancer

1. Introduction

Colon cancer has always been a hot topic, and a revolution has come about in its surgical management in the past 20 years with the introduction of laparoscopic surgery. This progress has culminated with the advent of robotic surgery.

Robotic surgery came about in an attempt to overcome the limitations of laparoscopy mainly because of long rigid instruments, poor ergonomics, and two-dimensional visualization [1–3].

Robotic system was introduced in the surgical field more than 25 years ago [4].

Laparoscopic and robotic surgeries have walked along a parallel path. When Semm reported the first laparoscopic appendectomy in 1983, the "Arthrobot" was first applied in orthopedic operations, which marked the beginning of robotic surgery [5].

Robotic technology applied to surgical procedures has had a rapid growth since then. PUMA (Programmable Universal Machine for Assembly), SARP (Surgeon-Assistant Robot for Prostatectomy) systems, PROBOT (Prostate robot), VRobot (Urology robot), and SPUD (Surgeon Programmable Urological Device) have been introduced and applied in urologic surgery [6–9].

The first robotic device approved by the US Food and Drug Administration (FDA) in 1994 was the AESOP (Automated Endoscopic System for Optimal Positioning) system followed by the ZEUS system (Computer Motion Inc.) in 1998 [10].

The ZEUS robotic system consisted of two separate components: a surgeon control center and three robotic arms attached to the operating table that provided four degrees of freedom and were able to hold various instruments, telemanipulated with joysticks at distance from the surgical console [11].

In 1998, this system was the one used for the first abdominal robotic procedure for fallopian tube anastomosis at Cleveland Clinic [12].

In 2001, Jacques Marescaux used the ZEUS system to perform the transatlantic robot-assisted cholecystectomy known as "Operation Lindbergh", between New York and Strasburg giving a great demonstration of telepresence surgery [13].

In 2001, 10 years after the first laparoscopic colectomy, Weber described the first robot-assisted colectomy [14].

The first fully robotic system that was approved by FDA in 2000 for its application in laparoscopic surgery was the da Vinci™ Surgical System.

It derives its name from military medical research and was initially developed in a project funded by the Pentagon's Defense Advanced Research Projects Agency with the aim of allowing remote operations on wounded soldiers [15].

This system was developed by Intuitive Surgical (Mountain View, CA). Later, Intuitive Surgical introduced the da Vinci S system, the da Vinci Si system, and the da Vinci Xi system in 2006, 2009, and 2014, respectively [16].

The da Vinci Si system consists of a remote surgeon's console, a patient cart, and a vision cart.

The console is composed of a stereo viewer, which provides a three-dimensional visualization of the operative field with 10× magnification, a touchpad, which allows for arms and control selection, and joysticks to control the instrument arms remotely. The footswitch panel is located at the base of the console and is composed of two groups of footswitches. The three switches on the left control the functions of the system such as camera control, master clutch, and arm swap. The four pedals on the right side of the footswitch panel are used for power supply.

The four arms of the column hold the robotic instruments.

They are wrapped in sterile drapes for operations and have clutch buttons used to vary arm joint angulation to adjust the instrument arms even during the procedure.

EndoWrist instruments are installed onto the instrument arms after the system is docked to ports that are inserted into the patient's abdominal wall. Most instruments offer seven degrees of freedom and 90° of articulation in the wrist.

The system provides for tremor filtration and scaled motion, translating larger movements of the surgeon's hands into finer motions of the instruments.

The vision cart includes a 24-inch touch screen monitor and provides shelves for optional surgical equipment such as insufflators and electrosurgical generators [16–18].

2. Right colectomy

This procedure is carried out in a three-arm technique.

The patient is placed in the supine position under general anesthesia with the arms alongside the body and in a mild reverse Trendelenburg position with a left tilt. This position allows the surgeon to expose the patient's right and transverse colon by moving the small bowel aside under gravity. Final positioning is adjusted according to the operative field exposure before robot docking.

Pneumoperitoneum is induced with a supraumbilical incision and the pressure is maintained between 12 and 15 mmHg.

A 12-mm port for the air sealer is positioned on the left midclavicular line, on transverse umbilical line. A 30° laparoscope is used in this procedure.

Once the 12-mm port for the laparoscope and the camera is inserted in the supraumbilical incision, the other port is placed under vision.

A total of four ports (three robotic ports and one assistant port) are set.

We usually place an 8-mm port for instrument arm 1 on the axillary line, 2 cm below the left costal margin, and another suprapubic 8 mm port for instrument arm 2. An assistant 10–12 mm port is placed on the left of the camera port.

The surgical cart is positioned cranial to the patient's head.

The bipolar vessel sealer, used to coagulate and dissect tissues, and the fenestrated grasper are mounted on arms 1 and 2.

The bed-assistant surgeon introduces a laparoscopic grasper used to give tension and facilitate the dissection.

The ileocolic vessels are identified, and the peritoneum is opened just below their prominence. Ileocolic vessels are divided, and the dissection is continued in an avascular plane under the right colon flexure to expose the duodenum between Gerota's fascia posteriorly and Toldt's fascia anteriorly.

Right colic vessels (if present), right colic veins, and the right branch of the middle colic artery are dissected with a bipolar vessel sealer. Parietal peritoneum is incised, and the dissection is carried out in a craniocaudal way till the cecum is reached. Once the specimen is totally mobilized, the transverse colon is resected with a mechanical stapler. In the case of intracorporeal anastomosis, the ileum is approximated to the transverse colon, and one sero-serosal stitch of suspension is positioned between the ileal loop and the transverse colon where the isoperistaltic side-to-side anastomosis is confectioned (**Figure 1**).

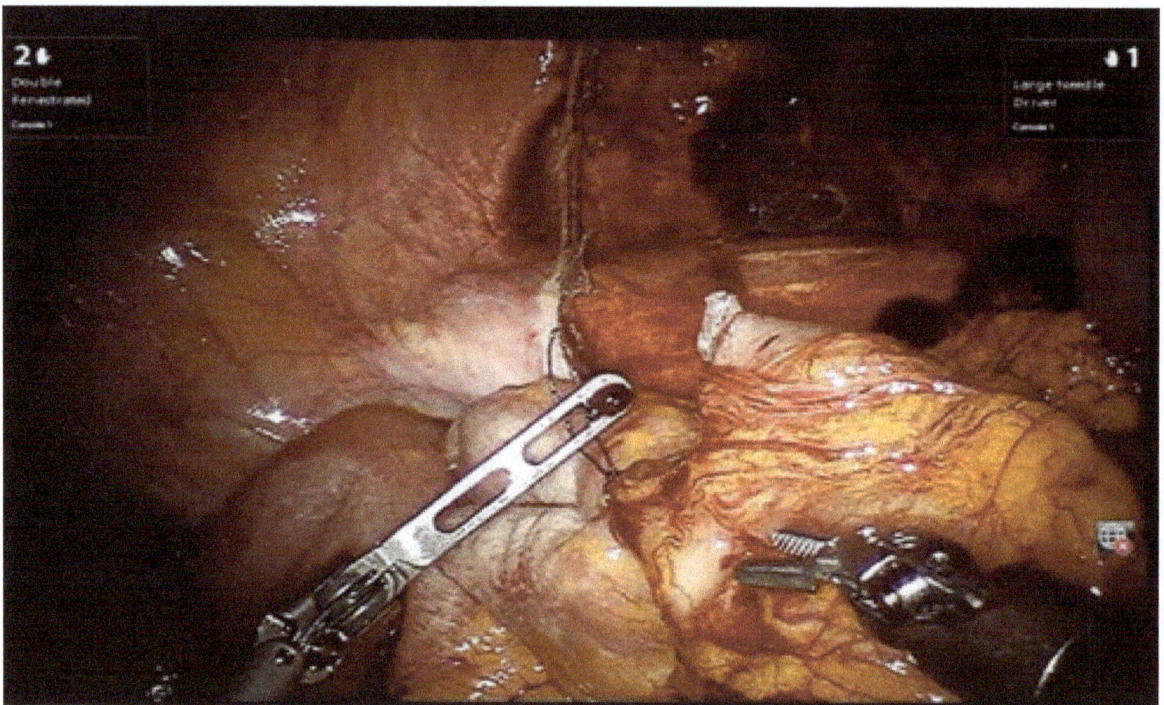

Figure 1. Suspension stitch between the ileal loop and the transverse colon.

Monopolar scissors are mounted on arm 1 and used to create enterotomies.

The surgeon-assistant introduces the larger part of the cartridge inside the colostomy and then the smaller part into the ileum (**Figure 2**). Intracorporeal latero-lateral isoperistaltic anastomosis is done. The enterotomies are then closed with a two-layer suture: the first layer of continuous suture and a second layer of interrupted sero-serosal suture with Vicryl 3/0 (**Figure 3**). A surgical specimen is extracted through the McBurney incision in the right iliac fossa.

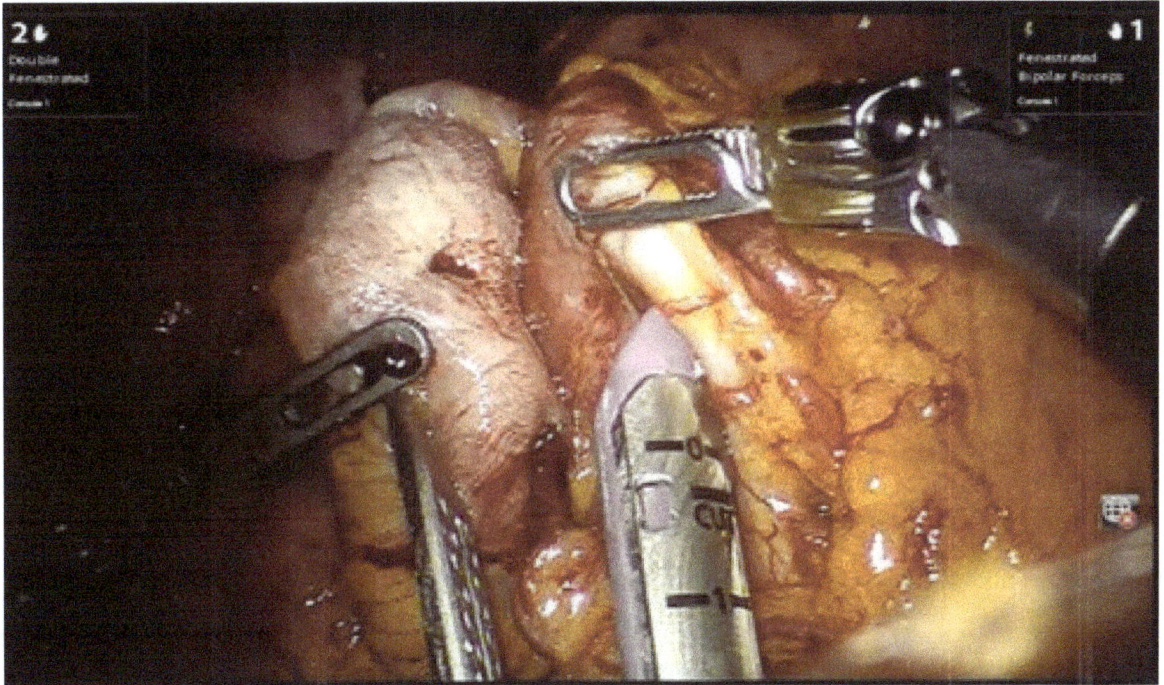

Figure 2. Insertion of the mechanical cartridge into the enterotomies.

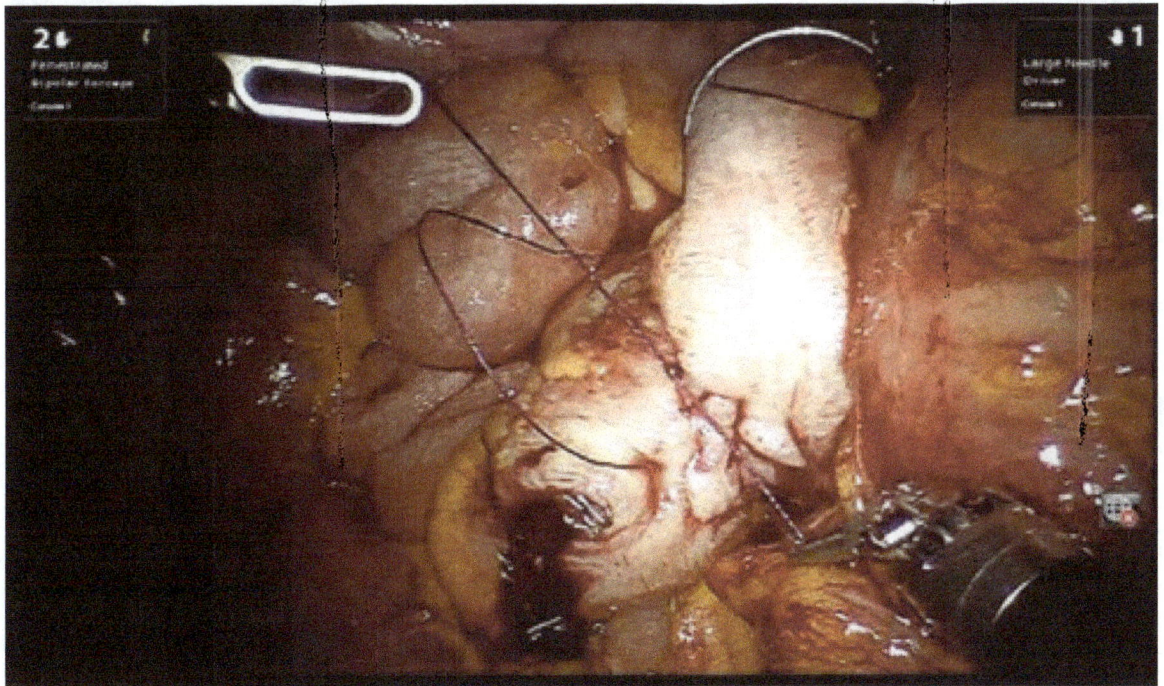

Figure 3. Closure of the enterotomies with a double layer manual suture with Vicryl 3/0.

3. Left colectomy

The patient is placed in a lithomy position with the left arm adducted.

A mild Trendelenburg position and a right tilt are set to expose the operative field. A 12-mmHg pneumoperitoneum is induced through a supraumbilical incision, and the 12-mm port for the camera is placed.

The other three 8-mm robotic ports are positioned under the vision, one on the right midclavicular line 2 cm below the right costal margin and the other in the midline under the xiphoid process. Two 10 mm trocars for the bed-assistant surgeon are added. A total of five ports are positioned. The robotic cart is on the patient's left side. The bipolar vessel sealer is mounted on arm 1. Arm 2 hosts the double fenestrated forceps. The dissection begins from the inferior mesenteric vein that is dissected by a bipolar vessel sealer once it is identified at the level of the inferior border of the pancreas.

The gastrocolic, splenocolic, and coloepiploic ligaments are dissected (**Figure 4**).

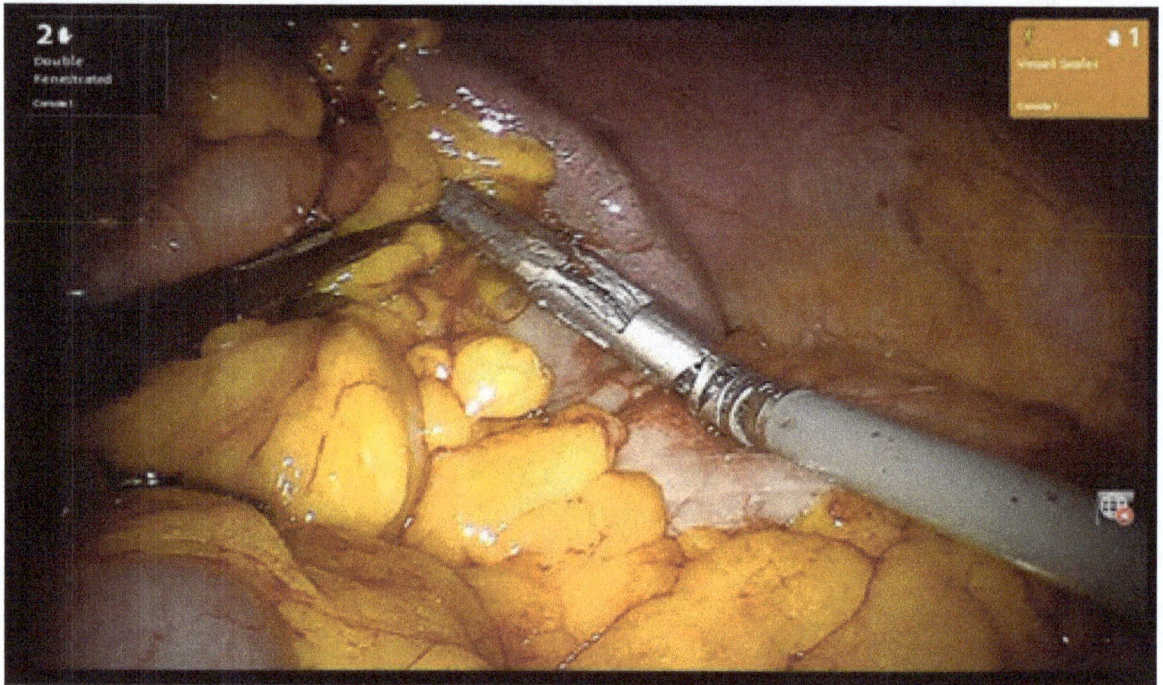

Figure 4. Division of the splenocolic ligament with electothermal bipolar vessel sealer.

The root of the transverse mesocolon is exposed by the assistant and dissected by bipolar electrocautery to expose the pancreas and allow for a full mobilization of the splenic flexure.

Then, the parietal peritoneum is incised, and the dissection is made on the avascular plane between the two folds of Toldt's fascia.

The assistant pulls up the dissected inferior mesenteric vein with a grasper, and the arch of the inferior mesenteric artery is lifted up.

Once the artery is identified, it is divided between the clips placed by the assistant.

A careful locoregional lymphadenectomy is carried out by preserving the paraaortic nerves and the superior hypogastric plexus.

The colon is resected at the level of the promontory with a mechanical stapler (**Figure 5**).

The anastomosis is fashioned according to the Knight & Griffen technique.

During this step, the robot is usually undocked.

The surgical specimen is extracted through a minilaparotomy in the left iliac fossa. The descending colon is extracted through the protected incision and transected proximally. The anvil of a circular stapler is inserted into the colon stump and fixed by a manual purse-string suture. The colon is then reintroduced into the abdomen and the minilaparotomy is closed. A laparoscopy is carried out to perform the transanal end-to-end mechanical colorectal anastomosis.

Sometimes, we did not undock the robot, and once the colon is reintroduced into the abdomen, robotic instruments are used to perform the end-to-end anastomosis (**Figure 6**).

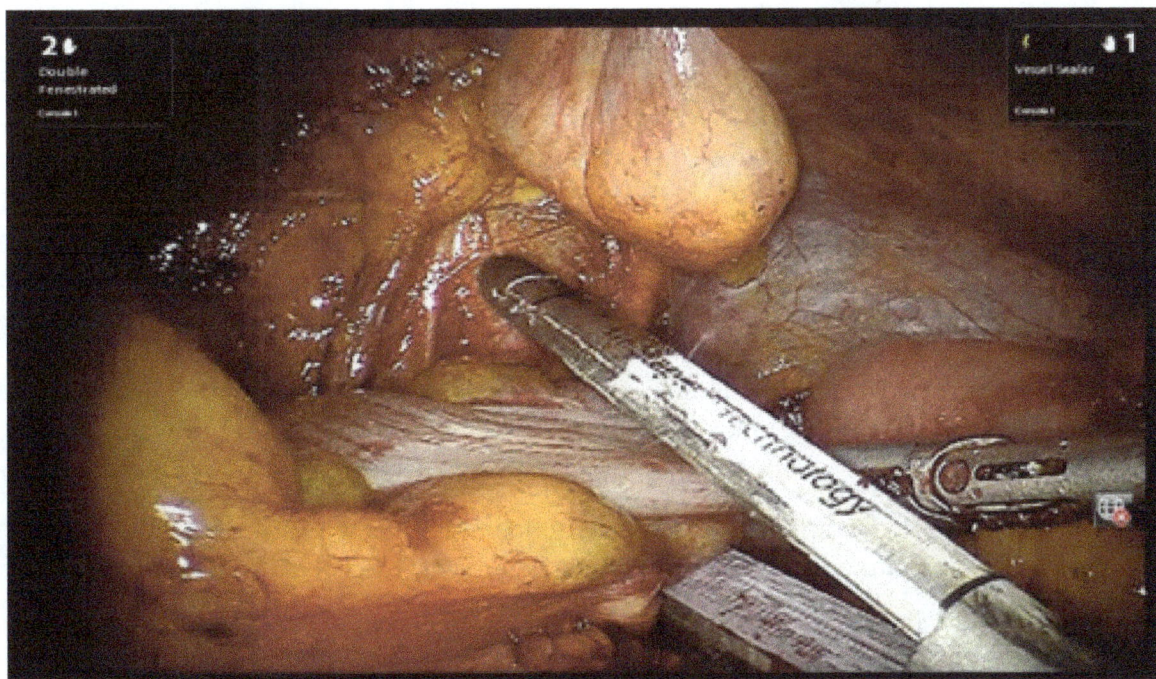

Figure 5. Section of the sigmoid colon at the level of the promontory with the mechanical cartridge.

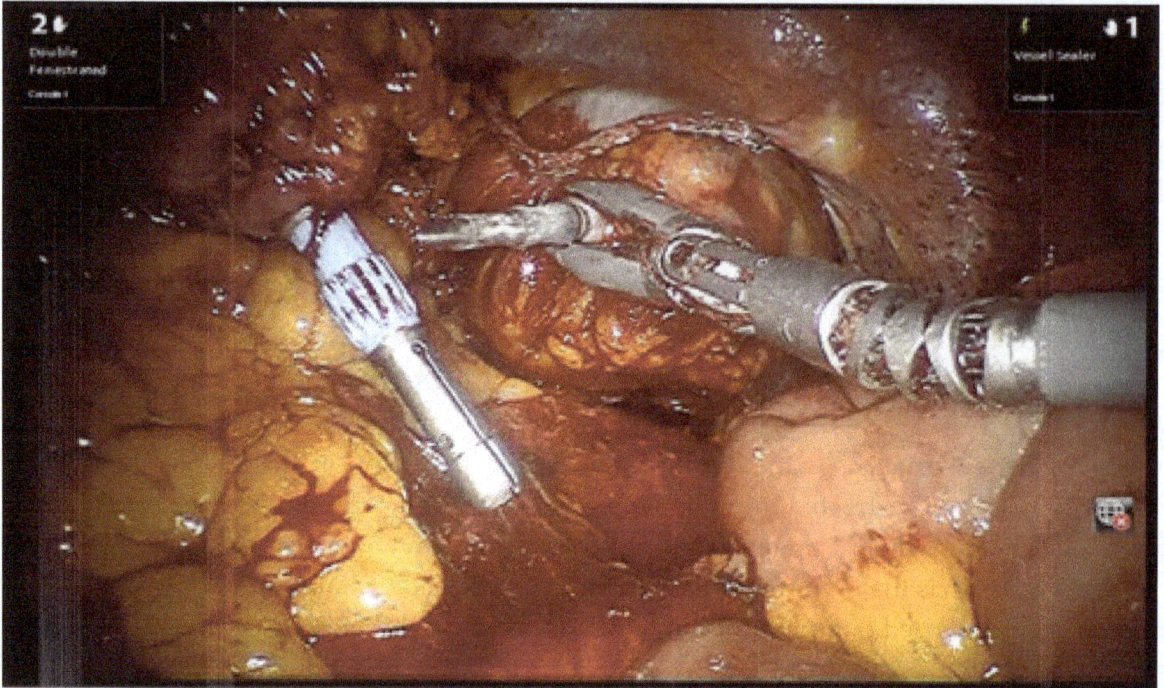

Figure 6. Confection of the end-to-end anastomosis without undocking the robotic system.

4. Advantages

Findings from the literature show how robot-assisted right and left hemicolectomies are comparable to conventional laparoscopic procedures in terms of short-term post-operative outcomes [18].

Patients undergoing robotic procedures typically return to normal activity faster and experience very low mortality and morbidity events [19–25].

The indications for robotic colectomy are well described and include benign conditions, such as inflammatory bowel disease, volvulus, diverticular disease, arteriovenous malformations, ischemic colitis, and polyps not amenable to endoscopic removal [26]. There are also emergent indications such as nearly obstructing lesions, ischemic colitis, and hemorrhage [27, 28].

Patients with contraindications for pneumoperitoneum, with an advanced disease invading adjacent organ and tumor greater than 8 cm in diameter, are contraindicated for robotic colectomy [26].

Colorectal robotic surgery also seems to be feasible for malignant disease comparable results in terms of oncologic radicality and surgical accuracy and in terms of short-term outcomes with respect to standard laparoscopy [18].

In a study of 50 consecutive right colectomies for cancer, D'Annibale et al. did not notice any statistically significant difference between laparoscopic and robotic groups in pathologic parameters and lymph node harvest. They concluded that robotic right colectomy was safe and provided adequate oncologic resection with acceptable short-term results [29].

However, if laparoscopic and robotic colectomies could be compared in terms of post-operative course and oncological outcomes, the robotic system offers several undoubtable technical advantages in performing colon surgery.

Robotic surgery allows an enhanced stabilized three-dimensional stereoscopic vision of the operative field and depth perception beyond the standard two-dimensional laparoscopic monitor [29, 30].

The da Vinci Si system provides hand stabilization, eliminating surgeon tremor and allowing for the refinement of scaled movements [29, 30]. This gives the surgeon the possibility to obtain greater precision in the surgical field.

In addition, the surgeon can work in a more ergonomic position compared with laparoscopic procedures that sometimes require maintaining a difficult posture even in long-lasting procedures [3, 20].

This improved surgical dexterity makes the switch to an intracorporeal anastomosis easier, which may lead to a higher adoption rate for intracorporeal anastomosis for right colectomies.

The potential benefits of intracorporeal anastomosis have been described in several studies and were known from laparoscopy.

Hanna et al. [31] recently concluded that intracorporeal anastomosis in laparoscopic right hemicolectomy is associated with similar post-operative and non-inferior oncologic outcomes compared with extracorporeal anastomosis, but it offers several advantages including freedom of specimen extraction sites, smaller incisions, and a lower risk of conversion to open resection especially in morbidly obese patients.

Hellan et al. [32] have found similar outcomes with intracorporeal and extracorporeal anastomosis but shorter incisions with intracorporeal anastomosis. Grams et al. [33] have reported an earlier return of bowel function, shorter length of hospital stay, and fewer complications.

Better outcomes are achieved when an intracorporeal anastomosis is performed. This is probably because of less traction and tension applied to the colon and the mesentery during an intracorporeal anastomosis as well as because of less trauma to the incision, which may result in less post-operative ileus and fewer complications [31, 34].

Another advantage in performing an intracorporeal anastomosis is the possibility to choose where to make the incision for extraction. In fact, keeping the extraction site far from the midline results in decreased risk of incisional hernia [35, 36].

The three-dimensional vision also provides advantages in mobilizing the left colic flexure with an accurate identification of the flexure borders and its relation to the spleen, while a gentle traction on the spleen is granted by the robotic arm, avoiding the risk of splenic rupture or laceration [14, 27, 36–38, 42].

Authors (years)	Patients (n)	OT (min)	HLN (n)	IC (%)	CR (%)	HS (days)	PC (%)	MR (%)
Rawling et al. [23]	LRC: 15	169.2			13.3	5.5	13.3	
	RRC: 17	189.9			0	5.2	11.7	
Park et al. [19]	LRC: 35	130	30.8	0	0	8.3	17.1	0
	RRC: 35	195	29.9	0	0	7.9	20	0
Deutsch et al. [20]	LRC: 47	214.4	18.7		0	6.3	42.55	2.12
	RRC: 18	219.2	21.1		11.1	4.3	33.33	0
Halabi et al. [21]	LRC: 53413					6	0.04	0.51
	RRC: 670					6	0	0
Casillas et al. [22]	LRC: 110	79	24	0	9.90	29	35	1
	RRC: 52	143	28	0	4.17	19	17	0

LRC, laparoscopic right colectomy; RRC, robotic right colectomy; OT, operative time; IC, intraoperative complications; HLN, harvested lymph node; CR, conversion rate; HS, hospital stay; PC, post-operative complications; MR, mortality rate.

Table 1. Robotic right colectomy data review.

Authors (years)	Patients (n)	OT (min)	HLN(n)	IC (%)	CR (%)	HS (days)	PC (%)	MR (%)
Rawling et al. [23]	LLC: 27	199.4		0	0	6.6	15.38	
	RLC: 30	225.2		7.7	15.38	6	23.07	
Deutsch et al. [20]	LLC: 45	254.7	30		0	4.2	17.7	0
	RLC: 61	289.7	10		3.33	4.1	18.03	0
Casillas et al. [22]	LLC: 68	188	14	0	5.88	32	12	0
	RLC: 82		14	0	5.88	32	12	0
Halabi et al. [21]	LLC: 62235					6	0.04	0.51
	RLC: 1473					6	0	0
Lim et al. [24]	LLC: 34	217.6	16.5			6.2	10.3	0
	RLC: 146	252.5	12			5.5	5.9	0

LLC, laparoscopic left colectomy; RLC, robotic left colectomy; OT, operative time; IC, intraoperative complications; HLN, harvested lymph node; CR, conversion rate; HS, hospital stay; PC, post-operative complications; MR, mortality rate.

Table 2. Robotic left colectomy review data.

The improved dexterity of the instruments favors precise tissue dissection and facilitates lymph node dissection.

Some authors have also reported lower conversion rates for laparoscopic colonic resections [16, 35, 36, 43], ranging from 0 to 4%, compared with 16.7–25%.

In our experience of 42 robotic colectomies, conversion was needed in three patients (7.1%). Two patients, who underwent right colectomy, required conversion to open surgery, one for excessive visceral obesity and the other for adhesions because of previous abdominal surgery. The mean number of lymph nodes in right colectomies (34 cases) and left colectomies (8 cases) was 17.7 and 13.9, respectively. Leak rate and 30-day mortality were 0%.

We recently conducted a retrospective analysis to compare operative measures and post-operative outcomes between laparoscopic 3D and robotic colectomy for cancer.

There were no differences between robotic colonic resections and 3D laparoscopic ones in terms of the number of lymph nodes removed and post-operative outcomes, but we found intracorporeal anastomosis easier to perform in robotic right colectomies than in the laparo-scopic ones. In left colectomies, we observed that the robotic technique provided better outcomes, with earlier solid food intake registered in patients [39] (**Tables 1** and **2**).

5. Limitations

The high cost of robotic surgery because of the purchase and maintenance of the equipment is the main limitation to the widespread diffusion of this technology [39]. We estimated a cost of €4,950 for robotic procedures versus €1,950 needed for laparoscopic ones [36]. The cost factor can be prohibitive to the availability of robotic technology restricting it only to bigger centers.

Moreover, a higher number of complications have been observed in the low volume centers when compared with medium- and high-volume centers and surgeons [40].

Furthermore, robotic procedures are associated with a significantly longer operating time. Most of the authors have reported that the docking time was the main cause of longer operating time [3, 18, 41, 44].

There are also some practical and technical disadvantages. The major technical drawback of robotic surgery is the lower tensile feedback. The surgeon must rely on visual clues through the monitor to guide the instrumentation and ensure that appropriate and safe manipulation is preserved by trying to estimate the tension placed on tissues by da Vinci's powerful robotic arms [3, 38]. Performing robotic surgery requires two equally experienced surgeons, one working from the console and the other one staying at the operating table. The risk of system malfunction, inability to reposition the patient once the robot is docked, external and internal collision of the bulky robotic arms, and limited access to the patient by the anesthesia team when the tower is placed have also been observed [3, 20].

6. Conclusions

As was the case with laparoscopy, robotic technology will certainly undergo substantial development in the near future. It has proven to be safe and feasible also in the case of cancer and comparable to laparoscopy, but it still presents some drawbacks.

However, the real benefit to the patient must be carefully proven before this technology can become widely accepted in clinical practice.

Author details

Monica Ortenzi*, Giovanni Lezoche, Roberto Ghiselli and Mario Guerrieri

*Address all correspondence to: monica.ortenzi@gmail.com

Polytechnic University of Marche, Surgical Clinic, United Hospitals, Ancona, Italy

References

[1] Ballantyne GH. (2002). Robotic surgery, telerobotic surgery, telepresence, and tele-mentoring: review of early clinical results. Surg Endosc. 10: 1389–1402.

[2] Yohannes P, Rotariu P, Pinto P, Smith AD, Lee BR. (2002). Comparison of robotic versus laparoscopic skills: is there a difference in the learning curve? Urology. 1: 39–45.

[3] Corcione F, Esposito C, Cuccurullo D, Settembre A, Miranda N, Amato F, Pirozzi F, Caiazzo P. (2005). Advantages and limits of robot-assisted laparoscopic surgery: preliminary experience. Surg Endosc. 19(1): 117–119.

[4] Kwoh YS, Hou J, Jonckheere EA, Hayati S. (1988). A robot with improved absolute positioning accuracy for CT guided stereotactic brain surgery. IEEE Trans Biomed Eng. 35(2): 153–160.

[5] Semm K. (1983). Endoscopic appendectomy. Endoscopy. 15: 59–64.

[6] Davies BL, Hibberd RD, Coptcoat MJ, Wickham JE. (1989). A surgeon robot prostatec-tomy–a laboratory evaluation. I Med Eng Tech. 13: 273–277.

[7] Harris SJ, Arambula-Cosio F, Mei Q, Hibberd RD, Davies BL, Wickham JEA, Nathan MS, Kundu B. (1997). The Probot—an active robot for procedures. Proc Inst Mech Eng H. 211: 317–325.

[8] Ho G, Ng WS, Teo MY. (2001). Experimental study of transurethral robotic laser resection of the prostate using the laser Trode lightguide. J Biomed Opt. 6: 244–251.

[9] Ho G, Ng WS, Teo MY, Cheng WS. (2001). Computer-assisted transurethral laser resection of the prostate (CALRP): theoretical and experimental motion plan. IEEE Trans Biomed Eng. 48: 1125–1133.

[10] Unger SW, Unger HM, Bass RT. (1994). AESOP robotic arm. Surg Endosc. 8: 1131.

[11] Kalan S, Chauhan S, Coelho RF, et al. (2010). History of robotic surgery. JRS. 4(3): 141–147.

[12] Falcone T, Goldberg J, Garcia-Ruiz A, Margossian H, Stevens L. (1999). Full robotic for laparoscopic tubal anastomosis: a case report. J Laparoendosc Adv Surg Tech A. 9: 107–113.

[13] Marescaux J, Leroy J, Rubino F, et al. (2002). Transcontinental robot-assisted remote telesurgery: feasibility and potential applications. Ann Surg. 235(4): 487–492.

[14] Weber P, Merola S, Wasielewski A, Ballantyne GH. (2002). Telerobotic-assisted laparoscopic right and sigmoid colectomies for benign disease. Dis Colon Rectum. 45(12): 1689–1696.

[15] Ballantyne GH, Moll F. (2003). The da Vinci telerobotic surgical system: the virtual operative field and telepresence surgery. Surg Clin North Am. 6: 1293–1304.

[16] Spinoglio G, Marano A, Priora F, Melandro F, Formisano G. (2015). History of robotic surgery. In: Spinoglio G. Editor. Robotic Surgery: Current Applications and New Trends. Springer-Verlag Italia, 2–12.

[17] Hagen ME, Curet MJ. (2014). The da Vinci Surgical® Systems. In: Watanabe G. Robotic Surgery. Springer Edition, 9–19.

[18] Spinoglio G, Summa M, Priora F, Quarati R, Testa S. (2008). Robotic colorectal surgery: first 50 cases experience. Dis Colon Rectum. 51(11): 1627–1632.

[19] Park JS, Choi GS, Park SY, Kim HJ, Ryuk JP. (2012). Randomized clinical trial of robot assisted *versus* standard laparoscopic right colectomy. Br J Surg. 99: 1219–1226.

[20] Deutsch GB, Sathyanarayana SA, Gunabushanam V, Mishra N, Rubach E, Zemon H, Klein JD, Denoto G, 3rd. (2012). Robotic vs. laparoscopic colorectal surgery: an institutional experience. Surg Endosc. 26(4): 956–963.

[21] Halabi WJ, Kang CY, Jafari MD, Nguyen VQ, Carmichael JC, Mills S, Stamos MJ, Pigazzi A. (2013). Robotic-assisted colorectal surgery in the United States: a nationwide analysis of trends and outcomes. World J Surg. 37(12): 2782–2790.

[22] Casillas MA, Jr., Leichtle SW, Wahl WL, Lampman RM, Welch KB, Wellock T, Madden EB, Cleary RK. (2014). Improved perioperative outcomes of robotic versus conventional laparoscopic colorectal operations. Am J Surg. 208(1): 33–40.

[23] Rawlings AL, Woodland JH, Vegunta RK, Crawford DL. (2007). Robotic versus laparoscopic colectomy. Surg Endosc. 21(10): 1701–1708.

[24] Lim DR, Min BS, Kim MS, Alasari S, Kim G, Hur H, Baik SH, Lee KJ, Kim NK. (2013). Robotic versus laparoscopic anterior resection of sigmoid colon cancer: comparative study of long-term oncologic outcomes. Surg Endosc. 27(4): 1379–1385.

[25] Delaney CP, et al. (2003). Comparison of robotically performed and traditional laparoscopic colorectal surgery. Dis Colon Rectum. 46:1633–1639.

[26] NCCN Clinical Practice Guidelines in Oncology: Colon Cancer. (2013). The National Comprehensive Cancer Network. http://www.nccn.org. Accessed 10 December 2012.

[27] Mutch M, Cellini C. (2011). Surgical management of colon cancer. In: Beck DE, Roberts PL, Saclarides TJ, Senagore AJ, Stamos MJ, Wexner SD. Editors. The ASCRS Textbook of Colon and Rectal Surgery. Second Edition, New York, NY: Springer Science + Business Media, LLC. 711–720.

[28] Lujan HJ, Plasencia G. (2014). Robotic right colectomy: three-arm technique. In: Kim KC. Editor, Springer Edition.

[29] D'Annibale A, Pernazza G, Morpurgo E, Monsellato I, Pende V, Lucandri G, Termini B, Orsini C, Sovernigo G. (2010). Robotic right colon resection: evaluation of first 50 consecutive cases for malignant disease. Ann Surg Oncol. 17: 2856–2862.

[30] D'Annibale A, A, Morpurgo E, Fiscon V, Trevisan P, Sovernigo G, Orsini C, Guidolin D. (2004). Robotic and laparoscopic surgery for treatment of colorectal diseases. Dis Colon Rectum. 47(12): 2162–8.

[31] Hanna MH, Hwang GS, Phelan MJ, Bui TL, Carmichael JC, Mills SD, Stamos MJ, Pigazzi A. (2015). Laparoscopic right hemicolectomy: short- and log-term outcomes of intra-corporeal versus extracorporeal anastomosis. Surg Endosc. Dec 29

[32] Hellan M, Stein H, Pigazzi A. (2009). Totally robotic low anterior resection with total mesorectal excision and splenic flexure mobilization. Surg Endosc. 23: 447–451.

[33] Grams J, Tong W, Greenstein AJ, Salky B. (2010) Comparison of intracorporeal versus extracorporeal anastomosis in laparoscopic-assisted hemicolectomy. Surg Endosc. 24(8): 1886–1891.

[34] Scatizzi M, Kroning KC, Borrelli A, Andan G, Lenzi E, Feroci F. (2010). Extracorporeal versus intracorporeal anastomosis after laparoscopic right colectomy for cancer: a case controlled study. World J Surg. 34: 2902–2908.

[35] Samia H, Lawrence J, Nobel T, Stein S, Champagne BJ, Delaney CP. (2013). Extraction site location and incisional hernias after laparoscopic colorectal surgery: should we be avoiding the midline? Am J Surg. 205: 264–226.

[36] Campagnacci R, Baldoni A, Ghiselli R, Cappelletti-Trombettoni MM, Guerrieri M. (2015). Prevention of hernia incision in laparoscopic left colon resection. Minerva Chir. 70(3): 155–160.

[37] Anvari M, Birch DW, Bamehriz F, Gryfe R, Chapman T. (2004). Robotic-assisted laparoscopic colorectal surgery. Surg Laparosc Endosc Percutan Tech. 14: 311–315.

[38] Rawlings AL, Woodland JH, Crawford DL. (2006). Telerobotic surgery for right and sigmoid colectomies: 30 consecutive cases. Surg Endosc. 20: 1713–1718.

[39] Guerrieri M, Campagnacci R, Sperti P, Belfiori G, Gesuita R, Ghiselli R. (2015). Totally robotic vs 3D laparoscopic colectomy: a single centers preliminary experience. World J Gastroenterol. 21(46): 13152–13159.

[40] Keller DS, Hashemi L, Lu M, Delaney CP. (2013). Short-term outcomes for robotic colorectal surgery by provider volume. J Am Coll Surg. 217: 1063–1069.

[41] Cirocchi R, Cochetti G, Randolph J et al. (2014). Laparoscopic treatment of colovesical fistulas due to complicated colonic diverticular disease: a systematic review. Tech Coloproctol. doi:10.1007/s10151-014-1157-5

[42] DeSouza AL, Prasad LM, Park JJ, Marecik SJ, Blumetti J, Abcarian H. (2010). Robotic assistance in right hemicolectomy: is there a role? Dis Colon Rectum. 53: 1000–1006.

[43] Jayne DG, Thorpe HC, Copeland J, Quirke P, Brown JM, Guillou PJ. (2010). Five-year follow-up of the Medical Research Council CLASICC trial of laparoscopically assisted versus open surgery for colorectal cancer. Br J Surg. 97: 1638–1645.

[44] Zimmern A, Prasad L, Desouza A. (2010). Robotic colon and rectal surgery: a series of 131 cases. World J Surg. 34: 1954–1958.

2

Colorectal Cancer and Inflammatory Bowel Disease

Paul Mitrut, Anca Oana Docea, Adina Maria Kamal,
Radu Mitrut, Daniela Calina, Eliza Gofita,
Vlad Padureanu, Corina Gruia and Liliana Streba

Abstract

Inflammatory bowel disease (IBD) with its two entities, ulcerative colitis and Crohn's disease, is at increased risk of developing colorectal cancer (CRC). Risk factors for CRC are represented by the duration of the disease, extent of disease, the association of primary sclerosing cholangitis, family history, and early age at onset. In inflammatory bowel disease, colonic carcinogenesis appears on an inflamed colon, being determined by different genetic alterations. The main element of the process of carcinogenesis is the dysplasia, which is a neoplastic intraepithelial transformation, limited to the basal membrane surrounding the glands around which it appears. The stages of carcinogenesis process start with dysplasia of varying degrees as follows: indefinite dysplasia, low-grade dysplasia, high-grade dysplasia, and finally invasive adenocarcinoma.

Endoscopic surveillance in IBD is absolutely necessary for early detection of dysplastic lesions. The endoscopic surveillance process begins after 7–10 years of disease progression, performed every 1 or 2 years, depending on the severity of the disease.

General principles of endoscopic surveillance involve the use of modern diagnostic methods (high definition, chromoendoscopy, indigo carmine with high definition, high-definition narrow band imaging).

The current standard-of-care (colonoscopy plus randomized biopsies) to detect dysplasia in IBD patients is inadequate. Guidelines now support to use of chromoendoscopy with targeted biopsy in the detection of dysplasia and/or colorectal cancer in patients with IBD.

Chemopreventive drugs involve the administration of therapeutic agents such as 5-ASA derivatives, ursodeoxycholic acid and folic acid, and possibly statins.

As for future goals, understanding the mechanisms of colonic carcinogenesis in IBD can identify patients at high risk for developing CRC and thus chemoprevention can be initiated. The discovery of new therapeutic agents plays an important role in chemo-prevention and represents a significant desideratum among researchers.

Keywords: colorectal cancer, inflammatory bowel disease, carcinogenesis, colono-scopic surveillance, chromoendoscopy, high-definition narrow band imaging

1. Introduction

Inflammatory bowel diseases with its two separate entities (ulcerative colitis and Crohn's disease) are conditions considered at high risk for developing colorectal cancer. Because inflammatory bowel diseases are relatively rare in the general population, only about 1% of colorectal cancers are attributed to them. Meta-analyzes showed that the risk is 2% at 10 years, 8% at 20 years, and 18% at 30 years after onset [1]. Absolute cumulative frequencies of colorectal cancer to Crohn's disease and ulcerative colitis are almost identical 7% for the first to 8% for the second, after 20 years of evolution [2]. Most knowledge about the pathogenesis of colorectal cancer come from studies on sporadic cancers or those associated with in-creased risk of hereditary disease (familial adenomatous polyposis or non-polyposis colorec-tal cancer), this data being then extrapolated for inflammatory bowel diseases.

Eaden et al. [3] reviewed 116 studies involving 55,000 patients with ulcerative colitis. One thousand seven hundred of these patients developed colorectal cancer, having an incidence of 2% after 10 years of evolution, and of 8% after 20 years finally increasing to 18% after 30 years.

2. Risk factors for colorectal cancer in inflammatory bowel disease

In ulcerative colitis, onset of colorectal cancer is correlated with many factors. Thus, the duration of the disease is recognized as one of the leading risk factors for developing colorectal cancer in ulcerative colitis. Neoplastic risk occurs after 8 years of evolution and increases exponentially after 20 years [1].

A systematic colonoscopy surveillance can detect early dysplastic lesions, and the systematic use of 5-ASA therapy can lower the risk of developing colorectal cancer in patients with IBD. The reduced incidence of prophylactic colectomy for dysplastic lesions determines a high risk for colorectal cancer. This information is an argument for preventive colonoscopy surveillance of patients with IBD and surgical prophylaxis in case of dysplasia [4, 5].

Younger age at onset is in the opinion of some authors, an independent risk factor for colorectal cancer. Younger patients have a potentially greater lifespan and therefore higher risks, which may reflect the longer duration of the disease [1, 4–6]. The association of PSC increases the risk of colorectal cancer. Its incidence in patients with ulcerative colitis is 2–5% [1]. In 1992, Broome et al. reported an increased risk of colorectal cancer in patients with ulcerative colitis associating PSC. Subsequent studies have shown that the cumulative risk of colorectal cancer is higher in patients with combination of cholangitis and ulcerative colitis compared with the ones only known for ulcerative colitis, that is, 9% after 10 years compared to 2, 31% after 20 years compared to 5, and 50% after 25 years to 10% [7].

The extent of the disease is also an important risk factor for the risk of developing colorectal cancer. Pancolitis presents the highest risk of malignancy [1]. The extension of inflammatory areas is an independent risk factor involved in the carcinogenesis and Crohn's disease.

A family history of colon cancer cancer is associated with an increased risk of colorectal –2 or 3 times higher, in the general population, which remains increased in patients with ulcerative colitis. A case–control study conducted on 297 patients at the Mayo Clinic found that a family history of sporadic colorectal cancer represents an independent risk factor for malignancy in patients with ulcerative colitis [7].

An interesting finding is that patients with asymptomatic disease (therapeutically controlled) have higher risks of malignancy compared with fulminant forms of ulcerative colitis that often require colectomy before the onset of dysplasia. In centers where a large number of colectomies are performed, the incidence of colorectal cancer (CRC) is significantly lower because the procedure eliminates the risk [1].

In Crohn's disease, the risk factors involved in carcinogenesis are areas of stenosis, inflammatory extension areas, younger age at onset and age >45 years at diagnosis. Risk factors specific to patients with inflammatory bowel disease [8]:

- Coexisting primary sclerosing cholangitis
- Increasing cumulative extent of colonic inflammatory lesions
- Increasing duration of inflammatory bowel disease
- Active chronic inflammation endoscopically assessed
- Active chronic inflammation histologically assessed
- Anatomical abnormalities such as:
  - Foreshortened colon
  - Strictures
  - Pseudo polyps
- Personal history of flat dysplasia.

The severity of inflammatory colonic lesion correlates with the risk of colorectal cancer in patients with IBD. There is a correlation between the degree of inflammation and the risk of dysplastic lesions and indirectly with the colorectal cancer incidence. Various studies have shown the relationship between the risk of colorectal cancer in patients with IBD and the degree of inflammation, extent of lesions and coexistence of other sites of inflammation [9]. Involved in the colonic carcinogenesis in patients with IBD are, besides inflammation areas of various degrees, also genetic and immunological factors.

3. Molecular and genetic markers

Sporadic colon cancer

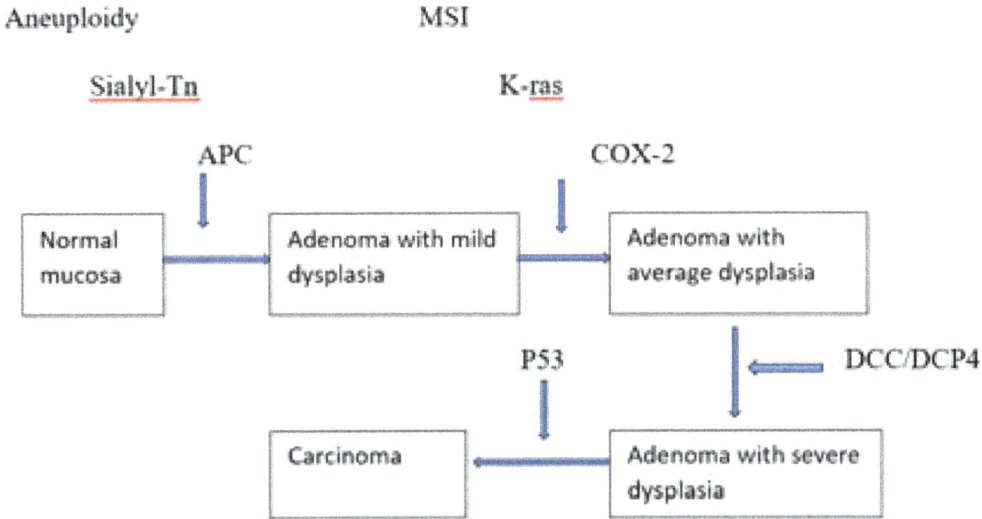

Aneuploidy   MSI

Sialyl-Tn   K-ras

APC   COX-2

| Normal mucosa | → | Adenoma with mild dysplasia | → | Adenoma with average dysplasia |

P53   DCC/DCP4

| Carcinoma | ← | Adenoma with severe dysplasia |

Colitis associated colon cancer [8]

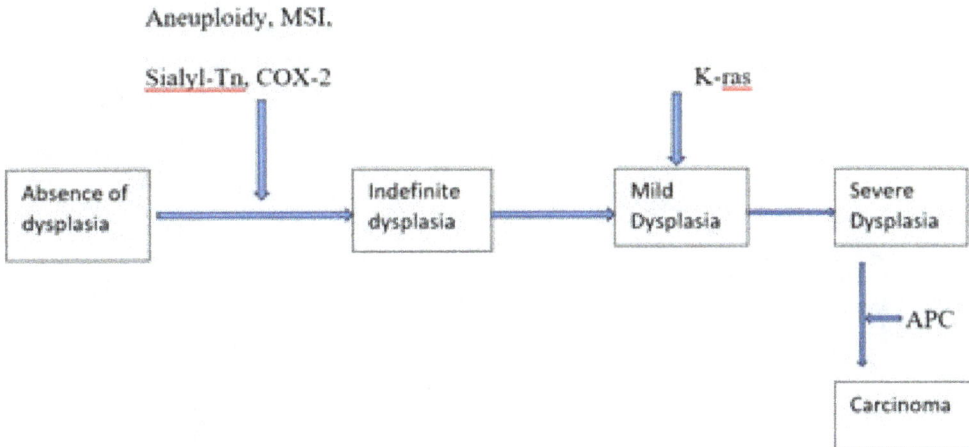

Aneuploidy, MSI,

Sialyl-Tn, COX-2   K-ras

| Absence of dysplasia | → | Indefinite dysplasia | → | Mild Dysplasia | → | Severe Dysplasia |

APC

| Carcinoma |

Pathogenesis of sporadic colon cancer and colitis-associated colon cancer [8].

Involved in the appearance of colorectal cancer associated with inflammatory bowel disease, are, on the one hand the chromosomal instability caused by abnormal chromosome separation (CRS) aneuploidy and loss of genetic material, and on the other hand, the microsatellite instability (MSI) mechanisms found in sporadic carcinogenesis. The trigger element for chromosomal instability is represented by impairing the function of APC associated with the induction of K-ras oncogene and inactivation of tumor suppressor gene on CRS 18q in DCC and DPC4 region. Adenoma–carcinoma transformation is a direct result of the loss of p53 gene function [1, 6, 8].

Microsatellite instability, which is absent on normal mucosa, is described as an early event in non-dysplastic mucosa in patients with ulcerative colitis.

It is important to understand what mechanisms and factors can contribute to dysplastic lesions and colorectal cancer in IBD. Inflammation and genetic mutations play a major role. The supervision and therapeutic intervention in these disorders depends on understanding of these pathological processes. Thus, some genes associated with inflammation such as cyclo-oxygenase-2, nitric oxide synthase-2, and 1–8 interferon inducible genes are increased in inflamed colonic mucosa and remain elevated in colonic neoplasms [10, 11].

Genetic changes, responsible for colorectal cancer in inflammatory bowel disease, are similar to those involved in sporadic colon cancer [8].

Oxidative stress and its role in cell destruction in inflamed tissue may also play an important role in the pathogenesis of colorectal cancer in IBD [12].

Figures 1 and **2** depict some pathology aspects of colon mucosa with inflammatory changes. The inflammatory context is suggested by an abundant lymphoplasmocitary infiltrate and polimorphonucleated within the mucosal corion.

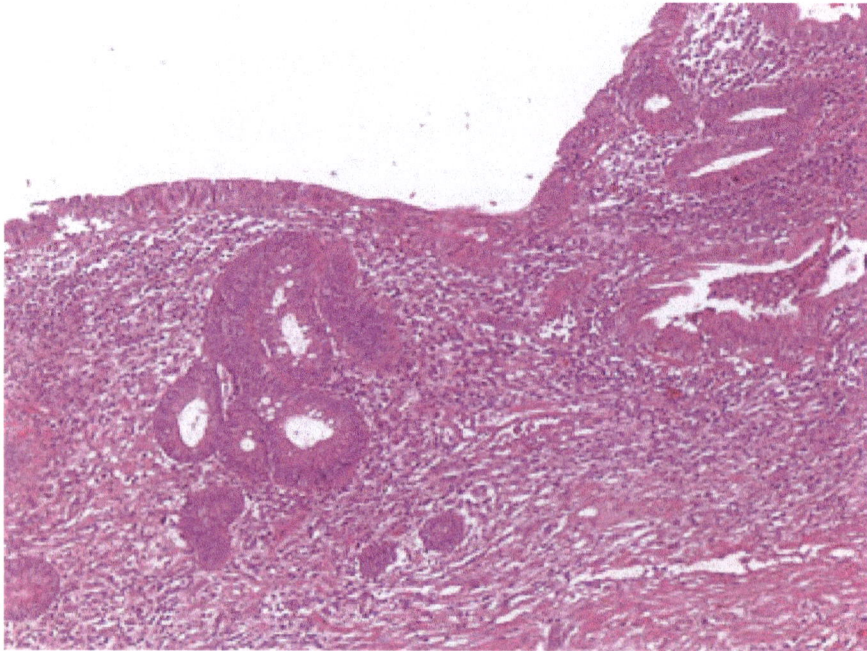

Figure 1. Inflammatory aspect of colonic mucosa. Modified cytoarchitectonics. Epithelial pseudostratification of the glandular tissue.

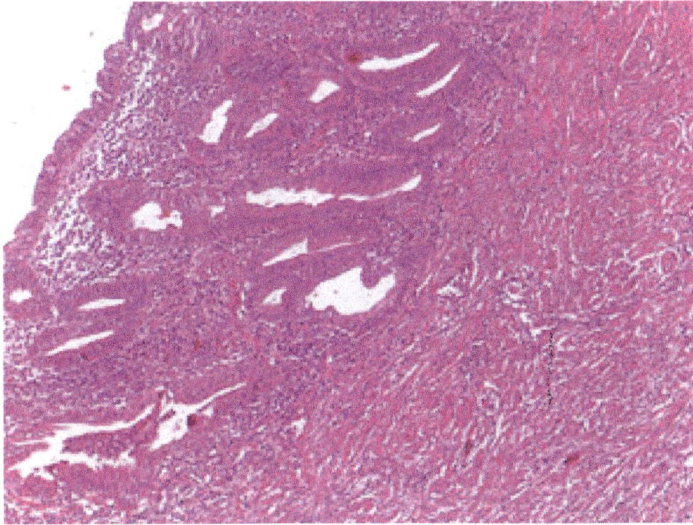

Figure 2. Inflammatory aspect of colonic mucosa. Nuclear pleomorphism. Mucus depletion, with a decreased number of secretory cells within normal glands.

4. Prevention of colorectal cancer in inflammatory bowel disease

4.1. Endoscopic surveillance in IBD

Endoscopic surveillance in IBD is designed to detect dysplastic lesions that can be treated surgically. As dysplastic lesions are difficult to recognize via endoscopic examination, their detection requires colectomy that prevents colorectal cancer (CRC). This fact is also determined by the risk of developing synchronous or metachronous cancer in IBD [13].

Colonoscopy surveillance reduces the risk of death from CRC in patients with long-term evolution of inflammatory disease. Given the cost–benefit ratio, this surveillance is especially recommended in patients with evolving active disease of over 7–10 years. The first colonoscopy screening program will be carried out in a remission period of the disease to avoid difficulties in identifying dysplasia in areas of increased inflammatory activity (**Figures 3** and **4**). The entire colonic mucosa will be examined and four biopsies will be taken from 10 to 10 cm. Any suspicious lesions will be biopsied. If the initial biopsy does not describe dysplastic foci, the colonoscopy is recommended to be repeated after 2 years or annually if the disease has more than 20 years of evolution when the risk of cancer increases exponentially. This interval is reduced to 6 months, 1-year maximum if the pathology result of the lesions comes back as indefinite dysplasia. The most controversial attitude is regarding mild dysplasia. In the case of dysplastic lesions associated with IBD, there are opinions saying that endoscopic resection can be done if the pathological examination of the fragments collected from the base of the polyp and also from the colon are negative for dysplasia [14]. The marking of the polypectomy site is recommended, and the colonoscopy should be repeated after 3–6 months. The confirmation of unifocal or multifocal dysplasia by a second expert requires that a colectomy should be performed. High-grade dysplasia is an absolute indication for colectomy.

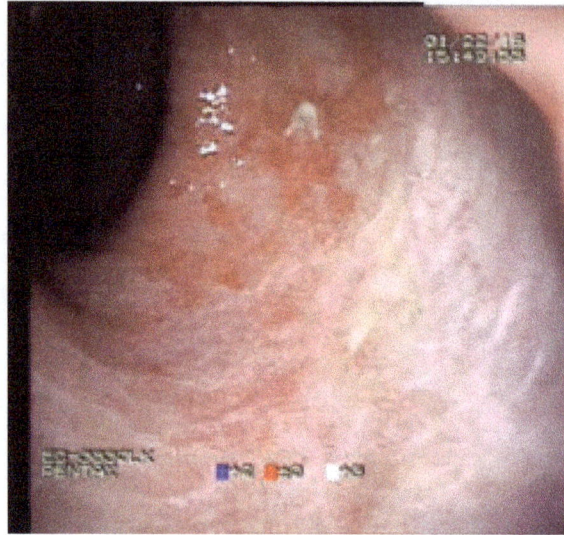

Figure 3. Ulcerative colitis with areas of low grade dysplasia.

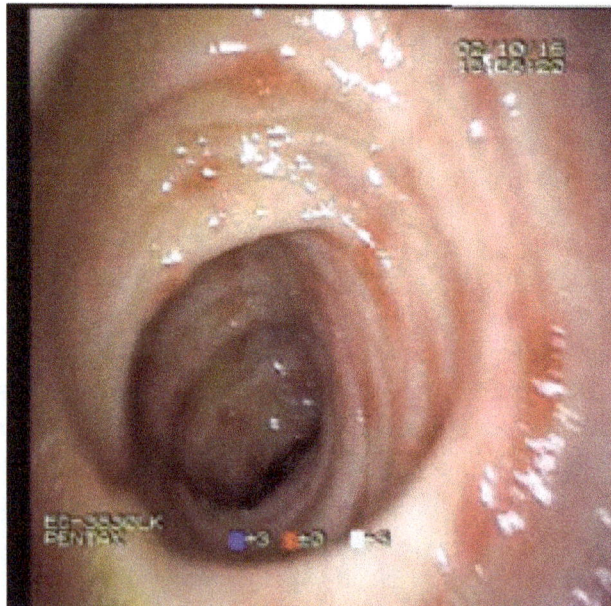

Figure 4. Ulcerative colitis with high grade dysplasia.

There is an evolution of the inflammatory lesions that either do not have dysplastic lesions or evolve from indefinite dysplasia to low-grade dysplasia, high-grade dysplasia, and finally carcinoma.

Dysplasia, detected at colonoscopic examination, represents an indication for colectomy. When low-grade dysplasia is detected, it is considered that the risk of developing colorectal cancer is nine times higher than in normal individuals and there is a 12 times higher risk of developing other advanced dysplastic lesions.

In patients with low-grade dysplasia, when colectomy is performed immediately, it was noted that 19% of the cases had high-grade dysplasia and 29–54% were at risk of developing advanced neoplasia in the following 5 years. High-grade dysplasia has a risk of 43% of combination with synchronous malignancy [14].

Dysplastic lesions are lesions that precede colorectal cancer development. Flat dysplasia can be discovered through microscopic examination of biopsy fragments, collected through random biopsies, sometimes from apparently normal mucosa. Often, flat dysplasia can be discovered with superior detection techniques such as chromoendoscopy, high-definition, and high magnification endoscopy [15–18].

Treatment for patients with dysplastic lesions and IBD depends on the degree of dysplasia. Patients presenting with multifocal flat low-grade dysplasia lesions or repetitive flat low-grade dysplasia should be advised to undertake prophylactic proctocolectomy.

Dysplasia-associated lesion or mass (DALM) is a specific endoscopic feature found in patients with ulcerative colitis. DALM is associated in a proportion of 40% with colorectal cancer; this

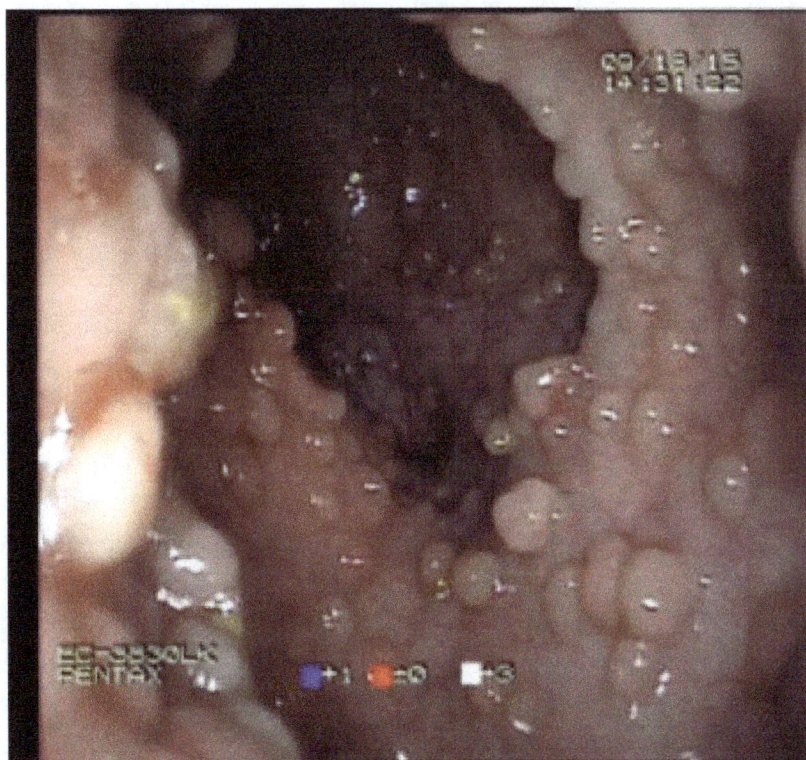

Figure 5. Polipoid lesions in a patient suffering from Crohn's disease.

association is enhanced by the presence of high-grade dysplasia lesions. DALM is an indication of proctocolectomy regardless of the degree of dysplasia.

Polypoid lesions identified in patients with IBD are not always malignant and can be treated with endoscopic polypectomy, especially if the polyps are adenomatous [19] (**Figure 5**).

Dysplastic lesions detected in biopsy samples from patients with IBD usually occur in areas of inflammation and can be polypoid, ulcerated lesions, or plague-like lesions (DALM). (**Figure 6** describes various instances of lesions in a patient with IBD).

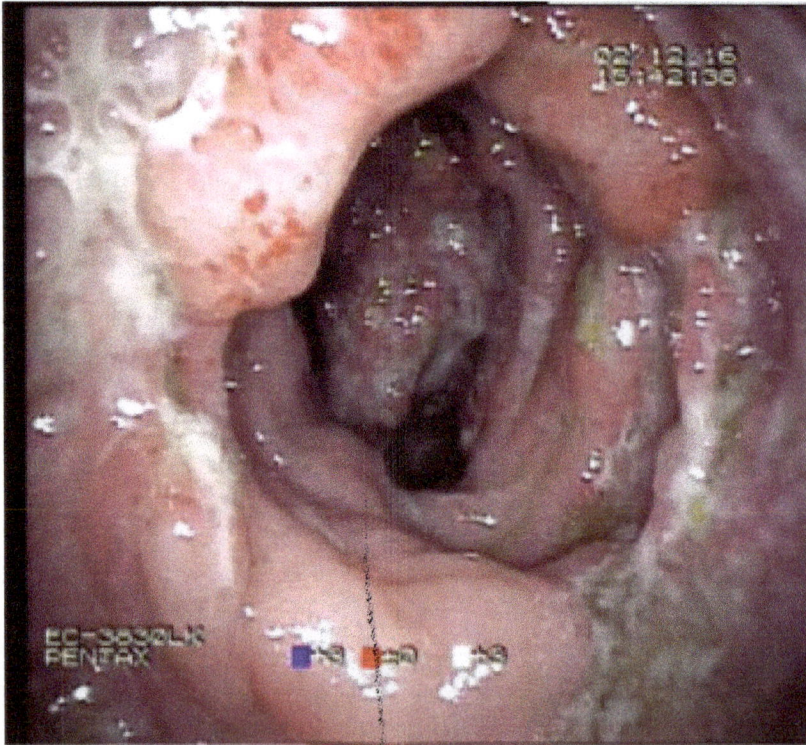

Figure 6. High grade dysplasia in a patient with Crohn's disease.

Although prophylactic proctocolectomy ensures the elimination of the risk of colon cancer (42% of cases in patients with high-grade dysplasia and 19% of cases in patients with low-grade dysplasia), there are practitioners who opt for a lifelong schedule of surveillance. They choose periodic examination at 6 months to 1 year by endoscopically investigating the entire colon, harvesting biopsy fragments and using preventive treatment with anti-inflammatory drugs and potentially chemopreventive agents. There are some major limitations to this attitude, namely the possibility of omission of malignant or dysplastic lesions during colonoscopy, especially if the number of biopsies is insufficient. Also, the lack of compliance of patients to colonoscopy surveillance programs is also an important risk factor for malignant lesions.

Guidelines from the Crohn's and Colitis Foundation of America (CCFA) and from European Crohn's and Colitis Organization (ECCO) mention the same methods for Crohn's colitis surveillance and ulcerative colitis as well due to the similar risk of developing colorectal. Colonoscopic screening is performed during remission of the disease, every 1 or 2 years, after 8–10 years of evolution. Screening interval may decrease with increasing duration of disease progression. Patients with proctosigmoiditis, who have a lower risk of malignancy compared to the general population, will be monitored using standard colorectal cancer prevention measures.

Patients with PSC, who have an increased risk of malignancy, should be monitored annually. Biopsy samples are collected from 10 to 10 cm (2–4 random biopsy specimens) and from suspect areas. In addition, in ulcerative colitis, biopsies are harvested from every 5 cm from the rectum and sigmoid, because the risk of developing colorectal cancer is higher in these regions. The degree of detection of dysplastic lesions is higher if a greater number of randomized biopsies are taken (90% if 33 and 95% if 56 random biopsies were taken) [20, 21].

4.2. New methods for early detection of dysplasia

To increase the rate of detection of dysplastic lesions, targeted biopsy represents an alternative. Guidelines now support the use of chromoendoscopy with targeted biopsy in the detection of dysplasia and/or colorectal cancer in patients with inflammatory bowel disease (IBD). Chromoendoscopy can see injuries that are not visible in the white light of standard endoscopy. Two substances are used, namely methylene blue and indigo carmine. High-magnification chromoendoscopy increases the detection of dysplastic lesions 3–4.5 times over [22–26].

Because of these arguments chromoendoscopy is used for routine surveillance of patients with IBD. With this method, the majority of dysplastic lesions can be discovered in patients with IBD during surveillance colonoscopy. Using only conventional colonoscopy is obviously insufficient in detecting dysplastic lesions [27–30].

Confocal laser endomicroscopy (CLE) is a modern technique for visualization of the histology of colonic mucosa in real time, being extremely useful for diagnosing intraepithelial neoplasia. With concomitant use of chromoendoscopic and CLE evaluation, the detection rate of dysplastic lesions was increased by 4.75 times compared to classical colonoscopy [21, 28–30].

Confocal chromoscopic endomicroscopy is superior to chromoscopy alone for the detection of intraepithelial neoplasia. Difficulties are caused by the high cost of exploration and biopsy interpretation difficulty that often requires an experienced pathologist.

The use of narrow band imaging (NBI) is not superior to conventional colonoscopy in detecting dysplastic lesions [31, 32].

Although many lesions can be identified by NBI, unfortunately equal numbers of dysplastic lesions can be missed by both conventional colonoscopy and this method. More studies are needed to clarify these issues.

We again underline that chromoendoscopy with targeted biopsy is indicated by all current guidelines for detecting dysplastic lesions in IBD.

4.3. Chemoprevention

Surveillance colonoscopy does not prevent colorectal cancer but allows early detection of dysplastic lesions and surgical therapeutic intervention.

Treatment of inflammatory lesions of IBD with specific anti-inflammatory therapy represents an important method of primary chemoprevention of colorectal cancer [33–36].

4.3.1. Aminosalicylates and other anti-inflammatory agents

IBD anti-inflammatory treatment in addition to relieving symptoms and improving lesions can prevent dysplastic lesions and colorectal cancer. Although studies are contradictory, most authors recommend administration of anti-inflammatory therapy for colorectal cancer prevention [37].

5-aminosalicylic acid preparations (5-ASA) are the main anti-inflammatory drugs used for the treatment of digestive tract inflammation in patients with IBD. Aminosalicylates inhibit cyclooxygenase and 5-lipoxygenase, thus inhibiting the synthesis of leukotriene B4, thromboxane A2 and prostaglandins and thus intervene in the immune response, reducing the production of antibodies and phagocytic activity. The administration of 5-ASA preparations reduces the risk of colorectal cancer, especially at higher doses of 2 g per day.

Mesalazine is effective in preventing colorectal cancer in IBD, proven experimentally on colon cancer cell lines [38].

4.3.2. Ursodeoxycholic acid

Ursodeoxycholic acid (UDCA) used for treating PSC has a preventive effect in colorectal cancer by decreasing the concentration of biliary acids in the colon and through its antioxidant properties. On the other hand, it is unclear whether ursodeoxycholic acid is effective in preventing colorectal cancer in patients with IBD without the association of primary sclerosing cholangitis. In IBD forms associated with PSC, UDCA can reduce mortality and prevent the evolution of dysplastic lesions [39].

Further studies are necessary to establish the dose of UDCA to be used for secondary chemoprevention.

4.3.3. Folic acid

There are numerous studies showing that as in sporadic CRC, folic acid supplementation would decrease the risk of CRC in patients with IBD. Although there is no consensus in this regard, given that it is a cheap drug, that offers long-term safety, folic acid is recommended in patients with IBD as chemopreventive purposes. The mechanism of action is possibly related to the process of maintenance of DNA methylation and maintenance of DNA precursors level.

4.3.4. Statins

There is little data on the protective effect of statins on the development of CRC. It seems that the protective effect is lower in sporadic colorectal cancer and more expressed in colorectal cancer associated with inflammatory bowel disease. Experimental studies on mice show the protective effect of statins in reducing colorectal Dysplasia by inhibiting DNA destruction. Also in experimental models simvastatin significantly reduced tumor development by inducing apoptosis and inhibiting angiogenesis [40, 41].

These experiments provide important arguments that statins could be a potential chemopreventive and therapeutic agent effective in CRC associated with IBD. Extensive studies over long periods of time are needed to bring new arguments and insights on these aspects.

Author details

Paul Mitrut*, Anca Oana Docea, Adina Maria Kamal, Radu Mitrut, Daniela Calina, Eliza Gofita, Vlad Padureanu, Corina Gruia and Liliana Streba

*Address all correspondence to: paulmitrut@yahoo.com

University of Medicine and Pharmacy of Craiova, Craiova, Romania

References

[1] Farraye FA, Odze RD, Eaden J, Itzkowitz SH. AGA technical review on the diagnosis and management of colorectal neoplasia in inflammatory bowel disease. Gastroenterology. 2010;138:746–774.

[2] Gillen CD, Walmsley RS, Prior B, et al. Primary sclerosing cholangitis and ulcerative colitis: evidence for increased neoplastic potential. Hepatology. 1995;22:1404–1408.

[3] Eaden JA, Abrams KR, Mayberry JF. The risk of colorectal cancer in ulcerative colitis: a metaanalysis. Gut. 2001;48:526–535.

[4] Lakatos PL, Lakatos L. Risk for colorectal cancer in ulcerative colitis: changes causes and management strategies. World J Gastroenterol. 2008;14(25):3937–3947.

[5] Ha F1, Khalil H. Crohn's disease: a clinical update. Ther Adv Gastroenterol. 2015;8(6): 352–9.

[6] Jiang D1, Zhong S2, McPeek MS. Retrospective Binary-Trait Association Test Elucidates Genetic Architecture of Crohn Disease. Am J Hum Genet. 2016;98(2):243–55.

[7] Nuako KW, Ahlquist DA, Mahoney DW, et al. Familial predisposition for colorectal cancer in chronic ulcerative colitis: a case control study. Gastroenterology. 1998;115:1079–1083.

[8] Beaugerie L, Itzkowitz SH. Cancers complicating inflammatory bowel disease. N Engl J Med. 2015;372:1441–1452.

[9] Gupta RB, Harpaz N, Itzkowitz S, Hossain S, Matula S, Kornbluth A, Bodian C, Ullman T. Histologic inflammation is a risk factor for progression to colorectal neoplasia in ulcerative colitis: a cohort study. Gastroenterology. 2007;133(4):1099–105.

[10] Cosnes J. Smoking and diet: impact on disease course? Dig Dis. 2016;34(1–2):72–77. [Epub ahead of print]

[11] Itzkowitz S. Colon carcinogenesis in inflammatory bowel disease: applying molecular genetics to clinical practice. J Clin Gastroenterol. 2003;36:S70–74.

[12] Clevers H. Colon cancer-understanding how NSAIDs work. N Engl J Med. 2006;354:761–763.

[13] Roessner A, Kuester D, Malfertheiner P, Schneider-Stock R. Oxidative stress in ulcerative colitis-associated carcinogenesis. Pathol Res Pract. 2008;204:511–524.

[14] Soetikno R, Kaltenbach T, McQuaid KR, Subramanian V, Laine L, Kumar R, Barkun AN. Paradigm shift in the surveillance and management of dysplasia in inflammatory bowel disease. Dig Endosc. 2016. doi:10.1111/den.12634. [Epub ahead of print]

[15] Wanders LK, Kuiper T, Kiesslich R, Karstensen JG, Leong RW, Dekker E, Bisschops R. Limited applicability of chromoendoscopy-guided confocal laser endomicroscopy as daily-practice surveillance strategy in Crohn's disease. Gastrointest Endosc. 2015. pii: S0016-5107(15)02834-5. doi:10.1016/j.gie.2015.09.001. [Epub ahead of print]

[16] Rubin PN, Friedman S, Harpaz N, et al. Colonosopicpolypectomy in chronic colitis: conservative management after endoscopic resection of dysplastic polyps. Gastroenterology. 1999;117:1295–300.

[17] Marion JF, Waye JD, Israel Y, Present DH, Suprun M, Bodian C, Harpaz N, Chapman M, Itzkowitz S, Abreu MT, Ullman TA, McBride RB, Aisenberg J, Mayer L. Chromoendoscopy is more effective than standard colonoscopy in detecting dysplasia during long-term surveillance of patients with colitis. Clin Gastroenterol Hepatol. 2015. pii: S1542-3565(15)01597-9. doi:10.1016/j.cgh.2015.11.011. [Epub ahead of print]

[18] Welman CJ. Crohn's disease imaging in the emergency department. J Gastroenterol Hepatol. 2016. doi:10.1111/jgh.13352. [Epub ahead of print]

[19] Aalykke C, Jensen MD, Fallingborg J, Jess T, Langholz E, Meisner S, Andersen NN, Riis LB, Thomsen OØ, Tøttrup A. Colonoscopy surveillance for dysplasia and colorectal cancer in patients with inflammatory bowel disease. Dan Med J. 2015;62(1):B4995.

[20] Triantafillidis JK, Nasivelos G, Kosmidis PA. "Colorectal cancer and inflammatory bowel disease: epidemiology, risk factors, mechanisms of carcinogenesis and prevention strategies". Auction Res. 2009;29(7):727–2737.

[21] Mattar MC, Lough D, Charabaty A. Current management of inflammatory bowel disease and colorectal cancer. Gastrointest Cancer Res. 2011;4(2):5361.

[22] Kiesslich R, Hoffman A, Neurath M-F. Colonoscopy, and inflamatory bowel disease. Tumors New Diagn Methods Endosc. 2006;38(1):5–10.

[23] Nakai Y, Isayama H, Shinoura S, IwashitaT, Samarasena J. Confocal laser endomicroscopy in gastrointestinal and pancreatobiliary diseases. Dig Endosc. 2014;26(Suppl 1): 86–94.

[24] Negrón ME1, Kaplan GG, Barkema HW, Eksteen B, Clement F, Manns BJ, Coward S, Panaccione R, Ghosh S, Heitman SJ. Colorectal cancer surveillance in patients with inflammatory bowel disease and primary sclerosing cholangitis: an economic evaluation. Inflamm Bowel Dis. 2014;20(11):2046–55.

[25] Lutgens M, van Oijen M, Mooiweer E, van der Valk M, Vleggaar F, Siersema P, Oldenburg B. A risk-profiling approach for surveillance of inflammatory bowel disease-colorectal carcinoma is more cost-effective: a comparative cost-effectiveness analysis between international guidelines. Gastrointest Endosc. 2014;80(5):842–8.

[26] Efthymiou M, Allen PB, Taylor AC, Desmond PV, Jayasakera C, De Cruz P, Kamm MA. Chromoendoscopy versus narrow band imaging for colonic surveillance in inflammatory bowel disease. Inflamm Bowel Dis. 2013;19(10):2132–8.

[27] Subramanian V, Bisschops R. Image-enhanced endoscopy is critical in the surveillance of patients with colonic IBD. Gastrointest Endosc Clin N Am. 2014;24(3):393–403.

[28] Rogler G. Chronic ulcerative colitis and colorectal cancer. Cancer Lett. 2014;345(2):235–41.

[29] Genta RM, Feagins LA. Advanced precancerous lesions in the small bowel mucosa. Best Pract Res Clin Gastroenterol. 2013;27(2):225–33.

[30] Beaugerie L, Svrcek M, Seksik P, Bouvier AM, Simon T, Allez M, Brixi H, Gornet JM, Altwegg R, Beau P, Duclos B, Bourreille A, Faivre J, Peyrin-Biroulet L, Fléjou JF, Carrat F. Risk of colorectal high-grade dysplasia and cancer in a prospective observational cohort of patients with inflammatory bowel disease. Gastroenterology. 2013;145(1): 166–175.

[31] Dekker E, van den Broek FJC, Reitsma JB, Hardwick JC, Johan Offerhaus G, van Deventer SJ, Hommes DW, Fockens P. "Narrow band imaging compared with conventional colonoscopy for the detection of dysplasia in patients with longstanding ulcerative colitis". Endoscopy. 2007;39(3):216–221.

[32] Moody GA, Jayanthi V, Probert CSJ, Mac Kay H, Mayberry JF. Long-term therapy with sulphasalazine protects against colorectal cancer in ulcerative colitis: a retrospective

study of colorectal cancer risk and compliance with treatment in Leicestershire. Eur J Gastroenterol Hepatol. 1996;8:1179–83.

[33] Qin X. Is colonic Crohn's disease more closely related to ulcerative colitis or Crohn's disease by nature? Inflamm Bowel Dis. 2016. [Epub ahead of print]

[34] Velayos FS, Loftus Jr. EV, Jess T, Scott Harmsen W, Bida J, Zinsmeister AR, Tremaine WJ, Sandborn WJ. Predictive and protective factors associated with colorectal cancer in ulcerative colitis: a case-control study. Gastroenterology. 2006;130:941–1949.

[35] Burman S, Hoedt EC, Pottenger S, Mohd-Najman NS, Ó Cuív P, Morrison M. An (anti)-inflammatory microbiota: defining the role in inflammatory bowel disease? Dig Dis. 2016;34(1–2):64–71.

[36] Herfarth HH. Methotrexate for inflammatory bowel diseases—new developments. Dig Dis. 2016;34(1–2):140–146.

[37] Megna BW, Carney PR, Kennedy GD. Intestinal inflammation and the diet: is food friend or foe? World J Gastrointest Surg. 2016;8(2):115–23.

[38] Gearry RB. IBD and environment: are there differences between east and west. Dig Dis. 2016;34(1–2):84–89.

[39] Sjooqvist U, Tribukait B, Öst A, Einarsson C, Oxelmark L, Lofberg R. Ursodeoxycholic acid treatment in IBD-patients with colorectal dysplasia and/or DNA-aneuploidy: a prospective, double-blind, randomized controlled pilot study. Anticancer Res. 2004;24(5B):3121–3127.

[40] Suzuki S, Tajima T, Sassa S, Kudo H, Okayasu I, Sakamoto S. Preventive effect of fluvastatin on ulcerative colitis-associated carcinogenesis in mice. Anticancer Res. 2006;26(6B):4223–4228.

[41] Cho S-J, Kim JS, Kim JM, Lee JY, Jung HC, Song IS. Simvastatin induces apoptosis in human colon cancer cells and in tumor xenografts, and attenuates colitis-associated colon cancer in mice. Int J Cancer. 2008;123:951–957.

3

Studies of Malaysian Plants in Prevention and Treatment of Colorectal Cancer

Yumi Z. H-Y. Hashim, Chris I. R. Gill, Cheryl Latimer,
Nigel Ternan and Phirdaous Abbas

Abstract

Incidence rates vary 10-fold globally for colorectal cancer (CRC). Asia has lower rates than Western countries, but as the Western life-style becomes more prevalent in economically developing Asian countries, rates are increasing. Clinical therapy has improved over the last few decades, and national screening programmes are a proven and effective means of reducing mortality; chemoprevention through diet and life-style choices may provide additional value. Diet has strong associations with the aetiology of CRC, considerable epidemiological evidence exist that fruits and vegetables are associated with reduced risk of CRC. There is also extensive experimental evidence that phytochemicals from fruit and vegetables can modulate pathways of carcinogenesis. In this chapter, we consider Malaysia specifically, with its rich ethnopharmacological heritage and megabiodiversity; Malaysian natural compounds may be a source of potentially chemo-protective with relevance to CRC.

Keywords: colon cancer, in vitro, Malaysia, plants, anticancer

1. Introduction

Botanically, Malaysia is one of the most bio-diverse countries in the world with more than 23,000 plant species recorded [1]. Many components of these plants are traditionally used for flavour and fragrances as well as for medicinal purposes. In line with bio-prospecting trend to find new pharmaceutical lead compounds for medical applications; researchers from local academic and research institutions within Malaysia have initiated investigations of the bioactive properties of various native plants. In Malaysia, colorectal cancer is the second most frequent cancer after breast cancer [2]. The aim of this review is to collate data and conclusions from recent studies undertaken on indigenous Malaysian plants with a view toward prevention and/or treatment of colorectal cancer (CRC).

2. Epidemiology of CRC

The geographical distribution of CRC differs significantly (~10-fold) across the world with the highest incidence rates in Australia/New Zealand (age-specific rate; ASR 44.8 and 32.2 per 100,000 in men and women, respectively), North America (ASR 30.1 and 22.7 per 100,000), Europe (ASR 37.3 and 22.7 per 100,000), and Japan (ASR 42.1 and 23.5 per 100,000). The lowest incidence rates occur in West Africa (ASR 4.5 and 3.8 per 100,000) although in this case, under-reporting is likely due to incomplete coverage by registries [2].

The global rise of incidence and mortality rates attributable to cancer is likely due to the ageing population, with incidence predicted to increase to 22.2 million cases globally by 2030 [3]. The cancer pattern among countries exhibits a strong societal and economic influence, where countries with a low human development index (HDI) (composite measure of life expectancy, education, and gross domestic product per head) tend to have higher levels of infection-related cancers (i.e., cervical) compared to medium and high HDI countries where the cancer burden is more commonly related to reproductive, dietary, and hormonal factors (e.g., lung, breast, and colorectal) [3]. As such, it is clear that CRC incidence rates increase in accordance with a country's income [4].

Asia as a whole consists mainly of developing countries and as such, incidence rates of CRC (ASR 16.5 and 11.1 per 100,000 in men and women, respectively) are noticeably lower than for the mainly developed countries of Europe—both in terms of incidence and in mortality (**Table 1**). However, cancer incidence and mortality in Asia is likely to rise over the next 20 years, due in part to a rapid population expansion that will not be experienced by Western countries. This increase will clearly impact on the health care burden associated with cancer, and also quality of life across Asia as a whole. Ng and colleagues [4] recently considered the wide variation in cancer incidence and mortality across Asia with respect to cancer survival, defining it in terms of mortality to incidence ratios (MIR = 1 no effect on survival). Although cancer incidence is lower in Asia, cancer survival is higher in Western countries as the MIRs are lower. Moreover, while Eastern and Western Asia have a higher incidence of CRC compared to South-Eastern and South-Central Asia, the pattern for survival is reversed in that the latter two regions have poorer survival than Western and Eastern Asia [4]. In Malaysia (South Eastern Asia), CRC is the second most common malignancy after breast cancer, while incidence rates exceed that of China, cancer survival is similar. By contrast, in Japan, both incidence and survival are higher.

2.1. CRC pathogenesis

The majority of colorectal malignancies occur as sporadic forms that appear to arise from benign adenomatous polyps, with carcinomas emerging slowly over a period of 10–20 years [6–9]. Epidemiological data indicate that incidence and mortality rates of colorectal cancers

(CRC) are greatly influenced by age rather than by gender. The majority of cases are detected in individuals over the age of 60 [10], with 55% of cases occurring in more developed regions in contrast to 52% of all CRC deaths which occur in the less-developed regions of the world, reflecting poorer survival. For individuals diagnosed with CRC, it has been determined that the 5-year survival rate is approximately 50–60% [11] and that survival among CRC patient is improved if WCRF/AICR lifestyle guidelines on physical activity, body fatness, and diet are adhered to [12]. The age-dependent increase in CRC development is associated with a multi-step oncogenesis process and a number of histological stages, reflecting the accumulation of genetic errors in somatic cells over time. Sporadic CRC is currently thought to arise via 1 of 3 identified molecular pathways (Micro Satellite instability—MSI, Chromosomal Instability—CIN and CpG island methylator phenotype—CIMP) depending upon the individual's complement of gene alterations [13]. Conversely, the inheritance of germline mutations may also result in development of neoplasms at an early age, with approximately 5% of CRC cases being due to inherited single-gene syndromes such as familial adenomatous polyposis (FAP) and hereditary non-polyposis colorectal cancer (HNPCC) [14]. It is estimated that as much as 12–35% of colon cancers can be explained by heritable factors, but known single-nucleotide polymorphisms appear to explain only a small proportion of these [15].

The high degree of molecular heterogeneity present in CRC is reflected by the effectiveness of chemotherapeutic regimes; however, the clinical significance of the majority of these individual molecular alterations is still to be fully determined [16]. From a treatment perspective, early-stage CRC is managed by surgical resection and advanced CRC with a combination of chemotherapy and surgery. Most chemotherapeutic regimes use 5-Fluorouracil (5-FU) as the main cytotoxic agent and this is commonly administered in conjunction with oxaliplatin for adjuvant therapy for high-risk stage II/stage III CRC, and with either oxaliplatin or irinotecan for metastatic CRC. Furthermore, the addition of bevacizumab-based chemotherapy (a vascular endothelial growth factor (VEGF)-targeted agent) has proven to be more effective than cytotoxic chemotherapy alone for the treatment of metastatic CRC [17].

While there is no doubt that CRC treatments have advanced over the last decade, improvement in disease outcome has been more modest relative to the increase in treatment costs. Thus, population screening is an important and cost-effective strategy given the improved prognosis with early detection [18]. The pathogenesis of CRC makes it very well suited to population screening especially given the correlation between disease stage and mortality. It is clear that the detection and the removal of cancer precursors can reduce CRC incidence and mortality and effective detection of CRC allows for less invasive treatment with a better prognosis. As is to be expected, a large variation exists globally in the implementation of screening programmes both in terms of strategy used (organised vs opportunistic) and standards applied (diagnostic test, detection threshold), with implementation more common in Western countries [19]. Europe for the most part has implemented an organized screening programme, while the USA operates an opportunistic approach. In Asia, several countries have already developed organized programmes including Japan, Korea and, to a lesser extent, China. As yet, however, Malaysia has no organized screening in place. As cancer incidences are likely to continue to rise, screening programmes will necessarily become more of an issue for low resource countries. Moreover, as cancer pattern types change, there will arise a need to developed tailored approaches [19].

Region	Incidence		Mortality		5-year prevalence	
	Number	ASR (W)	Number	ASR (W)	Number	Prop
Australian/New Zealand	18887	38.2	5489	10	54266	245.4
Europe	447136	29.5	214866	12.5	1203943	192.3
North America	158169	26.1	63465	9.4	486650	172.9
Asia	607182	13.7	331615	7.2	1493520	47
Asian region						
Eastern Asia (EA)	421343	18.4	207716	8.4	1130066	87.1
Western Asia (WA)	27140	14.8	15306	8.4	62162	37.5
South Eastern Asia (SEA)	69016	12.5	43234	7.9	158845	35.7
South Central Asia (SCA)	89683	6.1	65359	4.4	142447	11.3
Country						
Australia	15869	38.4	4168	9	45622	245.8
Japan (EA)	112675	32.2	49345	11.9	384877	350.8
UK	40755	30.2	16202	10.7	104047	200.5
Malaysia (SEA)	4539	18.3	2300	9.4	9714	47
China (EA)	253427	14.2	139416	7.4	583054	52.7
Saudi Arabia (WA)	2047	11.6	1094	6.6	4486	22.3
India (SCA)	64332	6.1	48603	4.6	86650	9.8

Incidence and mortality data for all ages. Five-year prevalence for adult population only. ASR (W) and proportions per 100,000 persons per year. The ASR is a weighted mean of the age-specific rates. Adapted from [5].

Table 1. Incidence and mortality rates (estimated, all sexes) for colorectal cancer, globally and within Asia and selected regions.

2.2. Diet and CRC

The relatively recent increase in CRC incidence in Japan (Eastern Asia) and in urbanized regions of China (Eastern Asia) is of significant concern [20] and is thought to be due to the adoption of a more a Western lifestyle and diet [21]. Diet plays a central role in CRC pathogenesis, as those rich in saturated animal fat, and red meat (especially processed meat) [22] together with alcohol intake [23] and smoking [24] have been positively associated with colorectal neoplasia. Fruit and vegetable consumption is associated with a reduction in the risk of CRC [25], and this concept is supported by a large body of case-control studies, although results from cohort or prospective studies are less convincing [26]. Nevertheless, the protective effects of fruits and vegetables against colorectal cancer are attributed to the large number of bioactive phytochemicals present within them [27], comprising mainly plant polyphenolic secondary metabolites [28] and plant structural and storage polysaccharides which make up dietary fiber [29, 30]. These various plant components or natural products are found within a range of indigenous Malaysian fruit and vegetables, and thus may potentially play a role in chemoprevention for CRC.

3. Natural product research in Malaysia

Natural products include a large and diverse group of substances produced by a variety of sources including marine organisms, bacteria, yeasts, fungi, and plants [31]. Research on natural products has focused primarily on the chemical properties, biosynthesis, and biological functions of secondary metabolites [32]. Natural products, in particular plants, have been used in traditional medicine and health practice. The World Health Organization has acknowledged traditional medicine as a contributor to achieve health care objectives [33] and Malaysia, blessed with its megabiodiversity and rich ethnopharmacological heritage, has been observed to elegantly capitalize on these attributes with a view toward boosting the wealth and wellness of its population [34].

In late 2010, the Malaysian government launched the Economic Transformation Programme (ETP), which focuses on 12 National Key Economic Areas (NKEAs). The Agriculture sector, under the purview of the Ministry of Agriculture (MoA) is one of the NKEA-identified areas where the Entry Point Project 1 (EPP1) is focused on high-value herbal products. The MoA has overseen the establishment of five R&D clusters, which focus on, respectively, discovery, crop production, and agronomy, standardization and product development, toxicology/pre-clinical and clinical studies, and processing technology. The initial phase of this EPP was focused on ensuring the supply of five main local herbs, namely Tongkat Ali (*Eurycoma longifolia* Jack), Misai Kucing (*Orthosiphon aristatus* (Blume) Miq.), Hempedu Bumi (*Andrographis paniculata* (Burm.f.) Nees), Dukung Anak (*Phyllanthus niruri* L.) and Kacip Fatimah (*Marantodes pumilum* (Blume) Kuntze (*syn. Labisia pumila* (Blume) Mez). Subsequently, six more herb species were added to the project, including Mengkudu (*Morinda citrifolia* L.), Roselle (*Hibiscus sabdariffa* L.), Ginger (*Zingiber officinale*), Mas Cotek (*Ficus deltoidea* Jack), Belalai Gajah (*Clinacanthus nutans* (Burm.f.) Lindau) and Pegaga (*Centella asiatica* (L.) Urb) [35]. In 2014, eight products developed through the EPP 1 underwent pre-clinical trials. It is estimated that commercialization of the identified herbs will contribute MYR2.2 billion to the Gross National Income (GNI) by 2020 [35].

In Malaysia, research on natural products including the EPP-listed local herbs described above is being undertaken by research centers and institutions of higher learning (**Table 2**). Nevertheless, research in this area is also being carried out by various independent research groups in the local academia.

Entities	Institutions
Advanced Medical and Dental Institute	Universiti Sains Malaysia (USM)
Atta-ur-Rahman Institute for Natural Product Discovery	Universiti Teknologi MARA (UiTM)
Bioresource and Drug Discovery Research Group (BDD), Faculty Science and Natural Resources (FSSA)	Universiti Malaysia Sabah (UMS)
Centre For Natural Products And Drug Research (CENAR)	Universiti Malaya (UM)
Drug Discovery and Development Research Group (under purview of the Natural Products Cluster)	Universiti Kebangsaan Malaysia (UKM)
Institute of Bioproduct Development (IBD)	Universiti Teknologi Malaysia
Laboratory of Natural products, Institute of Bioscience	Universiti Putra Malaysia (UPM)
Natural Medicine Products Centre (NMPC)	International Islamic University Malaysia (IIUM)
Natural Product and Drug Discovery Centre (NPDC)	Malaysian Institute of Pharmaceuticals and Nutraceuticals (IPharm)
Natural Product Lab, Institute of Marine Biotechnology	Universiti Malaysia Terengganu (UMT)
Natural Products Division	Forest Research Institute Malaysia (FRIM)

Table 2. Entities involved in natural product research and development in Malaysia.

4. Studies of the effect of Malaysian plants on colon cancer

It has been estimated that around 1200 medicinal plants have potential pharmaceutical value [1]. Many of these species have been scientifically investigated by researchers seeking to provide evidence of effectiveness toward different diseases such as cancer, diabetes, arthritis, heart diseases, and many others. However, work on the effects of Malaysian plants on colon cancer specifically has been very limited (**Tables 3** and **4**). Nonetheless, several observations may be made on work undertaken to date that allow trends to be identified for the future of such work.

It is clear that there is no focused approach on any particular species, and most of the studies were conducted at the early stage of screening for anti-cancer effects with little in the way of continued development thereafter. This work includes cytotoxicity screening of crude extracts or compounds derived from solvent fractions against several types of cancer using *in vitro* cell line-based experiments. While the species investigated are edible herbs and fruit plants, in several instances, the parts of the plant investigated may not be commonly consumed as food. For instance, Moghadamtousi et al. [36] studied the leaf of soursop plant, rather than the more commonly consumed fruits, while Aisha et al. [38] investigated the rind of mangosteen fruit instead of the flesh. To this end, selection of species seems to be based on ethnomedicinal evidence within local communities and capitalizing upon the novelty aspect in that the species (or parts of plants) have not been investigated by other groups. The use of inedible plant parts may be also be related to the zero waste and health to wealth concepts where all parts of plants are considered potential biomass to be exploited. As such, materials from inedible parts of plants may be more cost-effective to be used. Furthermore, the majority of studies appear to be "isolated studies" with lack of continuing development as stated above, which may perhaps be due to lack of funding and proper planning for future work including networking. The lack of funding may also correspond to lack of facilities and equipment required to do further in depth robust work.

Plant and part of plant used	Common name	Compound/ extract tested	Type of study	Details/IC_{50}	Reference
Annona muricata L. (Leaf)	Graviola, soursop; [a]durian belanda	Ethyl acetate extract	*In vitro* HCT 116, HT29 and CCD841 cell lines	*In vitro* cytotoxicity IC_{50} = 4.29 ± 0.24 μg/ml (HT29) IC_{50} = 3.91 ± 0.35 μg/ml (HCT116) IC_{50} = 34.24 ± 2.12 μg/ml (CCD841) 5-Fluorouracil (positive control) IC_{50} = 1.10 ± 0.11 μg/ml (HT29) IC_{50} = 0.90 ± 0.09 μg/ml (HCT116) The extract also showed cell cycle arrest at G_1, induction of apoptosis, anti-migration and anti-invasive effects.	[36]
Annona muricata L. (Leaf)	Graviola, soursop; [a]durian belanda	Ethyl acetate extract	*In vitro* HT29 and CCD 841 cell lines.	*In vitro* cytotoxicity HT29 IC_{50} = 5.72 ± 0.41 μg/ml (12 h) IC_{50} = 3.49 ± 0.22 μg/ml (24 h) IC_{50} = 1.62 ± 0.24 μg/ml (48 h) CCD 841 IC_{50} = 64.32 ± 3.76 μg/ml (12 h) IC_{50} = 47.10 ± 0.47 μg/ml (24 h) IC_{50} =32.51 ± 1.18 μg/ml (48 h)	[37]
			In vivo AOM-induced colon cancer in rats	Aberrant Crypt formation after 2 weekly injections of extract. 250 mg/kg = 61.2% inhibition 500 mg/kg = 72.5% inhibition 5-FU = 79.5% inhibition	
Garcinia mangostana (Fruit rind)	Mangosteen; [a]manggis	Xanthone (81% α-mangostin and 16% γ-	*In vitro* HCT 116 cell line *In vivo* Subcutaneous tumor of	*In vitro* cytotoxicity 1) IC_{50} = 6.5 ± 1.0 μg/ml 2) IC_{50} = 5.1 ± 0.2 μg/ml 3) IC_{50} = 7.2 ± 0.4 μg/ml IC_{50} of Cisplatin (positive	[38]

Plant and part of plant used	Common name	Compound/ extract tested	Type of study	Details/IC$_{50}$	Reference
		mangostin) from toluene extract of the fruit α-mangostin γ-mangostin)	HCT116 on nude mice	control) = 6.1 ± 0.2 μg/ml The extract also showed induction of apoptosis, anti-tumorigenicity and up-regulation of MAPK/ERK, c-Myc/Max, and p53 cell signalling pathways *In vivo* Xanthones extract caused significant growth inhibition of the subcutaneous tumor	
Garcinia mangostana (Fruit rind)	Mangosteen; [a]manggis	Hexane and ethyl acetate (Other extracts produced, butanol and methanol)	*In vitro* Caco-2 cell line (also tested on other cells KB and PBMC)	*In vitro* cytotoxicity IC$_{50}$ = 13.0 ± 3.8 μg/ml (Hexane) IC$_{50}$ = 8.1 ± 0.1 μg/ml (Ethyl acetate) IC$_{50}$ of Tamoxifen positive control = 4.0 ± 0.4 μg/ml	[39]
Garcinia mangostana (Fruit rind)	Mangosteen; [a]manggis	α-mangostin β-mangostin γ-mangostin hexane extracts	*In vitro* DLD-1 cells	All three extracts showed anti-proliferative effects at 20 μM.	[40]

Table 3. Studies of anticancer effects of plant materials obtained from fruit trees in Malaysia.

Plant and part of plant used	Common name	Compound/extract tested	Type of study	Details/IC$_{50}$	References
Alpinia mutica (Rhizome)	[a]Tepus	Methanol and fractionated extracts (hexane, ethyl acetate and water)	*In vitro* HT 29 and HCT 116 cell line (also tested on other cell lines; KB, CasKi, MCF-7, A549 and MRC-5)	Hexane extracts showed IC$_{50}$ of 36.1 ± 1.1 μg/ml (HCT116) and 47.4 ± 1.6 μg/ml (HT29) Ethyl acetate extracts showed IC$_{50}$ of 20.4 ± 3.2 μg/ml (HCT116) and 24.2 ± 0.04 μg/ml (HT29) Methanol and water extracts showed IC$_{50}$ of more than 100 μg/ml IC$_{50}$ of doxorubicin (positive control) = 0.24 ± 0.04 μg/ml (HCT116) and 0.33 ± 0.03 μg/ml	[41]

Plant and part of plant used	Common name	Compound/extract tested	Type of study	Details/IC$_{50}$	References
				(HT29)	
Casearia capitellata (Leaf) *Baccaurea motleyana* (fruits and peel) *Phyllanthus pulcher* (Leaf, stem and root) *Strobilanthus crispus* (Leaf, flower)	[a]Simmilit matangi [a]Rambai [a]Naga buana [a]Pecah kaca/Pecah beling/ Pokok pecah/Jin batu/	Hexane, dichloromethane, ethyl acetate and methanol extracts, respectively	*In vitro* HT29 cell line (also tested on other cell lines; MCF-7, DU-145 and H460)	DCM extract of *P.pulcher* root showed the lowest IC$_{50}$ among the extracts tested against HT29 cells (IC$_{50}$ = 8.1 ± 0.5 µg/ml)	[42]
Curcuma mangga (Rhizome)	[a]Temu pauh/ Kunyit mangga	Crude methanol and fractionated extracts (hexane, ethyl acetate)	*In vitro* HT 29 and HCT 116 cell line(also tested on other cell lines; KB, CasKi, MCF-7, A549 and MRC-5)	Extracts showed the IC$_{50}$ between 29.4 ± 0.2 and 36.8 ± 3.8 µg/ml against HCT116 cells Extracts showed the IC$_{50}$ between 17.9 ± 0.3 and 22.0 ± 1.1 µg/ml against HT29 cells IC$_{50}$ of doxorubicin (positive control) = 0.24 ± 0.04 µg/ml (HCT116) and 0.33 ± 0.03 µg/ml (HT29) Isolated compounds from the extracts also showed high cytotoxicity effects towards both cell lines (between 6.3 ± 0.26 and 14.9 ± 0.40 µg/ml) Several isolated compounds from the extracts also showed considerable cytotoxicity effects against the cancer cells	[43]
Curcuma mangga (Rhizome)	[a]Temu pauh/	Hexane and ethyl acetate extracts.	*In vitro* HT29 and CCD-18Co	*In vitro* cytotoxicity (72 h) Hexane: IC$_{50}$ = 17.9 ± 1.2 µg/ml (HT29)	[44]

Plant and part of plant used	Common name	Compound/extract tested	Type of study	Details/IC_{50}	References
	Kunyit mangga			IC_{50} = 45.7 ± 1.0 μg/ml (CCD-18Co) Ethyl acetate: IC_{50} = 15.6 ± 0.8 μg/ml (HT29) IC_{50} = 46.5 ± 0.1 μg/ml (CCD-18Co)	
Pereskia bleo (Kunth) DC. (Cactaceae) (Leaf)	[a]Jarum tujuh bilah	Compounds from ethyl acetate fraction • Dihydroactinidiolide • β-sitosterol • 2,4-di tert butyl phenol • α-tocopherol • Phytol	*In vitro* HCT 116 cell line (also tested on other cell lines; KB, CasKi, MCF-7, A549 and MRC-5)	Dihydroactinidiolide showed the lowest IC_{50} at 5 μg/ml against HCT116 cells Dihydroactinidiolide showed IC_{50} of 91.3 μg/ml against MRC-5 cells IC_{50} of doxorubicin (positive control) = 0.36 μg/ml (HCT116) and 0.55 μg/ml (MRC-5)	[45]
Piper betle (Leaf)	[a]Sirih	Aqueous extract	*In vitro* HCT 116 and HT29 cell lines	In the presence of the extract, a lower dosage of 5-FU is required to achieve the maximum drug effect in inhibiting the growth of HT29 cells. However, the extract did not significantly reduce 5-FU dosage in HCT116 cells	[46]
Strobilanthus crispus (part of plant used not stated)	[a]Pecah kaca/Pecah beling/ Pokok pecah/Jin batu/	Crude ethanol extract and fractions obtained from column chromatography	In vivo Sprague Dawley (SD) male rats *In vitro* HT29, CCD841	*S. crispus* ethanol extract protects against CRC formation (azoxymethane-induced aberrant crypt foci) in rats Exposure of HT29 and CCD-841 to extract and several fractions (tested between 0 and 500 μg/ml) induced a concentration dependent decrease in cell viability	[47]
Zingiber officinale (rhizome)	Ginger; [a]halia	Ginger: Water-based ultrasonic assisted extraction Honey: Packaged in plastic containers and	*In vitro* HT29 cell lines	*In vitro* cytotoxicity IC_{50} = 5.2 mg/ml (ginger alone) IC_{50} = 80 mg/ml (Gelam honey alone) The combinations of 3 and 4 mg/ml of ginger with 27 and 10 mg/ml	[48]

Plant and part of plant used	Common name	Compound/extract tested	Type of study	Details/IC$_{50}$	References
		sterilized using gamma radiation		of Gelam honey showed combination index (CI) values of 0.92 and 0.90, respectively, indicating synergistic effects. Cell death in response to the combined ginger and Gelam honey treatment was associated with the stimulation of early apoptosis	
Zingiber officinale (rhizome)	Ginger; [a]halia	Ethanol extract	*In vitro* HCT 116 and HT29 cell lines	Inhibition of proliferation IC$_{50}$ (HCT116) = 496 ± 34.2 µg/ml IC$_{50}$ (HT29) = 455 ± 18.6 µg/ml Induction of apoptosis at 500 µg/ml extract 35.05% (HCT116) and 19.81% (HT29) Ginger extract arrested HCT 116 and HT 29 cells at G0/G1 and G2/M phases with corresponding decreased in S-phase	[49]

[a]Local name in Malay language.
Cell lines: A549 (and human lung carcinoma cell line); CasKi (human cervical carcinoma cell line); CCD841 (normal human colon epithelial cell line); DU-145 (prostate cancer cell line); H460 (lung cancer cell line); HCT116 (colon cancer cell line); HT29 (colon cancer cell line); KB (human nasopharyngeal epidermoid carcinoma cell line); MCF-7 (hormone-dependent breast carcinoma cell line; MRC-5 (non-cancer human fibroblast cell line).

Table 4. Studies of anticancer effects of plant materials obtained herbs and spices in Malaysia.

Some species investigated for their effects against colon cancer in the listed studies have also been investigated for other biological effects. For example, prior to the report by Abdul Malek et al. [43], *Alpinia mutica* was previously reported to have inhibitory activity towards lipid oxidation [50] and anti-bacterial effects against *Bacillus subtilis* and methicillin-resistant *Staphylococcus aureus* (MRSA) [50] in addition to anti-platelet aggregation activities [51].

For *in vitro* work, two types of commercially available colon cancer cell lines, HT29 and HCT116, were used in the majority of studies. However, there is no consistency in the positive controls used in the empirical studies. Some studies include work on CCD841 normal human colon epithelial cells [36, 47], while others include work on 5-Fluorouracil [46, 47], doxorubicin [45], or cisplatin [38] as positive control. Cytotoxic screening results from the studies listed in **Table 3** and **Table 4** showed that effects on colon cancer were only moderate as compared to other cells lines tested. The follow-up study by Moghadamtousi et al. [37] demonstrated significant decreases in aberrant crypt foci counts in an AOM-induced CRC animal model supporting prior observation *in vitro*. The limited success of *in vitro* studies excluding the aforementioned study may explain the lack of in-depth studies on the effects of the extracts on colon cancer following the screening phase.

The colon cancer cell lines used in the studies differ in their origin, mutation status and metabolic requirements [52]. For example, HT29 cells utilize glucose through the pentose phosphate pathway [53], whereas HCT116 cells have higher requirements for glutamine [52, 54]. In terms of gene expression, HT29 is deficient in expression of p53 [55], while HCT116 cells possess mutations in PI3KCA and KRAS genes which confer constitutive activation of PI3K/AKT and KRAS pathways [56]. Since the two cells lines have different characteristics, the use of such cell lines in preliminary studies is substantial as it can set forth the mechanistic investigations on the effects of the plants against colon cancer.

Although the majority of work was *in vitro*-based preliminary work, Al-Henhena et al. [47] reported both *in vitro* and *in vivo* studies on *Strobilanthus crispus*. Meanwhile, some studies investigated the cytotoxic effects of not only the crude extracts and fractions, but also tested the isolated compounds [38, 40, 45]. Among the studies reported, the same group showed a more thorough investigation of the species selected. Other researchers have combined the selected species with other components to determine their combined effects on colon cancer cells. For instance, Ng et al. [46] looked at the potential effects of *Piper betle* leaf extract to reduce the 5-Fluorouracil dosage required to exert the same cytotoxicity in HT29 and HCT116 cells. Tahir et al. [48] studied the combined effects of *Zingiber officinale* extracts and Gelam honey on viability of HT29 cells. Some researchers have also studied the potential mechanism of the selected species beyond cytotoxicity tests. *Garcinia mangostana* rind extracts showed induction of apoptosis, anti-tumorigenicity, and upregulation of MAPK/ERK, c-Myc/Max, and p53 cell signaling pathways [38] while *Annona muricata* leaf extracts showed cell cycle arrest at G1, induction of apoptosis, anti-migration, and anti-invasive effects [36]. While the follow-up study by Moghadamtousi et al. [37] supports the previous *in vitro* observations with aberrant crypt foci counts significantly reduced by the treatment in an AOM induced CRC animal model. Taken together, studies on Malaysian plants against colon cancer are at different technological levels with, consequently, very limited data to enable a consensus to be made.

Compounding the lack of consensus and technical variability is the fact that choice of journals in which to publish is still very much dependent on funding; thus, publishing in the open access journals with high impact factors can only be afforded by certain groups of researchers. This clearly will have hampered the dissemination of research data as, while it may be beneficial for researchers to reach a wider audience at the early stage of work, this may correspond to having to publish in a low-cost, lower impact journals due to lack of funding. From another perspective, higher impact journals often require more conclusive data, which in turn means more experimental work—early stage work may not meet such journals' publication criteria and may be perceived to be low quality. Therefore, it would be more favorable to have a mechanism to help improve the dissemination of work in order to enhance the overall research and development in the subject area.

Based on the publications considered in **Tables 3** and **4**, it was also observed that authors did not always report the local names of species investigated. Since these are local plants that may not even have English names, it is to be recommended that this information is included together with full description of the species investigated. This could be one way to present the potential positive effects of the species to a wider scientific community thereby increasing the impact and scientific value of the work. Thus, the correct taxonomy including genus, species and family should be given for accuracy.

5. Conclusion

Some Malaysian plants that show anti-cancer effects towards colon cancer include *Alpinia mutica* (tepus), *Annona muricata* (soursop), *Baccaurea motleyana* (rambai), *Casearia capitellata* (simmilit mantangi), *Curcuma manga* (temu pauh), *Garcinia mangostana* (mangosteen), *Pereskia bleo* (Kunth) (jarum tujuh bilah), *Phyllanthus pulcher* (naga buana), *Strobilanthus crispus* (pecah kaca), *and Zingiber officinale* (ginger).

Nevertheless, much of the scientific evidence is preliminary at best despite the selection of plant species for study based upon ethnomedicinal practices. The introduction of the EPP by the Malaysian government is a commendable effort to raise the value of indigenous Malaysian plants in the pharmaceutical sector. However, a more concerted approach to the work is necessary including a comprehensive review of the existing data in order to fully exploit local plants toward prevention and treatment of colon cancer.

Acknowledgements

We wish to thank Dr. Rashidi Othman, Kulliyyah of Architecture and Environmental Design (KAED), International Islamic University Malaysia (IIUM) for his valuable comments.

Author details

Yumi Z. H-Y. Hashim[1*], Chris I. R. Gill[2], Cheryl Latimer[2], Nigel Ternan[2] and Phirdaous Abbas[1]

*Address all correspondence to: yumi@iium.edu.my

1 Department of Biotechnology Engineering, Kulliyyah of Engineering, International Islamic University Malaysia, Kuala Lumpur, Malaysia

2 School of Biomedical Sciences, Ulster University, Northern Ireland, United Kingdom

References

[1]   Aman R. Tumbuhan Liar Berkhasiat Ubatan (Wild Plants with Medicinal Properties). Kuala Lumpur: Dewan Bahasa dan Pustaka; 2006. 12-14. ISBN: 9789836281517

[2]   Ferlay J, Soerjomataram I, Dikshit R, Eser S, Mathers C, Rebelo M, Parkin DM, Forman D, Bray F. Cancer incidence and mortality worldwide: sources, methods and major patterns in GLOBOCAN 2012. Int J Cancer. 2015;136. doi:10.1002/ijc.29210

[3]   Bray F, Jemal A, Grey N, Ferlay J, Forman D. Global cancer transitions according to the Human Development Index (2008–2030): a population-based study. Lancet Oncol. 2012;13(8):790–801. doi:10.1016/S1470-2045(12)70211-5

[4]   Ng CJ, Teo CH, Abdullah N, Tan WP, Tan HM. Relationships between cancer pattern, country income and geographical region in Asia. BMC Cancer. 2015;15:613. doi:10.1186/s12885-015-1615-0

[5]   WHO (World Health Organization). GLOBOCAN 2012 v1.0, Cancer Incidence and Mortality Worldwide: IARC CancerBase No. 11. [internet]. 2012. Available from: http://globocan.iarc.fr.[Accessed:2016-01-20]

[6]   Peipins LA, Sandler RS. Epidemiology of colorectal adenomas. Epidemiol Rev. 1994;16(2):273–97.

[7]   Kinzler KW, Vogelstein B. Lessons from hereditary colorectal cancer. Cell. 1996;87(2):159–70. doi:10.1016/S0092-8674(00)81333-1

[8]   Brenner H, Hoffmeister M, Stegmaier C, Brenner G, Altenhofen L, Haug U. Risk of progression of advanced adenomas to colorectal cancer by age and sex: estimates based on 840 149 screening colonoscopies. Gut. 2007;56(11):1585–9. doi:10.1136/gut.2007.122739

[9]   Kuntz KM, Lansdorp-Vogelaar I, Rutter CM, Knudsen AB, van Ballegooijen M, Savarino JE, et al. A systematic comparison of microsimulation models of colorectal cancer: the role of assumptions about adenoma progression. Med Decis Mak. 2011;31(4):530–9. doi:10.1177/0272989X11408730

[10] Jemal A, Bray F, Center MM, Ferlay J, Ward E, Forman D. Global cancer statistics. CA Cancer J Clin. 2011;61(2):69–90. doi:10.3322/caac.20107

[11] WCRF. Food, nutrition and the prevention of cancer: a global perspective [comprehensive report]. World Cancer Research Fund/American Institute for Cancer Research, Washington, DC; 2006.

[12] Romaguera D, Ward H, Wark PA, Vergnaud AC, Peeters PH, van Gils CH, Ferrari P, Fedirko V, Jenab M, Boutron-Ruault MC, Dossus L, Dartois L, et al. Pre-diagnostic concordance with the WCRF/AICR guidelines and survival in European colorectal cancer patients: a cohort study. BMC Med. 2015;13:107. doi:10.1186/s12916-015-0332-5

[13] Carethers JM, Jung BH. Genetics and genetic biomarkers in sporadic colorectal cancer. Gastroenterology. 2015;149(5):1177–1190. doi:10.1053/j.gastro.2015.06.047

[14] Lang M, Gasche C. Chemoprevention of colorectal cancer. Dig Dis. 2015;33(1):58–67. doi:10.1159/000366037

[15] Jiao S, Peters U, Berndt S, Brenner H, Butterbach K, Caan BJ, et al. Estimating the heritability of colorectal cancer. Hum Mol Genet. 2014;23(14):3898–905. doi: 10.1093/hmg/ddu087

[16] Shiovitz S, Grady WM. Molecular markers predictive of chemotherapy response in colorectal cancer. Curr Gastroenterol Rep. 2015;17(2):431. doi:10.1007/ s11894-015-0431-7

[17] Saltz LB, Clarke S, Diaz-Rubio E, et al. Bevacizumab in combination with oxaliplatin-based chemotherapy as first-line therapy in metastatic colorectal cancer: a randomized phase III study. J Clin Oncol. 2008;26:2013–9. doi:10.1200/JCO.2007.14.9930

[18] Lansdorp-Vogelaar I, Knudsen AB, Brenner H. Cost-effectiveness of colorectal cancer screening. Epidemiol Rev. 2011;33:88–100. doi:10.1093/epirev/mxr004

[19] Schreuders EH, Ruco A, Rabeneck L, Schoen RE, Sung JJ, Young GP, Kuipers EJ. Colorectal cancer screening: a global overview of existing programmes. Gut. 2015;64(10):1637–49. doi:10.1136/gutjnl-2014-309086

[20] Sung JJ, Ng SC, Chan FK, et al. An updated Asia Pacific Consensus Recommendations on colorectal cancer screening. Gut. 2015;64:121–32. doi:10.1136/gutjnl-2013-306503

[21] Sung JJ, Lau JY, Goh KL, Leung WK. Increasing incidence of colorectal cancer in Asia: implications for screening. Lancet Oncol. 2005;6:871–6. doi:10.1016/ S1470-2045(05)70422-8

[22] Carr PR, Walter V, Brenner H, Hoffmeister M. Meat subtypes and their association with colorectal cancer: systematic review and meta-analysis. Int J Cancer. 2016;138(2):293–302. doi:10.1002/ijc.29423

[23] Fedirko V, Tramacere I, Bagnardi V, Rota M, Scotti L, Islami F, Negri E, Straif K, Romieu I, La Vecchia C. Alcohol drinking and colorectal cancer risk: an overall and dose-response meta-analysis of published studies. Ann Oncol. 2011;22:1958–1972. doi: 10.1093/annonc/mdq653

[24] Gong J, Hutter C, Baron JA, Berndt S, Caan B, Campbell PT, Casey G, Chan AT, Cotterchio M, Fuchs CS. A pooled analysis of smoking and colorectal cancer: timing of exposure and interactions with environmental factors. Cancer Epidemiol Biomark Prev. 2012;21:1974–1985. doi:10.1158/1055-9965.EPI-12-0692

[25] Bradbury KE, Appleby PN, Key TJ. Fruit, vegetable, and fiber intake in relation to cancer risk: findings from the European Prospective Investigation into Cancer and

Nutrition (EPIC). Am J Clin Nutr. 2014;100(Supplement 1):394S–8S. doi:10.3945/ajcn. 113.071357

[26] Leenders M, Siersema PD, Overvad K, Tjønneland A, Olsen A, Boutron-Ruault M-C, et al. Subtypes of fruit and vegetables, variety in consumption and risk of colon and rectal cancer in the European Prospective Investigation into Cancer and Nutrition. Int J Cancer. 2015;137(11):2705–14. doi:10.1002/ijc.29640

[27] Li YH, Niu YB, Sun Y, Zhang F, Liu CX, Fan L, Mei QB. Role of phytochemicals in colorectal cancer prevention. World J Gastroenterol. 2015;21(31):9262–72. doi:10.3748/wjg.v21.i31.9262

[28] Núñez-Sánchez MA, González-Sarrías A, Romo-Vaquero M, García-Villalba R, Selma MV, Tomás-Barberán FA, García-Conesa MT, Espín JC. Dietary phenolics against colorectal cancer—from promising preclinical results to poor translation into clinical trials: pitfalls and future needs. Mol Nutr Food Res. 2015;59(7):1274–91. doi:10.1002/mnfr.201400866

[29] Fung KY, Cosgrove L, Lockett T, Head R, Topping DL. A review of the potential mechanisms for the lowering of colorectal oncogenesis by butyrate. Br J Nutr. 2012;108(5):820–31. doi:10.1017/S0007114512001948

[30] van Dijk M, Pot GK. The effects of nutritional interventions on recurrence in survivors of colorectal adenomas and cancer: a systematic review of randomised controlled trials. Eur J Clin Nutr. 2016. doi:10.1038/ejcn.2015.210. [Epub ahead of print]

[31] NCCIH (National Centre for Complementary and Integrative Health). [Internet]. 2015. Available from: https://nccih.nih.gov/grants/naturalproducts [Accessed: 2015-12-04]

[32] Editorial. All natural. Nat Chem Biol. 2007;3:351. doi:10.1038/nchembio0707-351

[33] WHO (World Health Organization). 1991. Report on the intercountry expert meeting of traditional medicine and primary health care. WHO-EMTRM/1-E/L/12.92/168, November 30–December 3, 1991, Cairo, Egypt.

[34] Akarasereenont P, Datiles MJR, Lumlerdkij N, Yaakob H, Prieto JM and Heinrich M. A South-East Asian Perspective on Ethnopharmacology. In: Heinrich M, Jager A, editors. Ethnopharmacology. Wiley-Blackwell; 2015. pp. 317–328. doi: 10.1002/9781118930717.ch27

[35] Performance Management & Delivery Unit; PEMANDU. [Internet]. 2013. Available from http://etp.pemandu.gov.my/Agriculture-@-Agriculture_-_EPP_1-;_High-Value_Herbal_Products.aspx#sthash.YK0kpNR8.dpuf. [Accessed: 2015-12-04]

[36] Moghadamtousi SZ, Karimian H, Rouhollahi E, Paydar, Fadaeinasab M, Abdul Kadir H. *Annona muricata* leaves induce G1 cell cycle arrest and apoptosis through mitochondria-mediated pathway in human HCT-116 and HT-29 colon cancer cells. J Ethnopharmacol. 2014;156:277–289. doi:10.1016/j.jep.2014.08.011

[37] Moghadamtousi SZ, Rouhollahi E, Karimian H, Fadaeinasab M, Firoozinia M, Abdulla MA, Kadir HA. The chemopotential effect of *Annona muricata* leaves against azoxyme-thane-induced colonic aberrant crypt foci in rats and the apoptotic effect of acetogenin annomuricin E in HT-29 cells: a bioassay-guided approach. Plos One. 2015;10(4):e0122288. doi:10.1371/journal.pone.0122288

[38] Aisha AFA, Abu-Salah KM, Ismail Z, Majid AMSA. *In vitro* and *in vivo* anti-colon cancer effects of *Garcinia mangostana* xanthones extract. BMC Complement Altern Med. 2012;12(1):1–10. doi:10.1186/1472-6882-12-104

[39] Khonkarn R, Okonogi S, Ampasavate C, Anuchapreeda S. Investigation of fruit peel extracts as sources for compounds with antioxidant and antiproliferative activities against human cell lines. Food Chem Toxicol. 2010;48(8–9):2122–2129. doi:10.1016/j.fct.2010.05.014

[40] Matsumoto K, Akao Y, Ohguchi K, Ito T, Tanaka T, Iinuma M, Nozawa Y. Xanthones induce cell-cycle arrest and apoptosis in human colon cancer DLD-1 cells. Bioorganic Med Chem. 2005;13(21):6064–9. doi:10.1016/j.bmc.2005.06.065

[41] Abdul Malek SN, Phang CW, Ibrahim H, Abdul Wahab N, Sim KS. Phytochemical and cytotoxic investigations of *Alpinia mutica* rhizomes. Molecules. 2011;16:583–589. doi:10.3390/molecules16010583

[42] Ismail M, Bagalkotkar G, Iqbal S, Adamu HA. Anticancer properties and phenolic contents of sequentially prepared extracts from different parts of selected medicinal plant indigenous to Malaysia. Molecules. 2012;17:5745–5756. doi:10.3390/molecules17055745

[43] Abdul Malek SN, Lee GS, Hong SL, Yaacob H, Abdul Wahab N, Weber J-FF, Ali Shah SA. Phytochemical and cytotoxic investigations of *Curcuma mangga* rhizomes. Molecules. 2011;16:4539–4548. doi:10.3390/molecules16064539

[44] Hong GW, Hong SL, Lee GS, Yaacob H, Malek SNA. Non-aqueous extracts of *Curcuma mangga* rhizomes induced cell death in human colorectal adenocarcinoma cell line (HT29) via induction of apoptosis and cell cycle arrest at G0/G1 phase. Asian Pac J Trop Med. 2016;9(1):8–18. doi:10.1016/j.apjtm.2015.12.003

[45] Abdul Malek SN, Sim KS, Abdul Wahab N, Yaacob H. Cytotoxic components of *Pereskia bleo* (Kunth) DC. (Cactaceae) leaves. Molecules. 2009;14:1713–1724. doi:10.3390/molecules14051713

[46] Ng PL, Rajab NF, Then SM, Mohd Yusof YA, Wan Ngah WZ, Pin KY, Looi ML. *Piper betle* leaf extract enhances the cytotoxicity effect of 5-fluorouracil in inhibiting the growth of HT29 and HCT116 colon cancer cells. J Zhejiang Univ Sci B Biomed Biotechnol. 2014;15:692–700. doi:10.1631/jzus.B1300303

[47] Al-Henhena N, Khalifa SAM, Poh YYR, Ismail S, Hamadi R, Shawter AN, Mohd Idris A, Azizan A, Al-Wajeeh NS, Abdulla MA, El-Seedi. Evaluation of chemopreventive

potential of *Strobilanthes crispus* against colon cancer formation *in vitro* and *in vivo*. BMC Complement Altern Med. 2015;15:419. doi:10.1186/s12906-015-0926-7

[48] Tahir AA, Sani NFA, Murad NA, Makpol S, Ngah WZW, Yusof YAM. Combined ginger extract & Gelam honey modulate Ras/ERK and PI3K/AKT pathway genes in colon cancer HT29 cells. Nutr J. 2015;14(1):1–10. doi:10.1186/s12937-015-0015-2

[49] Abdullah S, Zainal Abidin SA, Murad NA, Makpol S, Wan Ngah WZ, Mohd Yusof YA. Ginger extract (*Zingiber officinale*) triggers apoptosis and G0/G1 cells arrest in HCT 116 and HT 29 colon cancer cell lines. Afr J Biochem Res. 2010;4:134–142. ISSN: 1996-0778

[50] Mohamad H, Abas F, Permana D, Lajis NH, Alib AM, Sukaric MA, Hinc TYY, Kikuzakid H, Nakatanid N. DPPH free radical scavenger components from the fruits of *Alpinia rafflesiana* Wall. ex. Bak. (Zingiberaceae). Z. Naturforsch. 2004;59c:811–815.

[51] Jantan I, Pisar M, Sirat HM, Basar N, Jamil S, Ali RM, Jalil J. Inhibitory effects of compounds from Zingiberaceae species on platelet activating factor receptor binding. Phytother Res. 2004;18:1005–1007.

[52] Richard SM, Marignac MVL. Sensitization to oxaliplatin in HCT116 and HT29 cell lines by metformin and ribavirin and differences in response to mitochondrial glutaminase inhibition. J Cancer Res Ther. 2015;11:336–340. doi:10.4103/0973-1482.157317

[53] Vizán P, Alcarraz-Vizán G, Díaz-Moralli S, Solovjeva ON, Frederiks WM, Cascante M. Modulation of pentose phosphate pathway during cell cycle progression in human colon adenocarcinoma cell line HT29. Int J Cancer. 2009;124(12):2789–2796. doi:10.1002/ijc.24262

[54] Weinberg F, Hamanaka R, Wheaton WW, Weinberg S, Joseph J, Lopez M, et al. Mitochondrial metabolism and ROS generation are essential for Kras-mediated tumorigenicity. Proc Natl Acad Sci USA. 2010;107:8788–8793. doi:10.1073/pnas.1003428107

[55] Davidson D, Coulombe Y, Martinez Marignac V, Amrein L, Grenier J, Hodkinson K, et al. Irinotecan and DNA-PKcs inhibitors synergize in killing of colon cancer cells. Investig New Drugs. 2012;30:1248–56. doi:10.1007/s10637-010-9626-9

[56] Wang J, Kuropatwinski K, Hauser J, Ross MR, Zhou Y, Conway A, et al. Colon carcinoma cells harboring PIK3CA mutations display resistance to growth factor deprivation induced apoptosis. Mol Cancer Ther. 2007;6:1143–50. doi:10.1158/1535-7163.MCT-06-0555

4

Laparoscopy in the Management of Colon Cancer

Valentin Ignatov, Anton Tonev, Nikola Kolev,
Aleksandar Zlatarov, Shteryu Shterev, Dilyan Petrov,
Tanya Kirilova and Krasimir Ivanov

Abstract

The minimally invasive techniques in surgical practice have been well introduced and widely accepted for certain procedures, including surgery for colon cancer. The advantages of the laparoscopic approach in terms of early and late postoperative results and the oncological safety have been established by numerous reports, including randomized controlled trials. The application of laparoscopic colon surgery for cancer has been adopted in various institutions. This chapter reviews the available literature data regarding the use of minimally invasive surgery for colon cancer, including early and late surgical and oncological results and new trends. Retrospective and prospective trials published in the last 20 years are reviewed to address the issues. Technological advantages such as intracorproreal anastomosis, single incision, and natural orifice surgery are commented in the chapter.

Keywords: minimally invasive surgery, laparoscopy, colon cancer, hemicolectomy, colectomy, sigma resection

1. Introduction

The mainstay of treatment of colon cancer is the multidisciplinary approach. The advances of medical technology in various areas have led to improvement of cancer staging, surgical technique, medical oncology, and cancer biology. The logical consequence led to better treatment options. It was well stated in the article by Dinu et al. that a multidisciplinary team consisting of oncologists, surgeons, radiologists, physicists, and pathologists should provide the patient with a specific elaborate protocol of treatment, given the generally accepted treatment guidelines that are based on the efficacy of the multimodal treatment [1].

Reference	Procedure	Conversion to open surgery, % (number of total)		Operating time, min		Length of hospital stay, days		Postoperative morbidity, % (number of total)	
		HALS	LAC	HALS	LAC	HALS	LAC	HALS	LAC
HALS Study Group[*] [3]	All	14% (3/22)	22% (4/18)	152 ± 66	141 ± 54	7 (2–12)	6 (2–10)	5% (1/22)	22% (4/18)
Hassan[*] [6]	All	15% (16/109)	11% (17/149)	277 ± 96[*]	211 ± 108[*]	6 ± 3[*]	5 ± 3[*]	20% (18/109)	17% (11/149)
Segmental colectomy									
Targarona [10]	Left and right colectomy	7% (2/27)	7% (2/27)	140 ± 56 (70–300)	152 ± 34 (109–240)	6.5 ± 3.7	7.2 ± 3.9	26% (7/27)	22% (6/27)
Chang [14]	Sigmoidectomy/ left colectomy	0% (0/66)[*]	13% (11/85)[*]	189 ± 40 (120–290)	205 ± 60 (90–380)	5.2 ± 3.0 (3–22)	5.0 ± 2.4 (2–17)	21% (11/66)	16% (14/85)
Yano [16]	Low anterior resection	0% (0/5)	12.5% (1/8)	211 ± 48[*]	311 ± 78[*]	–	–	–	–
Lee [18]	Sigmoidectomy diverticulitis	4.8% (1/21)	14% (3/21)	171 ± 34[*]	197 ± 42[*]	6.7 ± 2.1	7.5 ± 8.2	24% (5/21)	19% (4/21)
Anderson [24]	Sigmoidectomy diverticulitis	6.1% (6/98)	23.5% (4/17)	142 ± 46.5	153 ± 40.4	5.0 ± 3.0	5.1 ± 3.3	14.6% (14/98)[*]	29.4% (5/17)[*]
Ringley[*] [26]	Left and right colectomy	–	–	120 (78–181)[*]	156 (74–300)[*]	4 (2–11)	4 (2–14)	–	–
Tjandra[*] [28]	Ultralow anterior resection	0% (0/32)	0% (0/31)	170 ± 20[*]	188 ± 16[*]	5.9 ± 0.8	5.8 ± 1.2	22% (7/32)	26% (8/31)
Total (procto)colectomy									
Nakajima [29]	Total (procto-)colectomy	0% (0/12)	9.1% (1/11)	217 ± 63[*]	281 ± 62[*]	7.6 ± 2.7	8.1 ± 2.4	33% (4/12)	45% (5/11)
Rivadeneira [30]	Proctocolectomy	10% (1/10)	0% (0/13)	265 ± 57 (210–390)[*]	311 ± 40 (240–400)[*]	6.1 ± 3.3 (3–13)	7.2 ± 3.9 (4–17)	40% (4/10)	31% (4/13)
Boushey[*] [31]	Total (procto-) colectomy	2% (1/45)[*]	7% (6/85)[*]	TAC: 240 ± 49 TPC: 297 ± 52	271 ± 60 315 ± 70	TAC: 6 (3–34) TPC: 5 (4–14)	5 (4–25) 5 (3–24)	TAC: 24% (4/17) TPC: 32% (9/28)	35% (18/52) 24% (8/33)
Polle [32]	Total restorative proctocolectomy	0% (0/30)	0% (0/35)	231 ± 60 (149–400)	297 ± 38.5 (235–375)	11.8 ± 5.7 (5–31)			

Table 1. Characteristics of HALS and LAC in several studies included in the metaanalysis on hand-assisted and laparoscopic assisted approach in colorectal surgery by Aalbers et al. [33].

Laparoscopic approach is used with increased frequency for many surgical procedures. The laparoscopic colectomy follows the principles of open oncological surgery – low ligation of the blood vessels at their origin and no-touch isolation [2]. Usually the anastomosis for right-colon tumors is performed extracorporally, and thus minimal laparotomy is required. The laparoscopic technique decreases length of hospital stay and pain and allows sooner restoration of food intake. Laparoscopy can be safely used if the following criteria are absent: severe adhesions, advanced tumor (e.g., T4),and/ or complicated colon cancer. The similarity between oncological results and the defined short-term clinical advantages of laparoscopic and open surgery for colon cancer have been proven in various multicenter studies. [14]. The patients with previous abdominal surgery (PAS) are at risk due to severe adhesions. The laparoscopic adhesiolysis is more technically challenging and time consuming. The study of Zanghi et al. reviews that matter and concludes that laparoscopic adhesiolysis increases the risk of bowel injury [7]. PAS is not universally accepted as contraindication for laparoscopic surgery, although it complicates the procedure as a whole. Law et al. reported patients with PAS who did not develop short-term postoperative complications such as ileus, prolonged hospital stay, or conversion rate after colorectal surgery [4]. In contrast, Yamamoto et al. described relatively higher rates of intraoperative intestinal injury and postoperative complications, including ileus and delayed time to diet in patients with a history of abdominal surgery [5] (**Table 1**).

2. Laparoscopy for colon cancer

2.1. Patients

In results from a single-center study from Tajima et al., patients were compared according to their age, gender, and tumor location between the hand-assisted laparoscopy (HALS) and CL groups [8] (**Table 2**). Less bleeding during surgery, faster postoperative recovery, and shorter stay are some of numerous advantages of laparoscopic resection of colon. After all, there are doubts of the radical curative effect of complete tumor resection, lymph node dissection, and puncture implantation metastasis by laparoscopic surgery. However, the most important indicator for the radical curative effect of laparoscopic surgery is the number of dissected lymph nodes. CRM is significant for the assessing of the prognosis of colorectal cancer surgery. The long-term survival rate of colorectal cancer patients undergoing laparoscopic surgery compared to open surgery procedures is also analyzed. No statistical difference in 3- or 5-year OS and 3-or 5-year DFS between the two procedures was reported (P>0.05) [8].

Surgical time of colorectal cancer laparoscopic surgery is longer compared to open surgery, and laparoscopic surgery requires a more skilful surgeon. The surgeons undergo rigorous training and development for a period of time, which improves the surgical procedure [9]. Also the nonneoplasm technique is important, which is the same as the open surgery is. The previously used method for the quality assessment with digital score may cause deviation.

Surgical methods	HALS, % (n)	CL, % (n)	P-value
Right hemicolectomy	26.5 (26)	24.6 (28)	0.743
Transverse colectomy	2.0 (2)	7.0 (8)	0.088
Left hemicolectomy	8.2 (8)	7.0 (8)	0.753
Anterior resection	27.6 (27)	33.3 (38)	0.363

Table 2. Comparison of stage I/II/III patients (n = 145) who underwent HALS (n = 63) or CL (n = 82).

2.2. Hand-Assisted Laparoscopic Surgery

Over the last years, minimally invasive laparoscopic surgery is being used more and more. Additional bowel resection for stage I rectal cancer, radical resection of stage II or III rectal cancer, and palliative surgery in patients with stage IV rectal cancer are among the indications of laparoscopic surgery. Traditional laparotomy for rectal cancer makes it difficult to visualize certain areas, including the pelvic floor, the ventral part of the bladder, and the posterior to apical regions of the prostate.

The traditional laparoscopic approach has been well established. In some cases a hybrid approach is required, e.g., rectal cancer surgery. The traditional laparotomy may reveal certain anatomical areas. On the other hand, the laparoscope provides magnified view of the structures and allows for safer approach. Laparoscopy-assisted colorectal surgery (LACS) is used in Japan and several drawbacks are reported – is more time consuming and requires specific experience and technical equipment, which makes it more challenging. In Europe and the United States, the so-called hybrid-hand assisted laparoscopic surgery (HALS) is more widespread, which allows for direct vision. The advantages of HALS include direct safe palpation and grasping with the hand, shorter operative time, and shorter learning-curve.

2.3. Outcomes

2.3.1. Short-term benefits of laparoscopic surgery

Laparoscopic procedures have several short-term benefits that are well described in all reports on the topic of minimally invasive procedures. Those include earlier restoration of bowel function, oral food intake, smaller incision, and less operative trauma (therefore less need for analgesia) and were proven in various randomized control trials. In the case of cancer surgery, the laparoscopic approach allows for faster recovery, which may influence the oncological results by sooner initiation of systemic therapy. The hospital stay is shorter in comparison to open surgery. In elderly and comorbid patients, the laparoscopic surgery may lead to cardio-vascular and pulmonary complications, although the mortality and morbidity rates are lower than in open surgery.

2.3.2. Long-term outcomes

Oncological outcomes of LS and OS for colorectal cancer patients were similar in most randomized studies. The random trial conducted by Lacy et al. [11] showed excellent long-term oncologic outcomes following LS, when compared with OS in patients with curable colon cancer. This study had a median follow-up of 95 months, but there was only one difference between the two techniques including the higher survival rate of patients with stage III colon cancer.

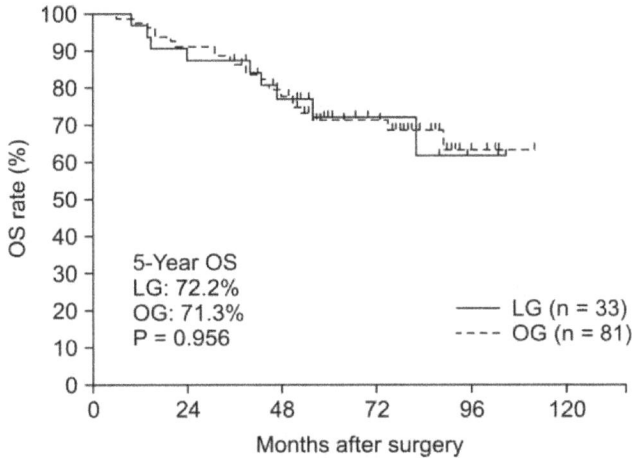

Figure 1. Overall survival (OS) of stage III colon cancer patients. LG, laparoscopic surgery group; OG, open surgery group [11].

The oncologic outcomes after performing LS instead of OS are still being analyzed when treating colorectal cancer patients. Recurrences and disease-free and overall survivals following LS compared to OS for stage III colorectal cancer patients are shown on **Figure 1** [11].

The long-term results are similar for laparoscopy and open surgery. On the contrary, a study made by Lacy et al. [11] has noted some oncological benefits for stage III colon cancer, including better local recurrence rates and higher rates of long-term and overall survival. For stage I and II, there were no significant oncological differences. Those results could be explained by patient's immunity response, dissemination of cancer cells, and earlier start of systemic treatment. The rates of local and distant metastases are found to be lower after laparoscopic surgery [12]. Despite that peritoneal carcinomatosis rates remain the same. The local recurrence rate of right colon cancer is relatively higher in compared to the left localization, although this is not confirmed by randomized studies [13].

3. New trends

3.1. SILS

The increasing patients' interest in cosmetic results has led to the more frequent use of single-incision surgery, even for colon cancer. The ultimate goal of "scarless surgery" could be achieved only when oncological results are proven to be equivalent to standard laparoscopic surgery. SILS ports are placed at the umbilicus or in case of rectal cancer at the planned site of a stoma. SILS reduces the abdominal incision trauma, provides better cosmesis, and reportedly, shorter hospital stay. SILS approach is successfully applied in laparoscopic colorectal procedures. For last few years, there are more data about this approach, which confirmed benefits of and interests in this technique. The SILS technique is administered to patients and the achieved results are promising. The development of SILS went from simple surgical procedures to the first colorectal resections in 2008. The first sigmoidectomy for benign disease was performed by Bucher et al. [17]. This approach was also used for anterior rectal resection, proctocolectomy, and total proctocolectomy. Lu C-C et al. as well as some other authors suggested that SILS could be applied both for benign and malignant cases [17, 20, 22, 23].

The operative time compared to conventional laparoscopic surgery is varying, and according to some retrospective studies the difference is not statistically significant. The operative time yet is longer, regardless of the procedure according to a study by Kwag et al [20]. The difference of operative times could be explained also by the fact that this techniques is not that widely used and the learning curve is steeper. Other criteria such as pain are reported to be more severe after SILS [20], although other authors report decrease of pain [22, 23].

4. NOTES

The first human colorectal natural orifice endoscopic surgery (NOTES) procedure was initiated with the reports of Bernhardt et al. [19] and Palanivelu et al. [25], who performed appendectomy in 2008. Performance of more complex procedures was limited by the instrumentation. In addition the colorectal procedures require restoration of continuity, which is a major limitation for NOTES. The hybrid NOTES procedures such as trans- anal total mesocolic excision (TEM) broaden the possibilities for this technique (**Figure 2**).

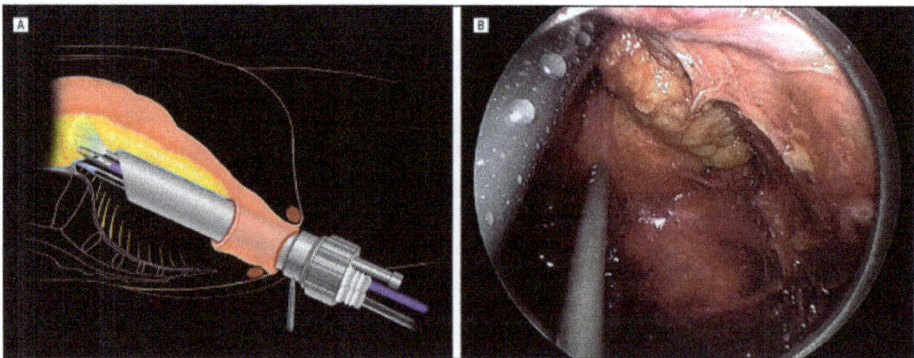

Figure 2. Schematic of retroperitoneal dissection with the transluminal transanal endoscopic operation device (A) and intraoperative view of the retroperitoneal approach at the sacral promontory (B) [24].

SILS evolved starting with cadavers and swines [25]. Sylla et al. [15] reported successful total mesorectum excision (TME) with laparoscopic assistance in a human. Two cases of laparoscopically assisted transanal TME were reported by Dumont et al. [21]. The clinical and oncological advantages are yet to be analyzed [2, 27–29].

Alternative technique is the mini-laparoscopy-assisted natural orifice surgery (MA-NOS), which includes additional laparoscopic ports less than 5mm and main port inserted in the natural orifice. The largest port is placed in the natural orifice. Lacy et al. [27] has pioneered this technique and presented a case of total colectomy. The authors suggest that the lack of dedicated NOTES instruments requires laparoscopic assistance.

5. Summary

Laparoscopic colon resection for cancer can be performed safely and accurately with many short-term benefits to the patients while resulting in at least equivalent long-term results as open surgery procedures. Other potential benefits may include better preservation of cell-mediated immune function and reduced tumor cell proliferation. The scientific confirmation of the efficacy of laparoscopic surgery is needed to implement it further in the practice and accept it as a worldwide standard. The available level 1 data support safety, patient-related benefits, and oncological similarity. Innovative approaches are being tested, including less abdominal wall trauma. Mastering the laparoscopic approach still has a steep learning curve, although the even more available laparoscopic courses will diminish that issue.

Author details

Valentin Ignatov, Anton Tonev*, Nikola Kolev, Aleksandar Zlatarov, Shteryu Shterev, Dilyan Petrov, Tanya Kirilova and Krasimir Ivanov

*Address all correspondence to: teraton@abv.bg

Department of General and Operative Surgery, Medical University of Varna, Varna, Bulgaria

References

[1] Therapeutic strategies in colonic cancer. Chir Buchar Rom 1990. 2014 Dec;109(6):741–6.

[2] García- Valdecasas JC, Delgado S, Castells A, Taurá P, Piqué JM,. Laparoscopy-assisted colectomy versus open colectomy for treatment of non-metastatic colon cancer: a randomised trial. The Lancet. 2002 Jun 29;359(9325):2224–9.

[3] HALS Study Group (2000) Hand-assisted laparoscopic surgery vs. standard laparoscopic surgery for colorectal disease: a prospective randomized trial. Surg Endosc 14:896–901 CrossRef

[4] Law WL, Lee YM, Chu KW. Previous abdominal operations do not affect the outcomes of laparoscopic colorectal surgery. Surg Endosc Interv Tech. 2005;19(3):326–30.

[5] Yamamoto M, Okuda J, Tanaka K, Kondo K, Asai K, Kayano H, . Effect of Previous Abdominal Surgery on Outcomes Following Laparoscopic Colorectal Surgery: Dis Colon Rectum. 2013 Mar;56(3):336–42.

[6] Hassan I, Nancy You Y, Cima RR, Larson DW, Dozois EJ, Barnes SA, Pemberton JH (2007) Hand-assisted versus laparoscopic-assisted colorectal surgery: practice patterns and clinical outcomes in a minimally-invasive colorectal practice. Surg Endosc Aug [Epub ahead of print]

[7] Zanghì A, Cavallaro A, Piccolo G, Fisichella R, Di Vita M, Spartà D, . Dissemination metastasis after laparoscopic colorectal surgery versus conventional open surgery for colorectal cancer: a metaanalysis. Eur Rev Med Pharmacol Sci. 2013 May;17(9):1174–84.

[8] Tajima T, Mukai M, Noguchi W, Higami S, Uda S, Yamamoto S, . Comparison of hand-assisted laparoscopic surgery and conventional laparotomy for rectal cancer: Interim results from a single center. Mol Clin Oncol [Internet]. 2015 Feb 9 [cited 2016 Feb 5]; Available from: http://www.spandidos-publications.com/10.3892/mco.2015.508

[9] Lee S. Laparoscopic Procedures for Colon and Rectal Cancer Surgery. Clin Colon Rectal Surg. 2009 Nov;22(04):218–24.

[10] Targarona EM, Gracia E, Garriga J, Martinez-Bru C, Cortes M, Boluda R, Lerma L, Trias M (2002) Prospective randomized trial comparing conventional laparoscopic colectomy with hand-assisted laparoscopic colectomy: applicability, immediate clinical outcome, inflammatory response, and cost. Surg Endosc 16:234–239 PubMed Cross Ref.

[11] Lacy AM, Delgado S, Castells A, Prins HA, Arroyo V, Ibarzabal A, . The long-term results of a randomized clinical trial of laparoscopy-assisted versus open surgery for colon cancer. Ann Surg. 2008 Jul;248(1):1–7.

[12] Baek J-H, Lee G-J, Lee W-S. Comparison of long-term oncologic outcomes of stage III colorectal cancer following laparoscopic versus open surgery. Ann Surg Treat Res. 2015;88(1):8.

[13] Guerrieri M, Campagnacci R, De Sanctis A, Lezoche G, Massucco P, Summa M, . Laparoscopic versus open colectomy for TNM stage III colon cancer: results of a prospective multicenter study in Italy. Surg Today. 2012 Nov;42(11):1071–7.

[14] Chang YJ, Marcello PW, Rusin LC, Roberts PL, Schoetz DJ (2005) Hand-assisted laparoscopic sigmoid colectomy: helping hand or hindrance? Surg Endosc 19:656–661 PubMed CrossRef.

[15] Sylla P, Bordeianou LG, Berger D, Han KS, Lauwers GY, Sahani DV, . A pilot study of natural orifice transanal endoscopic total mesorectal excision with laparoscopic assistance for rectal cancer. Surg Endosc. 2013 Sep;27(9):3396–405.

[16] Yano H, Ohnishi T, Kanoh T, Monden T (2005) Hand-assisted laparoscopic low anterior resection for rectal carcinoma. J Laparoendosc Adv Surg Tech A 15:611–614 PubMed CrossRef.

[17] Bucher P, Pugin F, Morel P. Single port access laparoscopic right hemicolectomy. Int J Colorectal Dis. 2008 Oct;23(10):1013–6.

[18] Lee SW, Yoo J, Dujovny N, Sonoda T, Milsom JW (2006) Laparoscopic vs. hand-assisted laparoscopic sigmoidectomy for diverticulitis. Dis Colon Rectum 49:464–469 PubMed CrossRef.

[19] Bernhardt J, Gerber B, Schober H-C, Kähler G, Ludwig K. NOTES--case report of a unidirectional flexible appendectomy. Int J Colorectal Dis. 2008 May;23(5):547–50.

[20] Kwag S-J, Kim J-G, Oh S-T, Kang W-K. Single incision vs conventional laparoscopic anterior resection for sigmoid colon cancer: a case-matched study. Am J Surg. 2013 Sep; 206(3):320–5.

[21] Dumont F, Goéré D, Honoré C, Elias D. Transanal endoscopic total mesorectal excision combined with single-port laparoscopy. Dis Colon Rectum. 2012 Sep;55(9):996–1001.

[22] Kim S-J, Ryu G-O, Choi B-J, Kim J-G, Lee K-J, Lee SC, . The short-term outcomes of conventional and single-port laparoscopic surgery for colorectal cancer. Ann Surg. 2011 Dec;254(6):933–40.

[23] Lu C-C, Lin S-E, Chung K-C, Rau K-M. Comparison of clinical outcome of single-incision laparoscopic surgery using a simplified access system with conventional laparoscopic surgery for malignant colorectal disease: Single-incision laparoscopic colectomy. Colorectal Dis. 2012 Apr;14(4):e171–6.

[24] Anderson J, Luchtefeld M, Dujovny N, Hoedema R, Kim D, Butcher J (2007) A comparison of laparoscopic, hand-assist and open sigmoid resection in the treatment of diverticular disease. Am J Surg 193:400–403 PubMed CrossRef.

[25] Palanivelu C, Rajan PS, Rangarajan M, Parthasarathi R, Senthilnathan P, Prasad M. Transvaginal endoscopic appendectomy in humans: a unique approach to NOTES-- world's first report. Surg Endosc. 2008 May;22(5):1343–7.

[26] Ringley C, Lee YK, Iqbal A, Bocharev V, Sasson A, McBride CL, Thompson JS, Vitamvas ML, Oleynikov D (2007) Comparison of conventional laparoscopic and hand-assisted oncologic segmental colonic resection. Surg Endosc 24: Epub ahead of print.

[27] Lacy AM, Adelsdorfer C, Delgado S, Sylla P, Rattner DW. Minilaparoscopy-assisted transrectal low anterior resection (LAR): a preliminary study. Surg Endosc. 2013 Jan; 27(1):339–46.

[28] Tjandra JJ, Chan MKY, Yeh CH (2007) Laparoscopic-vs. hand-assisted ultralow anterior resection: a prospective study. Dis Colon Rectum Dec [Epub ahead of print]

[29] Nakajima K, Lee SW, Cocilovo C, Foglia C, Sonoda T, Milsom JW (2004) Laparoscopic total colectomy: hand-assisted vs. standard technique. Surg Endosc 18:582–586 PubMed CrossRef

[30] Rivadeneira DE, Marcello PW, Roberts PL, Rusin LC, Murray JJ, Coller JA, Schoetz DJ Jr (2004) Benefits of hand-assisted laparoscopic restorative proctocolectomy: a comparative study. Dis Colon Rectum 47:1371–1376 PubMed CrossRef

[31] Boushey RP, Marcello PW, Martel G, Rusin LC, Roberts PL, Schoetz DJ Jr (2007) Laparoscopic total colectomy: an evolutionary experience. Dis Colon Rectum 50: 1512–1519 PubMed CrossRef

[32] Polle SW, van Berge Henegouwen MI, Slors FM, Cuesta MA, Gouma DJ, Bemelman WA (2008) Total laparoscopic restorative proctocolectomy: are there any advantages compared with the open and hand-assisted approach? Dis Colon Rectum [Epub ahead of print]

[33] Aalbers AGJ, Biere SSAY, van Berge Henegouwen MI, Bemelman WA. Hand-assisted or laparoscopic-assisted approach in colorectal surgery: a systematic review and meta-analysis. Surg Endosc. 2008;22(8):1769–80.

5

Current Immunotherapeutic Treatments in Colon Cancer

Zodwa Dlamini, Thandeka Khoza, Rodney Hull,
Mpho Choene and Zilungile Mkhize-Kwitshana

Abstract

The immune system is able to act against cancer cells and consequently these cells have developed a range of responses to evade or suppress the immune systems anticancer responses. The concept of cancer immunotherapy is based on techniques developed to restore or boost the ability of the immune system to recognize and target tumor cells. It is known that colon cancer does initiate an immune response and that this type of cancer initiates pathways and responses to evade or suppress the immune system. This chapter will discuss some of the dominant therapies being developed to treat colon cancer based on the concept of cancer immunotherapy. Cancer vaccines are based on the concept of providing the immune system with antigen targets derived from tumor-specific molecules, while monoclonal antibodies involve the development of antibodies specifically targeting proteins expressed on the surface of tumor cells. Antibody-based immunotherapy has further applications in the use of bispecific antibodies (BsAb), which are synthetic antibodies designed to be able to recognize two different antigens or epitopes and in this way can increase the immunoresponse and limit immune evasion observed in mono-targeted therapy. Immune checkpoint inhibitors target proteins that are responsible for keeping immune responses in check. Tumor cells overexpress these proteins in order to evade the immune response. Blocking these proteins will lead to an increased immune response against these cells. Cytokine-based immunotherapies involve the use of the immune systems' own molecular messengers that are responsible for a robust immune response, to boost the antitumor response of the immune system. Oncolytic viral therapy is based on the use of viruses that selectively infect and replicate in cancer and associated endothelial cells and subsequently kills these cells. Adoptive immunotherapy involves the use of immune cells from the patient to be cultured and altered in the laboratory and then reintroduced to boost the immune response. This is normally performed with T cells. Immunotherapy may be the next logical step in the development of an effective therapy for colon cancer and other cancers. The combination of these therapies with traditional chemotherapy or radiotherapy has shown promise in cancer treatment.

Keywords: Cancer vaccines, Monoclonal antibodies, Bispecific antibodies, Cytokines, Immune checkpoint inhibitors, Adoptive therapy, Immunotherapy

1. Introduction: immunotherapy

Tumor-associated antigens (TAAs) are antigens that can elicit a specific immune response. Immune cells and immune-related components such as macrophages, neutrophils, complement components, γδ T cells, natural killer (NK) cells, NKT cells, and certain cytokines (interleukin (IL)-12, interferon gamma (IFN-γ)) and cells of the adaptive immune system, including B lymphocytes, helper T cells (Th cells), and cytotoxic T lymphocytes (CTLs), are all active against cancer cells [1]. TAAs are presented to the cells of the adaptive immune system by cells such as dendritic cells (DCs) or other antigen-presenting cells (APCs). These antigens are processed and presented by major histocompatibility complex (MHC) class I and class II molecules leading to the activation of antigen-specific lymphocytes, resulting in antibody production [1].

Colon cancer evades the immune system through the shift from Th1 to Th2 immune responses [2] loss/downregulation of human leukocyte antigen (HLA) class I antigen processing and presentation [3], defective DC function [4, 5], T-cell loss of signaling molecules [6, 7], escaping death receptors, HLA G expression, alterations in transforming growth factor (TGF) beta signaling [8], Increased vascular endothelial growth factor (VEGF) expression, impaired NK activity, regulatory T-cell downregulation [9], and complement decay accelerating factor CD55 [2]. A shift is known to occur in the white blood cell composition with elevated numbers of CD8 T cells in the initial stages, but an overall reduction in the numbers of circulating immune-related cells. At the same time the levels of cytokines such as IFN-γ and tumor necrosis factor-α (TNFα) are reduced during vascular invasion [10]. Antitumor T cells can be inhibited through NO production by the enzyme arginase [11].

Immunotherapy can be divided into two main categories: passive and active immunotherapy. Passive immunotherapy makes use of *in vitro* produced immunologic effectors that are capable of influencing tumor cell growth. This includes monoclonal antibody (mAb) therapy and adaptive transfer of antigen-specific effector cells. Active immunotherapy aims at inducing or boosting immune effector cells [1].

2. Cancer vaccines

Cancer vaccines are active immunotherapeutic approaches that are intended to activate and expand tumor-specific T cells to induce an antitumor response. Conventional vaccines are preventative in nature, but current cancer vaccines activate the immune system to destroy tumors once present. A range of tumor antigens have been identified. These include T-cell epitope peptides, defined carbohydrates of glycoproteins and glycolipids, antibody-based anti-idiotype vaccines, plasmid DNA and recombinant viral vector vaccines, allogeneic or autologous whole tumor cell vaccines, DC-based vaccines, oncolysates, or autologous heat-shock protein (HSP)-peptide complex vaccines. An ideal prophylactic cancer vaccine would be affordable, stable, and safe. It would induce effective immunity rapidly and require few immunizations (ideally one) to induce protection [12]. This section aims to address advances made in developing vaccines against colon cancer. This will include vaccines that are currently in use and vaccines still undergoing clinical trials. It will report on the safety, side effects, and efficacy of these vaccines.

Colon cancers express multiple immunogenic proteins, all of which may serve as targets for the development of T-cell-mediated adaptive immune responses [10]. It is also known that colorectal cancers do activate the immune system, leading to the attenuation of metastasis and increasing the survival of patients [10]. In order to evade the immune response, colorectal cancer suppresses the immune response or displays only weak immunogenicity. Additionally, studies have shown that restoration or supplementation of the immune function toward these tumors is possible [10, 13, 14]. Peptides used to inoculate a patient suffering from colon cancer will be degraded and the resulting fragments will be endocytosed by APCs. These cells will then present the antigen to the T cells. CTLs or CD8+ T cells induce apoptosis in tumor cells through the release of granzymes and perforins and through the Fas death receptor pathway. Type 1 CD4+ T cells and T-helper cells secrete cytokines leading to the recruitment of CTLs, macrophages, and NK cells. These secrete cytokines that activate cytotoxic pathways [11] (**Figure 1**). It is also known that colorectal cancers do activate the immune system, leading to the attenuation of metastasis and an increase in the survival rate and time of patients [10]. The effectiveness of peptide vaccines can be enhanced by altering the amino acid sequence of the peptide to enhance the interaction with the T-cell receptor (TCR), to improve binding to MHC, and finally to improve biostability and reduce degradation by proteases [11].

2.1. Evasion of the immune system by altered ligand expression

One mechanism utilized by cancer cells to evade the immune system involves the expression of FasL. This ligand binds to the Fas receptor present on CTL, leading to the CTL to undergo apoptosis. The expression of FasL leads to the increased resistance to Fas-induced apoptosis. Altered peptide ligands (APLs) are analogs of immunogenic peptides which are ligands for TCRs. These altered ligands bind the TCR, but does not lead to lysis of the tumor cell [11]. Regulatory T cells can inhibit antitumor immunity by upregulating cell membrane molecules that lead to the inhibition of effector T-cell activation and function. Cancer cells have defective antigen presentation allowing them to avoid recognition by the immune system. This is accomplished by reduced expression of MHC I, antigen-processing machinery, or Tumor-associated antigens themselves [11].

2.2. Tumor-associated antigens (TAAs)

Defined TAA epitopes can be used to vaccinate cancer patients. The peptide fragments are presented by the two MHC proteins, MHC classes I and II (HLA I and II) to the TCRs. MHC class I presents the vaccine-derived peptide to naive CTLs. Primed CTLs recognize the tumor antigen on the surface of the tumor and send out a death signal to the tumor. Helper T cells are generated by MHC class II proteins [11] (**Figure 1**). However, there are not many specific peptides that can be targeted as cancer specific. In order to increase uptake and presentation of the antigens by APCs, an adjuvant is added [1]. Another strategy is to inject the DNA sequences coding for specific TAAs to be taken up. The target ill be transcribed into mRNA, translated into a protein, and processed into peptides by APCs. This can be done by using viruses engineered to express TAAs. However, the immune system may preferentially react to the viral antigens rather than the TAAs, leading to the attenuation of the antitumor immune response [1]. The earliest example of the therapeutic use of tumor antigens was in the form of crude tumor lysates being administered to patients. These lysates are still used as a means to prime DCs, facilitating peptide presentation [11]. This is because the ideal source of TAAs is all the TAAs the tumor itself expresses. By incubating DCs with dead tumor cell lysate, these antigens will all be presented by MHC class I (cross-presentation) and MHC class II pathways. This will result in a diversified immune response involving CTLs as well as CD4+ T-helper cells [1].

The use of tumor lysates has largely been superseded by the use of synthetic peptides. These have certain advantages over tumor lysates. They provide a higher amount of specific antigen and allow for modification of the target peptide. It is also easy to monitor the immune response to vaccination with a single peptide as only one CTL type requires evaluation [11]. Tumor-specific antigens (TSAs) are mutated or virus-derived epitopes and contain unique immuno-genic neo-antigens that can be recognized by the immune system. These include N-RAS and p53 [1].

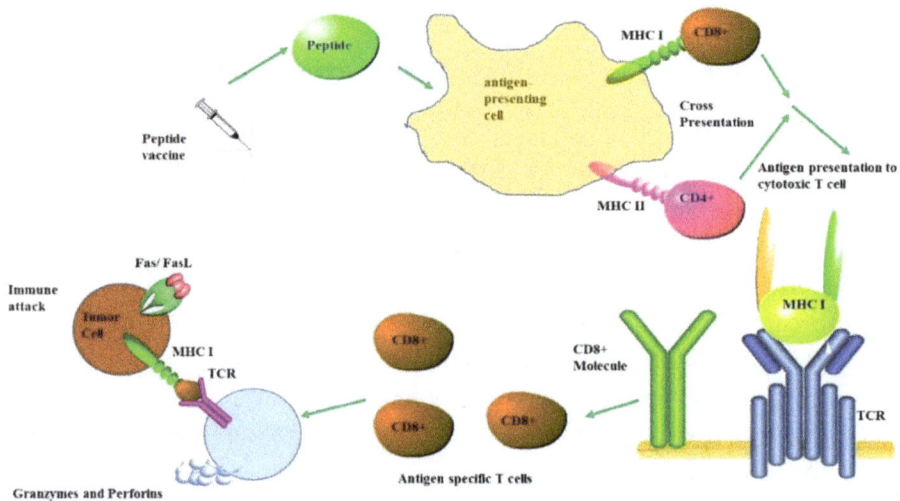

Figure 1. Antitumor effect of peptide vaccine therapy: following introduction of peptide vaccine to the bloodstream, it is processed and presented by the APC leading to the activation of CD4+ helper T cells and CD8+ cytotoxic T cells. Interaction between MHC I molecules on APC and TCR during antigen presentation facilitated by CD8 molecule leads to the generation of tumor-specific CTLs capable of lysing tumor cells.

Peptides	Mechanism	Study details	References
Tyrosine kinase receptor ephrin type-A receptor 2 (EphA2-derived peptide)	EphaA2 EphA2-specific CTL	High level of immunity against colorectal cancer in murine model	[15]
RNF43-721		Phase 1 clinical trial	[16]
ABT-737	Inhibition of antiapoptotic Bcl-2 family	Sensitized cancer cells in mouse colon cancer model	[17]
Epitopes of HER2, MVF, GMP, and n-MDP	Multiple targets	Phase 1 clinical trial	[18]
Endoglin	Inhibition of angiogenesis	Inhibition of tumor growth in mouse model	[19]
CEA CEA691	Induction of tumor-specific CTLs	Increase in survival rate in colon carcinoma mouse model	[20]
OX40L – TNF family protein		Inhibition of tumor growth in mouse model	[21]
Mucin 1: MUC1 a cell surface-associated protein		Stimulation of antigen-specific CTL, abundant secretion of IFN-γ. Tumor burden was significantly reduced in colon cancer mouse model	[22]
Heat-shock protein Gp96	Induction of tumor-specific CTLs	Two-year overall survival and disease-free survival were significantly improved	
SART3-tumor-rejection antigen	Induction of tumor-specific CTLs	Increased cellular immune responses to the tumor. No improved clinical outcome	[23, 24]
Lck-derived peptides	Induction of tumor-specific CTLs		[24]
Survivin-2B	Induction of HLA-A24-restricted cytotoxic T cells resulting in high toxicity against HLA-A24-positive survivin-2B-positive cancer in vitro	Increased proportion of peptide-specific CTL. No significantly improved clinical outcome	[25]
βHCG CTP37-DT (Avicine)		Phase II trials showed improved patient survival	[26]
CDX 1307	Fusion between βHCG and an antibody against the mannose receptor	Phase I trial. Inoculation leads to DC activation as well as cytotoxic T-cell activity against tumor cells	[27]
p53 (SLP)	p53-specific CD4+ Th cell SLP is a p53 synthetic long peptide	Antitumor response against p53-overexpressing tumors. The p53-SLP vaccine induces p53-specific T-cell responses	[10]

Peptides	Mechanism	Study details	References
EGFR2 gefitinib or erlotinib	EGFR mutations enhance tyrosine kinase activity in response to EGF, increasing the efficacy of anti-EGFR	In a phase I trial, the vaccine elicited antibody response phase II cancer	[28]
Gastrin: G17DT (gastroimmune)	Antigastrin-17 immunogen, raising antibodies that blockade gastrin-stimulated tumor growth	Phase II trials showed gastroimmune combined with irinotecan chemotherapy increased patient survival	[29]

Examples of peptide-based vaccine targets, their mechanism, as well as the current results of any trials performed using the vaccines to treat colon cancer.

Table 1. Peptide targets and mechanism of action.

Discussed below are examples of peptide-based vaccines and their targets that have been used to treat colon cancer. More examples are listed in **Table 1**. Beta human chorionic gonadotropin (βHCG) is not produced by normal colorectal cells. The increase in the expression of this antigen in colon cancer cells leads to an increase in tumor invasiveness, higher metastatic incidence and promotion of tumor growth, neovascularization, and immune system suppression. This makes it an attractive target for the development of an antibody-based vaccine [10]. Carcinoembryonic antigen (CEA) is an oncofetal antigen that can serve as a target for vaccine development. It is found overexpressed on the surface of colon cancer cells, with very low levels of expression on normal cells. Unfortunately this protein is normally expressed during fetal development and is therefore tolerated by the immune system. This led to the creation of an artificial CEA. CeaVac is based on anti-idiotypic antibodies and mimics CEA [10]. Another oncofetal protein 5T4 is a leucine-rich membrane glycoprotein. Once again it is nearly absent in normal tissues but is overexpressed in colon cancer cells and developing cells. Its presence is associated with poor survival. The drug TroVax uses 5T4 with a pox virus vector and a modified vaccinia virus. Preclinical trials in mouse models resulted in a 90% reduction of tumor burden [10].

Onyvax-105 is another anti-idiotype antibody mimicking the glycosylphosphatidylinositol-anchored protein CD55. CD55 regulates complement activation protecting cells against complement attack thereby enhancing tumor cell survival. The gastric acid–stimulating hormone gastrin is a hormone the precursors of which are overexpressed in colon cancer, where they act as growth factors. This leads to increases in angiogenesis and cell proliferation. Vaccines raised against this protein would therefore result in inhibition of cell growth, proliferation, and metastasis [10]. Onartuzumab is a mAb that targets human growth factor receptor (HGFR). It is a monovalent HGF antagonist antibody against MET Proto-Oncogene, Receptor Tyrosine Kinase that benefits patients who overexpress HGFR [30].

The FANG ™ vaccine consists of tumor cells from the patient and a plasmid expressing granulocyte-macrophage colony-stimulating factor (GM-CSF) and bifunctional short hairpin RNAfurin (bi-shRNAfurin). The growth and production of DCs are induced by GM-CSF. The enzyme furin transforms precursor proteins into active proteins and the presence of bi-shRNAi furin inhibits the production of active proteins. This particularly inhibits the production of TGF β1 and 2 (TGFβ). Overexpression of TGFβ is associated with cancer progression and immune suppression by inhibiting GM-CSF and the consequent production of dendritic and other APCs. The vaccine therefore prevents the overexpression of TGFβ and leads to immune cell activation and the inhibition of cancer cell proliferation [30]. The vaccine was manufactured using GM-CSF and IL-13 to generate DCs from monocytes. The DCs were loaded with 6HLA-A*0201-binding peptides derived, among others, from CEA, MAGE-2 (melanoma antigen overexpressed in gastrointestinal cancer), and HER2/neu [10, 30].

TroVax is an attenuated strain of vaccinia virus that encodes the 5T4 protein. This protein is an oncofetal antigen and is a transmembrane glycoprotein. It is highly expressed in colon cancers and is virtually absent in normal tissue. The receptor is thought to play a role in metastasis and the expression level increases with the advancement of the stage of the cancer. This vaccine is able to induce an effective immune response, as it results in the formation of antibodies for both the 5T4 antigen and the viral particle [31].

2.3. Heat-shock proteins (HSPs)

HSPs are widely expressed in tumors, where they promote cancer progression. HSP 72 and glucose-regulated protein 96 (gp96) are two of these proteins that are highly expressed in colon cancer [32]. These proteins are thought to play a role in cell growth and signal transduction and expression of these proteins is higher in tumors undergoing metastasis. This makes them useful as diagnostic and prognostic markers. However, this expression is not related to patient survival [32].

HSPs enhance antigen-specific tumor immunity as they play an important role in the presentation of antigens to CD8$^+$ T cells through the MHC I pathway. This is because of the roles HSP 70s play as chaperones and in the transport of peptides to the heterodimeric transporters associated with antigen processing [33]. Similarly gp96 is a major chaperone involved in the lumen of the endoplasmic reticulum (ER), where it facilitates the folding of the MHC Iβ-2 microglobulin-peptide complexes in the ER [34].

Vaccines based on HSPs have been tested in animal trials and been found to be highly effective in the treatment of cancers [32, 35]. The function of the HSP in transporting and presenting other peptides as surface antigens has led many researchers to propose that HSPs can be used to create a HSP target protein fusion. This booster strategy would therefore enhance the ability of the target protein to be used as an antigen by T cells [36]. Two of these proteins that can be coupled to HSPs to improve their immunogenicity and usefulness as a cancer vaccine are alpha-fetoprotein (AFP) in hepatocellular carcinoma and CD44 in colonic carcinomas [32].

3. Targeted therapy: monoclonal antibodies

Recently, a new class of targeted agents have been identified, which bind to the ligand or the extracellular domain of a receptor. This results in alteration of intracellular signal transduction pathways which will affect cell proliferation, dedifferentiation, inhibition of apoptosis, and stimulation of neoangiogenesis [37]. This section will look into VEGF-targeted drugs (e.g., ramucirumab (Cyramza®) and bevacizumab (Avastin®)), EGFR-targeted drugs (e.g., cetuximab (Erbitux®) and panitumumab (Vectibix®)), and others such as those that target kinases [37].

3.1. Bevacizumab and ramucirumab

VEGF is a potent angiogenic factor and functions by binding to one of three VEGF receptors located on endothelial cells and angioblasts. The VEGF receptor-2 is overexpressed on up to 50% of colorectal cancer cell surfaces. VEGF-A and other proangiogenic factors promote the degradation of the extracellular matrix. This enables proliferation and migration of endothelial cells [37]. The ligands of the VEGF family include VEGF-A, VEGF-B, VEGF-C, VEGF-D, and VEGF-E; and the receptors are VEGFR-1, R-2, and R-3. In colon cancer the ligand that is most abundant is VEGF-A [38]. Sustained angiogenesis is a hallmark of cancer; and targeted inhibition of blood vessel development is an established strategy for antitumor therapy [38]. Anti-VEGF therapies have been associated with a survival benefit across multiple malignancies including colon cancer [38].

Bevacizumab is a humanized mAb against VEGF and it acts by preventing ligand binding by binding to VEGF. This prevents downstream intracellular signal transduction; however, the response to bevacizumab appears to be independent of VEGF expression or high microvessel density (MVD) [37]. MVD assessment is a good predictor of metastasis, with selective antibodies, such as endoglin, distinguishing between tumor neovascularization and preexisting vessels. VEGF expression is highest in patients with metastatic tumors and the level is associated with cancer stage [38]. Bevacizumab is typically used in combination with other chemotherapeutic agents, and it is also indicated in improving the delivery of chemotherapy by changing tumor vasculature and decreasing the elevated interstitial pressure in tumors. The combination of therapies results in improved survival [38].

Ramucirumab is a fully humanized IgG1 mAb targeting the extracellular domain of VEGF receptor 2 (VEGFR2). Large-scale trials have indicated that ramucirumab shows promising antitumor effects and is well tolerated. The origin of this antibody was through the use of a large phage display library with tailored *in vitro* selection methods to identify a high-affinity antibody [39]. Measurement of VEGFA and soluble VEGFR1/2 during phase I trials of the antibody indicated that there is an increase in the expression of VEGF as well as a decrease in VEGFR1/2 levels. These changes were not dose related, which suggests that the receptor was saturated [39]. Phase I trial results were promising and phase II trials resulted in a high percentage of patients presenting with progression free survival at 6 months. Phase III trials showed an increase in overall patient survival [39]. Adverse reactions to ramucirumab included hypertension, vascular thrombotic events, and proteinuria [40].

Aflibercept is a recombinant fusion protein consisting of the second immunoglobulin (Ig) domain of VEGFR-1 and the third Ig domain of VEGFR-2, fused to human IgG1. It exhibits affinity for VEGF-A, VEGF-B, and PlGF. The antibody displayed effective activity against colon cancers with improvements in the primary endpoint of overall survival and overall response rate, as well as displaying a high degree of tolerability in patients [40]. VEGFR-1 also plays a role in colon cancer and inhibiting its signaling could also play a role in cancer treatment. An antibody developed to target this receptor named IMC-18F1 has been developed. This is a high-affinity human VEGFR-1-neutralizing antibody that specifically binds the extracellular domain of VEGFR-1. It exhibits antiangiogenic and antiproliferative activity [40].

3.2. Panitumumab and cetuximab

The epidermal growth factor receptor (EGFR) is a target for the therapeutic monoclonal antibodies panitumumab and cetuximab the treatment of metastatic colorectal cancer. Panitumumab is a fully human Ig G2 mAb that binds the EGFR extracellular domain with high affinity and inhibits ligand-induced EGFR tyrosine phosphorylation, tumor cell activation, and tumor cell proliferation (**Figure 2**). Cetuximab is a chimeric human-mouse IgG1 mAb [41]. Cetuximab and panitumumab are both Food and Drug Administration (FDA) approved for advanced colorectal cancer therapy, and both have clear benefits for colon cancer treatment of most patients. The exception is those patients that carry *KRAS* mutations at codons 12 and 13 [42]. *KRAS* mutations occur in approximately 35–40% of colorectal tumors, and *KRAS* is a member of the rat sarcoma virus (Ras) gene family of oncogenes and is involved in integrating the signaling cascades controlling gene transcription, including many EGFR-mediated pathways [41]. The ligands of the EGFR transmembrane tyrosine kinase receptor include EGF, TGFα, epiregulin, amphiregulin, β-cellulin, and heparin. EGFR activates downstream signaling pathways such as the Ras/Raf/mitogen-activated protein kinase (MAPK) pathway, the phosphatidylinositol 3-kinase (PI3K)/AKT pathway, and the signal transducer and activator of transcription (STAT) pathway. These downstream pathways activate cellular survival, proliferation, invasion, metastasis, and angiogenesis. Abnormal activation of the EGFR signaling network due to excessive overexpression is common in colon cancer (**Figure 2**). EGFR is composed of an extracellular ligand-binding domain, a hydrophobic transmembrane region, and an intracellular domain with tyrosine kinase activity [41, 43].

Cetuximab competes with EGFR ligands, such as EGF or TGFα, with a high affinity ($K_d = 1 \times 10^{-10}$ M). This results in the inhibition of cell cycle progression and arrest of cell cycle in G1 phase, inhibition of angiogenesis, inhibition of metastasis by reduction of production of matrix metalloproteinase, inhibition of apoptosis, and potentiation of antitumor activities of chemotherapy and radiotherapy [43]. Panitumumab treatment results in improved clinical outcomes in patients with chemotherapy-refractory colon cancer [41]. Panitumumab also has a high affinity for EGFR ($K_d = 5 \times 10^{-11}$ M) and acts to arrest cell cycle progression and block cancer growth; however, it is an IgG2 and does not act through antibody-dependent cell cytotoxicity [43].

Using a single type of mAb to block a single transduction pathway may only have a limited effect, as tumors can shift to other alternate pathways. One solution is to combine monoclonal antibodies to block two signaling transduction pathways [44]. Use of multiple monoclonal antibodies has other advantages including limited overlapping toxicity and few to no pharmacokinetic interactions between antibodies. However, some studies indicate that certain combinations such as bevacizumab with cetuximab or panitumumab lead to shorter survival and increased toxicity in advanced colorectal cancer compared to therapy with a single antibody [44]. The addition of panitumumab to chemotherapy improves clinical outcomes among patients with wild-type *KRAS* [41]. Other biomarkers that affect the efficacy of panitumumab include mutations in the *BRAF* and *PIK3CA* genes [41]. An important side effect of panitumumab treatment is the occurrence of skin toxicity; however, occurrences of skin toxicity correlate with favorable outcomes for patients [41, 43].

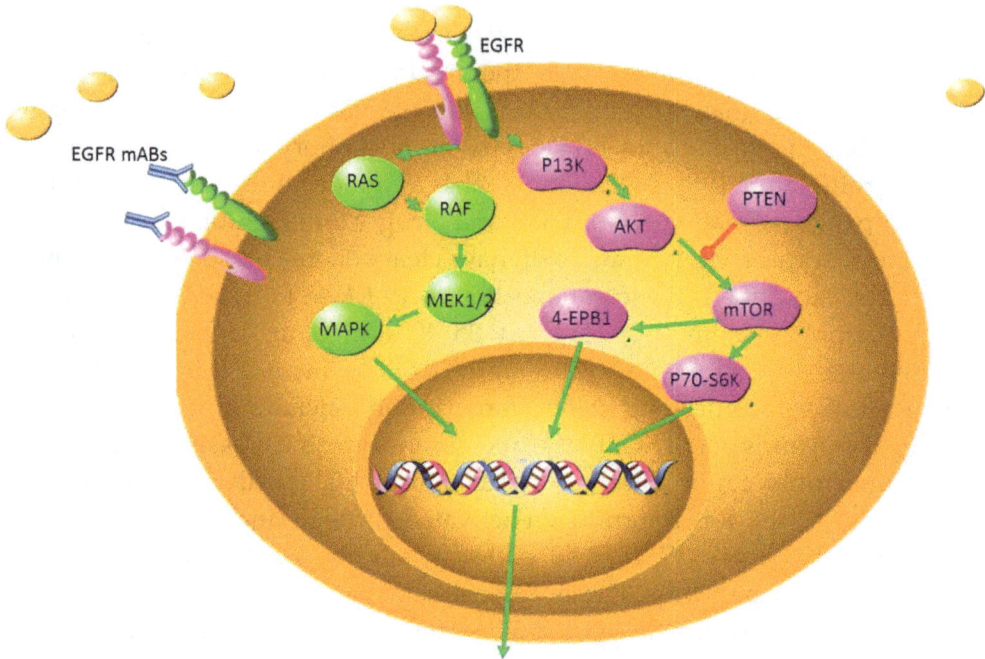

Figure 2. Mechanism of action of anti-EGFR mAbs. The binding of these mAbs on EGFR prevents the dimerization and the activation of EGFR.

4. Immune checkpoint inhibitors

During the progression of tumor development, the cancer cells undergo changes to escape immune surveillance. In order to accomplish this, a large enough number of the tumor cells must escape in order for there to be an equilibrium between tumor growth and tumor killing [1]. Normally, tumor-infiltrating lymphocytes (TIL) would control the progression of cancers; however, cancer cells can evade this response using a process known as T-cell exhaustion. This occurs due to the expression of inhibitory receptors. Blocking these receptors through the use of inhibitory molecules or monoclonal antibodies is known as immune checkpoint inhibition [45]. The immune system depends on multiple checkpoints to avoid overactivation in healthy cells. These inhibitory molecules expressed by the cancer cells take advantage of these checkpoints to escape detection by the immune system. They will often express molecules that serve as "immune checkpoints," by so doing; a message is sent to the immune system that an immune response is not necessary. Drugs are being developed to block immune checkpoint molecules from binding to their molecular partners, thus allowing the body to elicit an immune response and therefore attack cancer cells. An analysis of the expression patterns in colon cancers revealed a large overexpression of immune checkpoint-related proteins [46].

The programmed death-1 (PD-1) checkpoint is blocked in most cancers and blocking the pathway with antibodies to reactivate this checkpoint is a viable cancer therapy [47]. Recent insights indicate that blockade of the PD-1 checkpoint exists in many cancer patients and a repertoire of tumor-specific or tumor-selective T cells can be reactivated to achieve tumor therapy [48, 49]. Blocking the PD-1 pathway with antibodies results in durable tumor regression. Programmed death-ligand 1 (PD-L1) is a transmembrane receptor that plays a role in suppressing the immune system by suppressing the proliferation of CD8+ T cells and to lower the level of antigen particles by regulating apoptosis. PD-1, expressed on T cells, B cells, and other immune effector cells, interacts with this receptor, resulting in a negative signal to the T cell. Expression of PD-L1 in tumor biopsies shows that this pathway acts to block antitumor immune responses [46]. PD-1 has two ligands, PD-L1 and PD-L2. Tumor cells expressing PD-L1 are associated with poor outcomes for patients. Targeting these ligands prevent T-cell exhaustion and promotes T-cell recognition of tumors [45]. PD-L1 also binds to the co-stimulatory molecule CD80, implying that CD80 has the potential to facilitate antitumor immunity by inhibiting the PD-1 suppressive pathway [47].

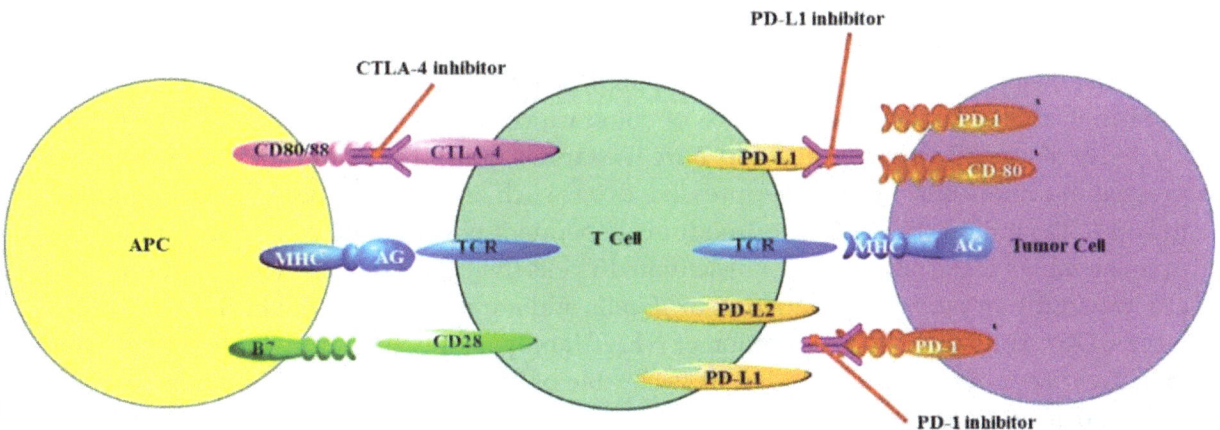

Figure 3. Immune checkpoint interactions and antibody-based inhibition on T cells. CTLA-4 inhibition can be performed by inhibiting CD28 co-stimulation (through binding with its ligands CD80 or CD86) that is required to complete T-cell activation. The PD-1/PD-L1 pathway can be inhibited by targeting its inhibitory role. Here it interacts with PD-L1 on the tumor cell. Inhibiting this interaction results in a more robust targeted antitumor immune response.

Ipilimumab is a mAb that targets CTLA-4 (cytotoxic T-lymphocyte-associated protein 4), which normally negatively regulates the activity of T cells. This antibody was the first checkpoint-blocking antibody to be approved by the US FDA for cancer treatment; CTLA-4 is a member of the Ig superfamily of receptors, which also includes PD-1, TIM-3 (T-cell Ig and mucin domain-containing protein 3), BTLA (B and T-lymphocyte attenuator), and VISTA (V domain Ig suppressor of T-cell activation). Use of this drug enhances the antitumor activity of

CD8 T cells and inhibits the suppressive function of Tregs [45]. This was followed by a second antibody, pembrolizumab, which targets the programmed death 1 (PD-1; CD279) molecule [50] (**Figure 3**). Trials of these antibody therapies have only shown modest clinical benefits, and this may indicate that tumors use multiple and nonoverlapping immunosuppressive mechanisms to evade the immune response [45]. Multiple studies indicate that effective therapy involves the targeting of multiple immunosuppressive pathways [51].

Tumor cells can also evade the immune system through the production of extracellular adenosine by CD73 which is expressed on lymphocytes and endothelial and epithelial cells. CD73 performs an endothelial cell barrier function, protecting cells from ischemia and regulating immune responses. This receptor is overexpressed in many types of cancer, with high CD73 expression being associated with poor outcomes for patients due to increases in tumor immune escape and metastasis [45]. Blocking CD73 can induce potent antitumor immune responses. Additionally the inhibition of molecular pathway components upstream of CD73 such as CD39 also has similar therapeutic effects. This treatment can also be used to supplement immune checkpoint therapies that make use of anti-CTLA-4 and anti-PD-1 mAbs, to increase the effectiveness of such therapies [45].

Another strategy to target immune checkpoints is the use of small molecule drugs that target critical survival pathways. These include Gleevec and ibrutinib, both of which are tyrosine kinase inhibitors. Ibrutinib is a covalent inhibitor of BTK (Bruton's tyrosine kinase), a key enzyme in B-cell receptor signaling [49].

Controlling the immune response to cancer cells through the use of anti-inflammatory drugs to control the inflammatory components reduces the risk of developing certain types of cancer. Aspirin is able to reduce the incidence of colon cancer and slow down tumor progression. Cyclooxygenase (Cox) enzymes 1 and 2 are the targets of aspirin. These enzymes are overexpressed in tumor cells. Immunosuppressive drugs such as cyclosporine A (CsA) and tacrolimus (FK506) inhibit the calcium/calmodulin-dependent phosphatase calcineurin, which acts upon members of the nuclear factor of activated T cells (NFAT) [52]. These transcription factors are important for cytokine production by T cells and are required for the normal function of B cells, DCs, and mast cells. Expression of NFAT family members leads to tumor suppression [53]. Treatment of tumor cells with CsA is capable of inducing necroptosis and a mild G0/G1 cell cycle arrest [52].

5. Cytokines

Cytokines are signaling proteins produced by white blood cells that help control the growth and activity of immune system cells. The two types of cytokines that are used in the treatment of cancer are IFNs and ILs. Cytokines stimulate a broad-based immune response as opposed to generating a targeted response to a specific antigen [54]. Tumors secrete factors to recruit inflammatory cells and/or activate stromal cells. Inflammation plays a major role in tumor promotion and progression. The soluble factors that drive inflammation are cytokines and chemokines produced by tumor cells themselves and by the cells recruited to the tumor microenvironment [55].

Several cytokines are capable of activating and recruiting specific immune cells that can enhance antitumor immunity; these include IL-2, IL-12, IL-15, TNFα, and GM-CSF. These cytokines can be used as single-agent therapies or in combination with other immunotherapeutic strategies. GM-CSF immunization leads to APC recruitment. Tumors activate Stat3 and Braf, which leads to the release of IL-10, inhibiting the tumoricidal activity of NK cells. Stat3 activation in DCs leads to these cells becoming tolerogenic DC [11].

Additionally, TNFα, hepatocyte growth factor, PDGF, and FGF19 activate Wnt/β-catenin signaling in tumor cells. This is the oncogenic pathway activated in the majority of colon cancers. This pathway results in β-catenin accumulation in the cytoplasm, which activates cell growth and differentiation pathways. IL-1β is a potent activator of Wnt signaling in colon cancer cells leading to increased survival of colon cancer cells [55].

Oncogenic signaling through the Wnt and NF-kB pathways is activated through TNFα. Pharmacological inhibition of TNFα by neutralizing TNFα antibodies has been used to treat both irritable bowel disorders and colon cancer. Results from trials using enbrel or remicade suggest that these neutralizing antibodies have activity against colon cancer cells. TNFα signaling initiates NF-kB signaling. NF-kB is continuously expressed in certain tumors, leading to enhanced survival by protecting the tumor cells from apoptosis. Treatment with the TNFα antagonist, etanercept led to inhibition of Wnt/β-catenin6 signaling as seen by the , reduced expression of active β-catenin [55].

5.1. Interleukins 1β, IL-6, and IL-1

The proinflammatory cytokine IL-1β is produced by activated macrophages. In turn, IL-1β induces the expression of TNFα, IL-6, IL-8, IL-17, Cox-2, and PGE2, promoters of tumor cell growth. Inducing the expression of IL-1β leads to increased incidence of cancer in wild-type mice. The IL-1β signaling pathway functions through the receptors IL-1RI and IL-1RII to induce NF-kB activity. The pathway involves the two adaptor proteins, MyD88 and IRAK. Macrophages are stimulated to release IL-1β and activate NF-kB and Wnt pathways, but IL-1β signaling requires STAT1. The silencing of STAT1 expression leads to decreased IL-1β release and prevented cancer cell growth [55].

IL-6 is secreted by stimulated monocytes, fibroblasts, and endothelial cells, macrophages, T cells, and B lymphocytes. Macrophages are stimulated by colon cancer cells to produce IL-6 and activate STAT3 in tumor cells. Inhibition of IL-6 signaling interferes with the growth of tumor cells and protects them from apoptosis. Research indicates that decreasing the expression or inhibiting the activity of STAT3 may have adverse effects on tumor promotion. Targeting STAT3 will affect the expression of β-catenin and the co-expression of STAT3 and β-catenin is associated with poor survival of colon cancer patients [55].

A subset of T-helper cells produces the cytokines IL-17, IL-22, and TNFα (Th17 cells). Paneth cells also produce IL-17. Th17 cells require IL-6, TGFβ, IL-1β, and IL-23, while IFN-γ and IL-4 negatively regulate differentiation of Th17 cells. IL-17 induces IL-6 and STAT3, promoting the survival of cancer cells. This cytokine may also have an anticancer function by enhancing antitumor immunity [55].

5.2. Tumor necrosis factor-related apoptosis-inducing ligand (TRAIL)

TRAIL (also known as Apo2L) activates the apoptotic cascade. Tumor cells can evade this apoptosis signal through the action of β-catenin. TRAIL's role in tumor surveillance has been confirmed in knockdown experiments and is a promising candidate to be used in cancer therapy, because it selectively kills cancer cells while leaving normal cells unharmed [55].

Sorafenib a Raf kinase inhibitor sensitized A TRAIL –resistant colon cancer line to TRAIL-induced apoptosis by preventing NF-kB-dependent expression of the antiapoptotic genes, IAP2 and MCl-1.

6. Oncolytic virus (OV) therapy

Over a century ago, researchers observed that viral infection both in human and animal models results in the expression of targets that can be recognized by T cells and/or antibodies. Subsequently, vaccination has been used to treat an array of diseases such as hepatitis B virus and human papillomavirus 15 which can cause liver and cervical cancer respectively. Vaccination against infections is used to induce neutralizing antibodies that act prophylactically. However, with regard to cancer vaccination, cancer vaccine candidates should induce and expand immune responses that can cause disruption of biological pathways that support cancer growth.

The concept of cancer immunotherapy is based on the ability of the immune system to recognize cancer cells and affect their growth and replication. Researchers have observed that cancer regression would occur spontaneously in patients after viral infection [56, 57]. For example, studies conducted by Lindeman and Klein 1967 showed that oncolysis of tumor cells by influenza virus increased immunogenicity of tumor cell antigens. The recent advances in successful sequencing of the cancer genome together with insights into how tumors evade the immune system have led cancer research to evolve from searching for a gene that causes individual cancer to one that blocks or disrupts biological pathways that support cancer growth [58, 59]. As a result, cancer vaccines are now being designed with the aim to boost the immune system to protect itself from carcinogenesis and progression of cancer. In 2010, the FDA approved Provenge which is a therapeutic vaccine for cancer [60]. It is designed to treat advances in prostate cancer and has shown to increase the survival rate. The success of Provenge resulted in stimulating the interest in the development of other therapeutic cancer vaccines.

In recent years, OV has been shown to be effective in treating cancer in both preclinical models and clinical trials. Toda and coworkers showed that genetically modified oncolytic HSV G207 is a potential cancer vaccine for induction of specific antitumor immunity in CT26 colon cancer cells [64, 61, 62]. This type of immunotherapy is largely dependent on the network of the host immune system to fight cancer by (i) boosting the patient's immune system, (ii) decreasing cancer-induced immunosuppression, and (iii) increasing the immunogenicity of the tumor itself [63, 64]; OVs can be RNA- or DNA-based virus derived from human or animals.

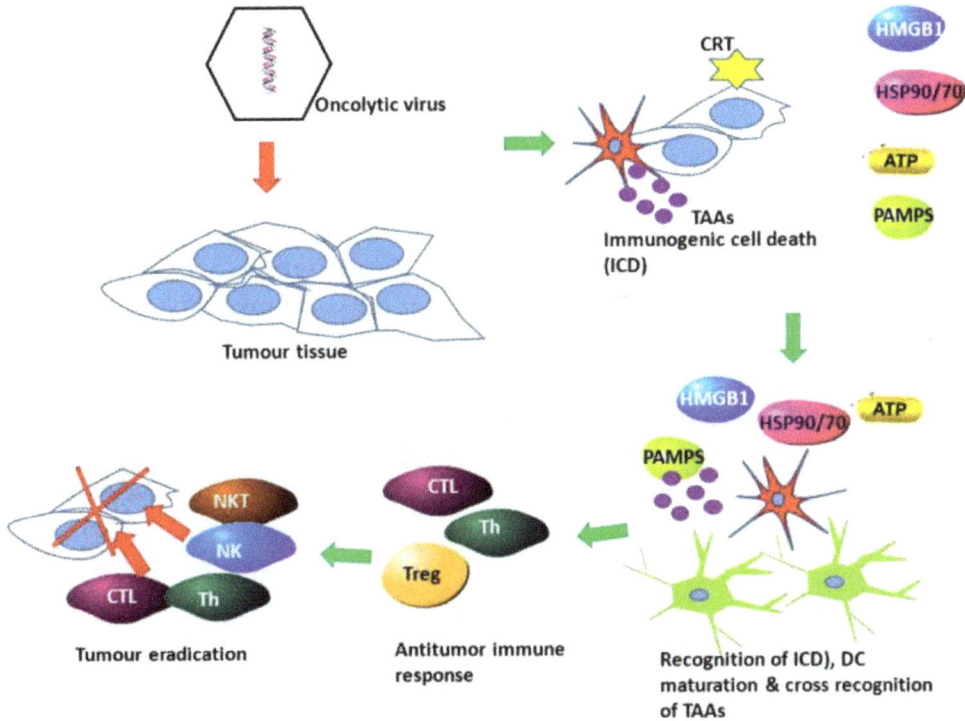

Figure 4. Immunogenic cell death of cancer cells induced by oncolytic viruses. An oncolytic virus selectively replicates in tumor cells, leading to induction of the death of these cells, presenting destruction signals on the cell surface and consequent release of danger signals from necrotic cells. Apoptotic bodies are engulfed by APC, and TAAs are processed and presented along with MHC complex and co-stimulatory molecules. The released DAMPs (and PAMPs) activate and mature DCs, and TAAs are cross-presented to naive T cells. This process can be further enhanced at different steps by other immunomodulatory agents (in a combination strategy). The resulting cytotoxic immune response against tumor and associated stromal cells, involving CD4+ and CD8+ T cells, may help in complete eradication of tumor mass. Additional immunotherapies targeting DCs, T cells, and the immunosuppressive TME can further enhance this antitumor immune response.

OV selectively infects and replicates in cancer and associated endothelial cells and subsequently kills these abnormal cells without harming the normal cells. The selectivity of OV can be an inherited feature of the virus or due to genetic engineering [56, 65]. OV therapy has multiple antitumoral activities including direct effect by cytotoxic cytokines released upon infection by tumor residents or infiltrating immune cells [66, 67]. The lysis-dependent cytoreductive activity activates innate immune receptors when immunogenic cell debris is taken up and cross presented by APCs (**Figure 4**).

OVs also directly affect various signaling pathways which are implicated in cancer such as Ras, Wnt, anti-apoptosis, and EGFR [66, 68, 69]. The altered signaling pathway creates a favorable environment for OV replication resulting in Cells infected with these viruses showing sustained proliferation, resisting cell death, evading growth suppressors and escaping immune surveillance. Cancer cells also show increased genomic instability and DNA damage stress, which is favorable to OV replication [70–72]. Genetic manipulation of OV enables these viruses to be (i) safe for use as a vaccine, (ii) highly selective for specific cancer type, and (iii) altering virus tropism. In comparison with current regimes for cancer treatment, OVs are advantageous because (i) they have a low chance for generation of resistance because they use multiple ways to exert cytotoxicity and (ii) virus dose in a tumor increases with time due to in situ virus replication whereas in the classical drug Pharmacokinetics, dose decreases with time [71, 73].

The major drawbacks in the use of OV include nonimmune human serum, development of anti-OV antibodies resulting from the use of human virus, and appropriate delivery into the tumor. Various delivery mechanisms have been explored to enable delivery of OV to tumor cells. For an example, cell carriers such as neural stem cells and myeloid-derived suppressor cells have been used to deliver OV to specific tumor cells. The cells protect the virus from anti-OV antibody neutralization, thereby facilitating virus deliver [71, 73]. In using OV to treat colon cancer, ONYX-015 has advanced to phase II clinical trials and is used in combination with chemotherapy [74, 75]. Recently, adenovirus 5 (PSE-EA1 and E deleted) has been approved to treat prostate cancer in China giving hope to development of OV as an alternative cancer treatment.

7. Bispecific antibody

Antibody-based therapy has been explored in treating a range of diseases and is promising to be a success with the FDA having approved more than 13 monoclonal antibodies for treatment of cancer (see Section 2). Furthermore, over 100 antibodies are at different stages of clinical trials. Medical researchers have explored the properties of antibodies which are (i) highly specific in binding their targets and (ii) are nontoxic for medical application using technologies such as hybridoma and phage display for antigen targeting [76–79]. Also, new technologies have been employed to manipulate antibodies for wide application. For example, the conventional antibody which is made up of two identical pairs of heavy and light chain linked together by disulfide bonds is monospecific and bivalent. Using a hybridoma technology, a fusion can be created between two hybridoma resulting in quadromas with two different heavy and light chains as a result of random pairing, thus forming molecules that do not occur in nature (**Figure 5A**). Antibodies produced by these methods have an ability to bind different species but could also be nonfunctional [77, 79, 80].

Conventional antibodies posed various challenges to therapeutic application due to inadequate exposure to the tumor as a result of their size (150 kDa) and impaired interactions with the immune system. Using enzyme-based antibody digestion, full antibodies may be truncated into Fc and Fab regions (**Figure 5A**). The Fab region which has the antigen-binding domain of the antibody is then used for therapeutic application. The drawback in using the Fab region of the antibody is its reduced half-life due to renal clearance [81, 82]. In addressing these challenges, bispecific antibodies (BsAb) were developed in 1961 [83]. Just as their name implies, this class of antibodies binds two different antigens or two different epitopes on the same region.

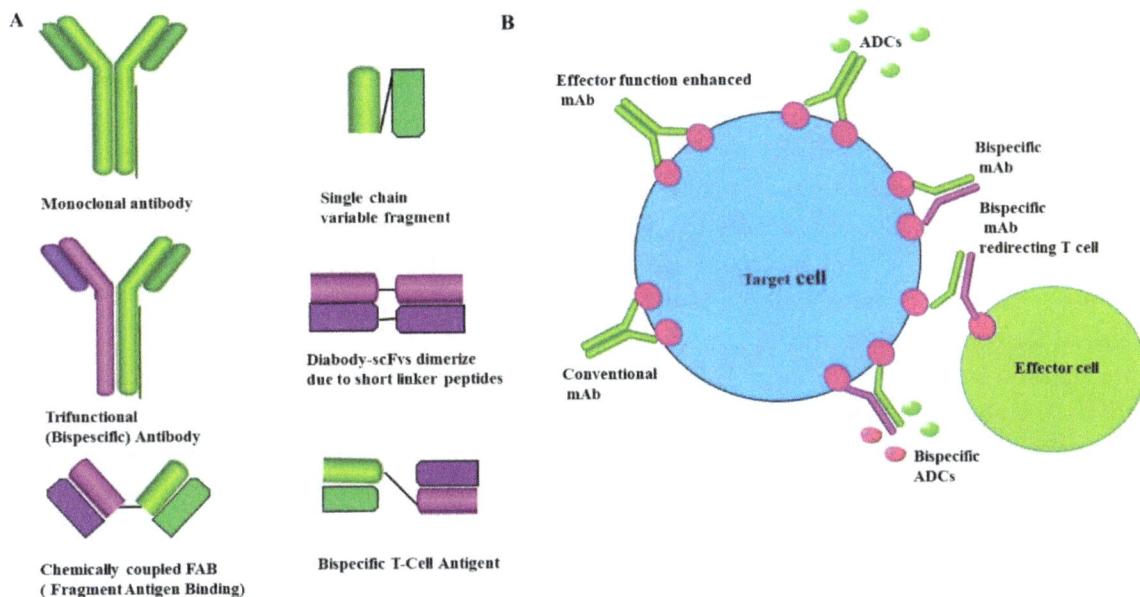

Figure 5. (A) Different forms of bispecific antibody. Trifunctional antibodies consist of two heavy and two light chains from two different antibodies. This results in an antibody with binding sites for two different antigens as well as an Fc region made up of two heavy chains forming a third binding site. A diabody consists of scFvs with very short linker peptides that force the closely positioned variable regions to fold together, forcing the scFvs to dimerize. Chemically coupled Fabs consist of the antigen-binding regions of two different monoclonal antibodies linked by a chemical means. Bispecific T-cell antigens are fusion proteins of two scFvs from four separate genes. (B) Development of bispecific compounds. Bispecific compounds enable simultaneous inhibition of two cell surface receptors, simultaneous blocking of two ligands, cross-linking of two receptors, and/or the recruitment of T cells to the proximity of tumor cells (redirected immune cell killing).

BsAb represent a class of antibodies that are yet to be fully explored in the treatment of cancer and other diseases. BsAb have a greater potential therapeutic efficiency than mono-targeted therapy, since they allow simultaneous engagements of two targets and limit potential escape pathways [84–86]. Numerous studies have shown that there is evidence of cross talk between receptor tyrosine kinases such as MET, VEGFR, and IGFR-IR which are known to promote cancer progression and drug resistance. And patients with colon cancer are known not to respond to anti-EGFR drugs with resistance emerging after initial usage [87, 88]. Engelman et al. showed that MET amplification leads to gefitinib resistance by activating the ERBB3 pathway, showing the complexity of tumor signaling pathways and a need to treat patients with drugs that target multiple targets [89].

In the use of BsAb, T cells are targeted because of their high cytotoxic retention, abundance in bloodstream, surveillance function, and proven ability to control malignant diseases [90, 91]. During cancer progression, cancer cells escape immune recognition by interfering with antigen presentation or T-cell activation or differentiation. In using the bispecific antibody, most targeted antigens for tumor therapy are differentiation antigens such as CD19, CD33, CEA, EpCAM Epithelial cell adhesion molecule, PMSA Prostate-specific membrane antigen , and EGF receptors. In most cases these antigens are overexpressed in cancer cells compared to the normal cells.

Blinatumomab is an example of a bispecific antibody that has shown great promise clinically in cancer patients. Blinatumomab is a 55 kDa-fusion protein comprised of two single-chain antibodies to CD19 and CD3, recombinantly joined by a flexible, non-glycosylated five-amino acid non-immunogenic linker that affords a very short distance between arms [92, 93]. Blinatumomab has high affinity for CD19 which is important in sustaining the malignant B-cell phenotype via mechanisms of proliferation, cell survival, and self-renewal [94, 95]. It draws malignant B cells in close proximity to CD3-positive T cells without regard to TCR specificity or reliance on MHC class I molecules on the surface of APCs for activation. The nonspecific binding of the polyclonal T-cell population prevents resistances to T-cell-based therapies as a result of downregulation of MHC molecules. CD19 and CD3 binding results in T-cell activation, marked by upregulation of T-cell activation markers CD25, CD69, CD2, IFN-γ, TNFα, and IL-2, IL-6, and IL-10 [96]. Cell lysis is mediated by secretion of perforin and various granzymes stored in the secretory vesicles of cytotoxic T cells [97]. In vitro data suggest that efficacy of blinatumomab is not compromised or dependent upon T cells, which may be limited in number in heavily pretreated patients [98]. Also blinatumomab-activated T cells appear to effectively induce serial target cell killing [92, 93].

8. Adoptive immunotherapy

In the wake of cancer treatment challenges or therapies, adoptive immunotherapy is one of the novel strategies being researched for cancer treatment. This concept was presented five decades ago [99–101] and is based on the transfer of ex vivo expanded antitumor CD8 T cells into affected patients (**Figure 6**). Delorme and Alexander [101] showed that the transfer of immune lymphocytes could inhibit the growth rate of carcinogen-induced sarcoma.

The immune system is responsible for the prevention of tumors or elimination of pathogens that can cause inflammation or an inflammatory environment for tumorigenesis or destroy tumor cells expressing TSAs or molecules induced by stress [102, 103]. Therefore, tumor development and progression are largely dependent on the patient's immune system to effectively inhibit cancer growth using its network of immune cell types. Each and every cell type has a specific function in inhibiting tumor growth (**Figure 7**). Consequently, the success of adoptive immunotheraphy depends on approaches which will target different immune subsets.

Adoptive immunotherapies have explored the use of infiltrating T cells (CD8+ effector T cells and CD8+ effector memory cells), NK cells, and IL-2 for cancer-targeted therapies. The T cells are able to destroy tumor cells using cytotoxic granules containing perforin and granzymes and by using cell surface receptor such as TNF-related apoptosis-inducing ligand [104, 105]. Studies using mice have shown that adoptive transfer of T cells successfully induces antitumor

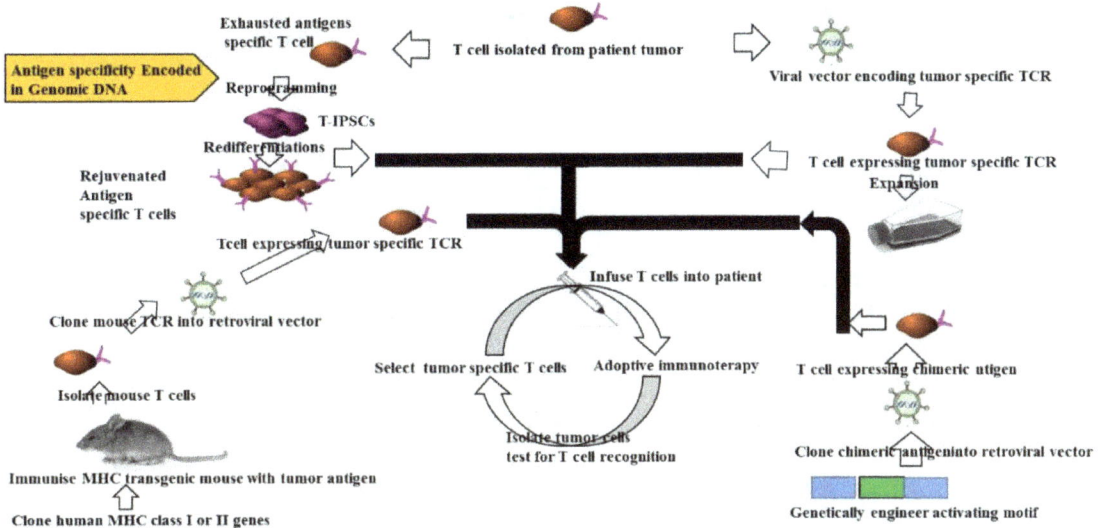

Figure 6. Different techniques used in adoptive immunotherapy. Adoptive immunotherapy with functional T cells can be performed in numerous ways. Exhaustion of antigen-specific T cells which can be a major problem in the practical application of this therapy can be solved through reprogramming clonally expanded antigen-specific CD8+ T cells and then redirecting their redifferentiation into CD8+ T cells possessing antigen-specific killing activity. T cells can be isolated from the patient. Isolated peptide antigens could be used to stimulate T cells that are already present in the patient's tumor or be used to prime tumor-specific T cells. If the T-cell populations generated are specific for the patient's tumor, they could be expanded and adoptively transferred if they are of human origin. T cells can be genetically engineered to recognize TAAs. TCRs from T cells that show a good antitumor response can be cloned and inserted into retroviruses, which are used to infect autologous T cells from the patient. Chimeric antigen receptors (CARs) can be generated through genetic engineering and then cloned into a retroviral vector and used to infect T cells from the patient. TCRs can also be isolated from humanized mice that express human MHC molecules and can be immunized with the tumor antigen of interest. Mouse T cells can then be isolated, and their TCR genes are cloned into recombinant vectors that can be used to genetically engineer autologous T cells from the patient.

response. Also, only a small number is required to mediate effective regression of tumor and survival [106–108]. Genetic modification of T cells has been successfully used to broaden their effective application by pairing with antigen receptors that recognize a range of different TAAs. Genetic engineering has also been employed to alter T cells so that they are able to avoid or be resistant to immune invasion strategies used by tumors such as the production of cytokines. Another modification of T cells involves attaching stimulatory signals for their activation [109, 110].

NK cells target and kill diseased cells using various mechanisms such as perforins and granzyme. The use of NK cells was first explored by Rosenberg et al. [111]. Lymphokine-activated killer cells were co-administered with IL-2 and resulted in a positive response in people with metastatic cancer [111]. Another combination of chemotherapy with transfer of allogeneic NK cells resulted in disease remission [112]. It is anticipated that a hybrid of T and NK cell will have great potential in the treatment of cancer using adoptive immunotherapy. However we are still a long way from the development of such a model treatment that can be developed for clinical trials and introduced into clinical practice.

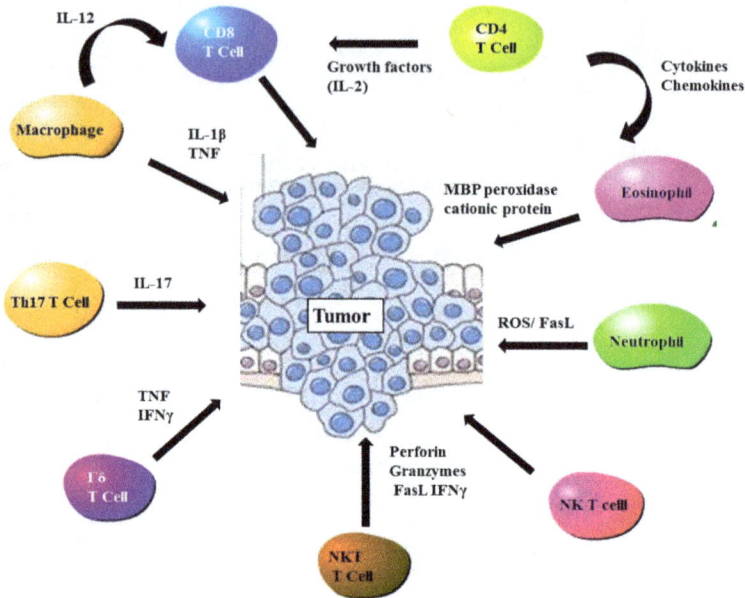

Figure 7. White blood cell types and mechanisms of response against tumors. The diagram illustrates all of the different immune-related cell types including T cells, NK, macrophages, eosinophils, and neutrophils that are able to respond against cancer cells. The method of response against the tumor cells is also indicated. In some cases these cell types can cooperate to produce additional responses.

9. Conclusion

The final goal of immunotherapeutic strategies to treat colon cancer would be the development of tumor-specific therapies that can be used in conjunction with standard chemotherapies with little side effects. The use of various combinations of different antibodies and OVs with synergistic antitumor activity and reduced toxicity will aim to achieve durable tumor eradication. One of the main obstacles is the identification of tumor-specific and essential tumor antigens. These antigens may differ with different tumors. In terms of checkpoint inhibition, it is important to establish the correct level of inhibition each patient requires to minimize toxicity. Another important goal is the identification and development of biomarkers to serve as prognostic markers for the monitoring of the individual patients response to immunotherapy, allowing for the identification of those patients who are most likely to benefit from these treatments. These goals require extensive further studies to refine immunotherapeutic strategies and combinatorial approaches.

Author details

Zodwa Dlamini*, Thandeka Khoza, Rodney Hull, Mpho Choene and
Zilungile Mkhize-Kwitshana

*Address all correspondence to: dlaminiz@mut.ac.za

Research, Innovation & Engagements Portfolio, Mangosuthu University of Technology, Durban, South Africa

References

[1] Cornelissen R, Heuvers ME, Maat AP, Hendriks RW, Hoogsteden HC, Aerts JG, Hegmans JP: New roads open up for implementing immunotherapy in mesothelioma. *Clinical and Developmental Immunology* 2012, 2012:927240.

[2] Evans C, Dalgleish AG, Kumar D: Review article: immune suppression and colorectal cancer. *Alimentary Pharmacology & Therapeutics* 2006, 24(8):1163–1177.

[3] Aptsiauri N, Cabrera T, Mendez R, Garcia-Lora A, Ruiz-Cabello F, Garrido F: Role of altered expression of HLA class I molecules in cancer progression. *Advances in Experimental Medicine and Biology* 2007, 601:123–131.

[4] Ma Y, Shurin GV, Peiyuan Z, Shurin MR: Dendritic cells in the cancer microenvironment. *Journal of Cancer* 2013, 4(1):36–44.

[5] Ma YJ, He M, Han JA, Yang L, Ji XY: A clinical study of HBsAg-activated dendritic cells and cytokine-induced killer cells during the treatment for chronic hepatitis B. *Scandinavian Journal of Immunology* 2013, 78(4):387–393.

[6] Roy S, Majumdar APN: Signaling in colon cancer stem cells. *Journal of Molecular Signaling* 2012, 7:11.

[7] Maccalli C, Pisarra P, Vegetti C, Sensi M, Parmiani G, Anichini A: Differential loss of T cell signaling molecules in metastatic melanoma patients' T lymphocyte subsets expressing distinct TCR variable regions. *Journal of Immunology* 1999, 163(12):6912–6923.

[8] Calon A, Espinet E, Palomo-Ponce S, Tauriello Daniele VF, Iglesias M, Céspedes María V, Sevillano M, Nadal C, Jung P, Zhang Xiang HF *et al*: Dependency of colorectal cancer on a TGF-β-driven program in stromal cells for metastasis initiation. *Cancer Cell* 2012, 22(5):571–584.

[9] Erdman SE, Poutahidis T: Cancer inflammation and regulatory T cells. *International Journal of Cancer* 2010, 127(4):768–779.

[10] Merika E, Saif MW, Katz A, Syrigos K, Morse M: Review. Colon cancer vaccines: an update. *In Vivo* 2010, 24(5):607–628.

[11] Bartnik A, Nirmal AJ, Yang S-Y: Peptide vaccine therapy in colorectal cancer. *Vaccines* 2013, 1(1):1.

[12] Beverley PCL: Immunology of vaccination. *British Medical Bulletin* 2002, 62(1):15–28.

[13] Heriot AG, Marriott JB, Cookson S, Kumar D, Dalgleish AG: Reduction in cytokine production in colorectal cancer patients: association with stage and reversal by resection. *British Journal of Cancer* 2000, 82(5):1009–1012.

[14] Galizia G, Lieto E, De Vita F, Romano C, Orditura M, Castellano P, Imperatore V, Infusino S, Catalano G, Pignatelli C: Circulating levels of interleukin-10 and interleukin-6 in gastric and colon cancer patients before and after surgery: relationship with radicality and outcome. *Journal of Interferon & Cytokine Research* 2002, 22(4):473–482.

[15] Yamaguchi S, Tatsumi T, Takehara T, Sasakawa A, Yamamoto M, Kohga K, Miyagi T, Kanto T, Hiramastu N, Akagi T *et al*: EphA2-derived peptide vaccine with amphiphilic poly(γ-glutamic acid) nanoparticles elicits an anti-tumor effect against mouse liver tumor. *Cancer Immunology, Immunotherapy* 2009, 59(5):759–767.

[16] Hazama S, Nakamura Y, Takenouchi H, Suzuki N, Tsunedomi R, Inoue Y, Tokuhisa Y, 7 Iizuka N, Yoshino S, Takeda K et al: A phase I study of combination vaccine treatment8 of five therapeutic epitope-peptides for metastatic colorectal cancer; safety, immuno–9 logical response, and clinical outcome. Journal of Translational Medicine 2014, 12:63.

[17] Begley J, Vo DD, Morris LF, Bruhn KW, Prins RM, Mok S, Koya RC, Garban HJ, Comin-Anduix B, Craft N *et al*: Immunosensitization with a Bcl-2 small molecule inhibitor. *Cancer Immunology, Immunotherapy* 2009, 58(5):699–708.

[18] Kaumaya PTP, Foy KC, Garrett J, Rawale SV, Vicari D, Thurmond JM, Lamb T, Mani A, Kane Y, Balint CR *et al*: Phase I active immunotherapy with combination of two chimeric, human epidermal growth factor receptor 2, B-cell epitopes fused to a promiscuous T-cell epitope in patients with metastatic and/or recurrent solid tumors. *Journal of Clinical Oncology* 2009, 27(31):5270–5277.

[19] Tan G-H, Li Y-N, Huang F-Y, Wang H, Bai R-Z, Jang J: Combination of recombinant xenogeneic endoglin DNA and protein vaccination enhances anti-tumor effects. *Immunological Investigations* 2007, 36(4):423–440.

[20] Saha A, Chatterjee SK, Foon KA, Celis E, Bhattacharya-Chatterjee M: Therapy of established tumors in a novel murine model transgenic for human carcinoembryonic antigen and HLA-A2 with a combination of anti-idiotype vaccine and CTL peptides of carcinoembryonic antigen. *Cancer Research* 2007, 67(6):2881–2892.

[21] Ali SA, Ahmad M, Lynam J, McLean CS, Entwisle C, Loudon P, Choolun E, McArdle SEB, Li G, Mian S *et al*: Anti-tumour therapeutic efficacy of OX40L in murine tumour model. *Vaccine* 2004, 22(27–28):3585–3594.

[22] Mukherjee P, Pathangey LB, Bradley JB, Tinder TL, Basu GD, Akporiaye ET, Gendler SJ: MUC1-specific immune therapy generates a strong anti-tumor response in a MUC1-tolerant colon cancer model. *Vaccine* 2007, 25(9):1607–1618.

[23] Miyagi Y, Imai N, Sasatomi T, Yamada A, Mine T, Katagiri K, Nakagawa M, Muto A, Okouchi S, Isomoto H *et al*: Induction of cellular immune responses to tumor cells and

peptides in colorectal cancer patients by vaccination with SART3 peptides. *Clinical Cancer Research* 2001, 7(12):3950–3962.

[24] Imai N, Harashima N, Ito M, Miyagi Y, Harada M, Yamada A, Itoh K: Identification of Lck-derived peptides capable of inducing HLA-A2-restricted and tumor-specific CTLs in cancer patients with distant metastases. *International Journal of Cancer* 2001, 94(2):237–242.

[25] Umansky V, Malyguine A, Shurin M: New perspectives in cancer immunotherapy and immunomonitoring. *Future Oncology* 2009, 5(7):941–944.

[26] Moulton HM, Yoshihara PH, Mason DH, Iversen PL, Triozzi PL: Active specific immunotherapy with a β-human chorionic gonadotropin peptide vaccine in patients with metastatic colorectal cancer: antibody response is associated with improved survival. *Clinical Cancer Research* 2002, 8(7):2044–2051.

[27] Morse MA, Bradley DA, Keler T, Laliberte RJ, Green JA, Davis TA, Inman BA: CDX-1307: a novel vaccine under study as treatment for muscle-invasive bladder cancer. *Expert Review of Vaccines* 2011, 10(6):733–742.

[28] Lynch TJ, Bell DW, Sordella R, Gurubhagavatula S, Okimoto RA, Brannigan BW, Harris PL, Haserlat SM, Supko JG, Haluska FG *et al*: Activating mutations in the epidermal growth factor receptor underlying responsiveness of non-small-cell lung cancer to gefitinib. *New England Journal of Medicine* 2004, 350(21):2129–2139.

[29] Watson SA, Gilliam AD: G17DT – a new weapon in the therapeutic armoury for gastrointestinal malignancy. *Expert Opinion on Biological Therapy* 2001, 1(2):309–317.

[30] Comeau JM, Labruzzo Mohundro B: From bench to bedside: promising colon cancer clinical trials. *American Journal of Managed Care* 2013, 19(1 Spec No):SP32–SP37.

[31] Rowe J, Cen P: TroVax in colorectal cancer. *Human Vaccines and Immunotherapeutics* 2014, 10(11):3196–3200.

[32] Wang X, Wang Q, Lin H, Li S, Sun L, Yang Y: HSP72 and gp96 in gastroenterological cancers. *Clinica Chimica Acta* 2013, 417:73–79.

[33] Walker KB, Keeble J, Colaco C: Mycobacterial heat shock proteins as vaccines – a model of facilitated antigen presentation. *Current Molecular Medicine* 2007, 7(4):339–350.

[34] Binder RJ, Han DK, Srivastava PK: CD91: a receptor for heat shock protein gp96. *Nature Immunology* 2000, 1(2):151–155.

[35] Liu B, Ye D, Song X, Zhao X, Yi L, Song J, Zhang Z, Zhao Q: A novel therapeutic fusion protein vaccine by two different families of heat shock proteins linked with HPV16 E7 generates potent antitumor immunity and antiangiogenesis. *Vaccine* 2008, 26(10):1387–1396.

[36]   Huang C, Zhao J, Li Z, Li D, Xia D, Wang Q, Jin H: Multi-chaperone-peptide-rich mixture from colo-carcinoma cells elicits potent anticancer immunity. *Cancer Epidemiology* 2010, 34(4):494–500.

[37]   Tol J, Punt CJ: Monoclonal antibodies in the treatment of metastatic colorectal cancer: a review. *Clinical Therapeutics* 2010, 32(3):437–453.

[38]   Martins SF, Reis RM, Rodrigues AM, Baltazar F, Filho AL: Role of endoglin and VEGF family expression in colorectal cancer prognosis and anti-angiogenic therapies. *World Journal of Clinical Oncology* 2011, 2(6):272–280.

[39]   Clarke JM, Hurwitz HI: Targeted inhibition of VEGF receptor 2: an update on ramucirumab. *Expert Opinion on Biological Therapy* 2013, 13(8):1187–1196.

[40]   Saif MW: Anti-VEGF agents in metastatic colorectal cancer (mCRC): are they all alike? *Cancer Management and Research* 2013, 5:103–115.

[41]   Peeters M, Cohn A, Köhne C-H, Douillard J-Y: Panitumumab in combination with cytotoxic chemotherapy for the treatment of metastatic colorectal carcinoma. *Clinical Colorectal Cancer* 2012, 11(1):14–23.

[42]   Vale CL, Tierney JF, Fisher D, Adams RA, Kaplan R, Maughan TS, Parmar MKB, Meade AM: Does anti-EGFR therapy improve outcome in advanced colorectal cancer? A systematic review and meta-analysis. *Cancer Treatment Reviews* 2012, 38(6):618–625.

[43]   You B, Chen EX: Anti-EGFR monoclonal antibodies for treatment of colorectal cancers: development of cetuximab and panitumumab. *Journal of Clinical Pharmacology* 2012, 52(2):128–155.

[44]   Henricks LM, Schellens JHM, Huitema ADR, Beijnen JH: The use of combinations of monoclonal antibodies in clinical oncology. *Cancer Treatment Reviews* 2015, 41(10):859–867.

[45]   Allard B, Pommey S, Smyth MJ, Stagg J: Targeting CD73 enhances the antitumor activity of anti-PD-1 and anti-CTLA-4 mAbs. *Clinical Cancer Research* 2013, 19(20):5626–5635.

[46]   Llosa NJ, Cruise M, Tam A, Wicks EC, Hechenbleikner EM, Taube JM, Blosser RL, Fan H, Wang H, Luber BS *et al*: The vigorous immune microenvironment of microsatellite instable colon cancer is balanced by multiple counter-inhibitory checkpoints. *Cancer Discovery* 2015, 5(1):43–51.

[47]   Ostrand-Rosenberg S, Horn LA, Alvarez JA: Novel strategies for inhibiting PD-1 pathway-mediated immune suppression while simultaneously delivering activating signals to tumor-reactive T cells. *Cancer Immunology, Immunotherapy* 2015, 64(10):1287–1293.

[48] Brahmer JR, Tykodi SS, Chow LQ, Hwu WJ, Topalian SL, Hwu P, Drake CG, Camacho LH, Kauh J, Odunsi K *et al*: Safety and activity of anti-PD-L1 antibody in patients with advanced cancer. *New England Journal of Medicine* 2012, 366(26):2455–2465.

[49] Brahmer JR, Pardoll DM: Immune checkpoint inhibitors: making immunotherapy a reality for the treatment of lung cancer. *Cancer Immunology Research* 2013, 1(2):85–91.

[50] Sagiv-Barfi I, Kohrt HEK, Czerwinski DK, Ng PP, Chang BY, Levy R: Therapeutic antitumor immunity by checkpoint blockade is enhanced by ibrutinib, an inhibitor of both BTK and ITK. *Proceedings of the National Academy of Sciences of the United States of America* 2015, 112(9):E966–E972.

[51] Curran MA, Montalvo W, Yagita H, Allison JP: PD-1 and CTLA-4 combination blockade expands infiltrating T cells and reduces regulatory T and myeloid cells within B16 melanoma tumors. *Proceedings of the National Academy of Sciences of the United States of America* 2010, 107(9):4275–4280.

[52] Werneck MB, Hottz E, Bozza PT, Viola JP: Cyclosporin A inhibits colon cancer cell growth independently of the calcineurin pathway. *Cell Cycle* 2012, 11(21):3997–4008.

[53] Mancini M, Toker A: NFAT proteins: emerging roles in cancer progression. *Nature Reviews Cancer* 2009, 9(11):810–820.

[54] Koido S, Ohkusa T, Homma S, Namiki Y, Takakura K, Saito K, Ito Z, Kobayashi H, Kajihara M, Uchiyama K *et al*: Immunotherapy for colorectal cancer. *World Journal of Gastroenterology : WJG* 2013, 19(46):8531–8542.

[55] Klampfer L: Cytokines, inflammation and colon cancer. *Current Cancer Drug Targets* 2011, 11(4):451–464.

[56] Kelly E, Russell SJ: History of oncolytic viruses: genesis to genetic engineering. *Molecular Therapy* 2007, 15(4):651–659.

[57] Lindenmann J, Klein PA: Viral oncolysis: increased immunogenicity of host cell antigen associated with influenza virus. *Journal of Experimental Medicine* 1967, 126(1):93–108.

[58] Bell J, McFadden G: Viruses for tumor therapy. *Cell Host & Microbe* 2014, 15(3):260–265.

[59] Hayden R, Pounds S, Knapp K, Petraitiene R, Schaufele RL, Sein T, Walsh TJ: Galacto-mannan antigenemia in pediatric oncology patients with invasive aspergillosis. *Pediatric Infectious Disease Journal* 2008, 27(9):815–819.

[60] Cheever MA, Higano CS: PROVENGE (Sipuleucel-T) in prostate cancer: the first FDA-approved therapeutic cancer vaccine. *Clinical Cancer Research* 2011, 17(11):3520–3526.

[61] Toda M, Martuza RL, Kojima H, Rabkin SD: In situ cancer vaccination: an IL-12 defective vector/replication-competent herpes simplex virus combination induces local and systemic antitumor activity. *Journal of Immunology* 1998, 160(9):4457–4464.

[62] Toda M, Rabkin SD, Kojima H, Martuza RL: Herpes simplex virus as an in situ cancer vaccine for the induction of specific anti-tumor immunity. *Human Gene Therapy* 1999, 10(3):385–393.

[63] Davis ID, Jefford M, Parente P, Cebon J: Rational approaches to human cancer immunotherapy. *Journal of Leukocyte Biology* 2003, 73(1):3–29.

[64] Bauzon M, Hermiston T: Armed therapeutic viruses – a disruptive therapy on the horizon of cancer immunotherapy. *Frontiers in Immunology* 2014, 5:74.

[65] Stanford MM, Barrett JW, Nazarian SH, Werden S, McFadden G: Oncolytic virotherapy synergism with signaling inhibitors: rapamycin increases myxoma virus tropism for human tumor cells. *Journal of Virology* 2007, 81(3):1251–1260.

[66] Prestwich RJ, Harrington KJ, Pandha HS, Vile RG, Melcher AA, Errington F: Oncolytic viruses: a novel form of immunotherapy. *Expert Review of Anticancer Therapy* 2008, 8(10): 1581–1588.

[67] Wongthida P, Diaz RM, Galivo F, Kottke T, Thompson J, Pulido J, Pavelko K, Pease L, Melcher A, Vile R: Type III IFN interleukin-28 mediates the antitumor efficacy of oncolytic virus VSV in immune-competent mouse models of cancer. *Cancer Research* 2010, 70(11):4539–4549.

[68] Guo ZS, Thorne SH, Bartlett DL: Oncolytic virotherapy: molecular targets in tumor-selective replication and carrier cell-mediated delivery of oncolytic viruses. *Biochimica et Biophysica Acta* 2008, 1785(2):217–231.

[69] Russell SJ, Peng K-W, Bell JC: Oncolytic virotherapy. *Nature Biotechnology* 2012, 30(7): 658–670.

[70] Cattaneo R, Miest T, Shashkova EV, Barry MA: Reprogrammed viruses as cancer therapeutics: targeted, armed and shielded. *Nature Reviews Microbiology* 2008, 6(7):529–540.

[71] Chiocca EA, Rabkin SD: Oncolytic viruses and their application to cancer immunotherapy. *Cancer Immunology Research* 2014, 2(4):295–300.

[72] Hanahan D, Weinberg Robert A: Hallmarks of cancer: the next generation. *Cell* 2011, 144(5):646–674.

[73] Casares N, Pequignot MO, Tesniere A, Ghiringhelli F, Roux S, Chaput N, Schmitt E, Hamai A, Hervas-Stubbs S, Obeid M et al: Caspase-dependent immunogenicity of doxorubicin-induced tumor cell death. *Journal of Experimental Medicine* 2005, 202(12): 1691–1701.

[74] Galanis E, Okuno SH, Nascimento AG, Lewis BD, Lee RA, Oliveira AM, Sloan JA, Atherton P, Edmonson JH, Erlichman C et al: Phase I–II trial of ONYX-015 in combination with MAP chemotherapy in patients with advanced sarcomas. *Gene Therapy* 2005, 12(5):437–445.

[75] Nemunaitis J, Khuri F, Ganly I, Arseneau J, Posner M, Vokes E, Kuhn J, McCarty T, Landers S, Blackburn A *et al*: Phase II trial of intratumoral administration of ONYX-015, a replication-selective adenovirus, in patients with refractory head and neck cancer. *Journal of Clinical Oncology* 2001, 19(2):289–298.

[76] Carter PJ: Potent antibody therapeutics by design. *Nature Reviews Immunology* 2006, 6(5):343–357.

[77] Hoogenboom HR: Selecting and screening recombinant antibody libraries. *Nature Biotechnology* 2005, 23(9):1105–1116.

[78] Kohler G, Milstein C: Continuous cultures of fused cells secreting antibody of predefined specificity. *Nature* 1975, 256(5517):495–497.

[79] Lonberg N: Human antibodies from transgenic animals. *Nature Biotechnology* 2005, 23(9):1117–1125.

[80] Staerz UD, Kanagawa O, Bevan MJ: Hybrid antibodies can target sites for attack by T cells. *Nature* 1985, 314(6012):628–631.

[81] Glennie MJ, McBride HM, Worth AT, Stevenson GT: Preparation and performance of bispecific F(ab' gamma)2 antibody containing thioether-linked Fab' gamma fragments. *Journal of Immunology* 1987, 139(7):2367–2375.

[82] Repp R, van Ojik HH, Valerius T, Groenewegen G, Wieland G, Oetzel C, Stockmeyer B, Becker W, Eisenhut M, Steininger H *et al*: Phase I clinical trial of the bispecific antibody MDX-H210 (anti-FcgammaRI × anti-HER-2/neu) in combination with Filgrastim (G-CSF) for treatment of advanced breast cancer. *British Journal of Cancer* 2003, 89(12):2234–2243.

[83] Nisonoff A, Rivers MM: Recombination of a mixture of univalent antibody fragments of different specificity. *Archives of Biochemistry and Biophysics* 1961, 93:460–462.

[84] Chan AC, Carter PJ: Therapeutic antibodies for autoimmunity and inflammation. *Nature Reviews Immunology* 2010, 10(5):301–316.

[85] Kontermann RE: Alternative antibody formats. *Current Opinion in Molecular Therapeutics* 2010, 12(2):176–183.

[86] Kontermann RE: Dual targeting strategies with bispecific antibodies. *MAbs* 2012, 4(2): 182–197.

[87] Dienstmann R, De Dosso S, Felip E, Tabernero J: Drug development to overcome resistance to EGFR inhibitors in lung and colorectal cancer. *Molecular Oncology* 2012, 6(1):15–26.

[88] Nahta R, Esteva FJ: HER2 therapy: molecular mechanisms of trastuzumab resistance. *Breast Cancer Research* 2006, 8(6):215.

[89] Engelman JA, Zejnullahu K, Mitsudomi T, Song Y, Hyland C, Park JO, Lindeman N, Gale CM, Zhao X, Christensen J et al: MET amplification leads to gefitinib resistance in lung cancer by activating ERBB3 signaling. Science 2007, 316(5827):1039–1043.

[90] Galon J, Costes A, Sanchez-Cabo F, Kirilovsky A, Mlecnik B, Lagorce-Pages C, Tosolini M, Camus M, Berger A, Wind P et al: Type, density, and location of immune cells within human colorectal tumors predict clinical outcome. Science 2006, 313(5795):1960–1964.

[91] Wahlin BE, Sander B, Christensson B, Kimby E: CD8+ T-cell content in diagnostic lymph nodes measured by flow cytometry is a predictor of survival in follicular lymphoma. Clinical Cancer Research 2007, 13(2 Pt 1):388–397.

[92] Hoffman L, Gore L: Blinatumomab, a bispecific anti-CD19/CD3 BiTE® antibody for the treatment of acute lymphoblastic leukemia: perspectives and current pediatric applications. Frontiers in Oncology 2014, 4.

[93] Hoffmann P, Hofmeister R, Brischwein K, Brandl C, Crommer S, Bargou R, Itin C, Prang N, Baeuerle PA: Serial killing of tumor cells by cytotoxic T cells redirected with a CD19-/CD3-bispecific single-chain antibody construct. International Journal of Cancer 2005, 115(1):98–104.

[94] Fujimoto M, Poe JC, Inaoki M, Tedder TF: CD19 regulates B lymphocyte responses to transmembrane signals. Seminars in Immunology 1998, 10(4):267–277.

[95] Rickert RC, Rajewsky K, Roes J: Impairment of T-cell-dependent B-cell responses and B-l cell development in CD19-deficient mice. Nature 1995, 376(6538):352–355.

[96] Brandl C, Haas C, d'Argouges S, Fisch T, Kufer P, Brischwein K, Prang N, Bargou R, Suzich J, Baeuerle PA et al: The effect of dexamethasone on polyclonal T cell activation and redirected target cell lysis as induced by a CD19/CD3-bispecific single-chain antibody construct. Cancer Immunology, Immunotherapy 2007, 56(10):1551–1563.

[97] Haas C, Krinner E, Brischwein K, Hoffmann P, Lutterbüse R, Schlereth B, Kufer P, Baeuerle PA: Mode of cytotoxic action of T cell-engaging BiTE antibody MT110. Immunobiology 2009, 214(6):441–453.

[98] Loffler A, Gruen M, Wuchter C, Schriever F, Kufer P, Dreier T, Hanakam F, Baeuerle PA, Bommert K, Karawajew L et al: Efficient elimination of chronic lymphocytic leukaemia B cells by autologous T cells with a bispecific anti-CD19//anti-CD3 single-chain antibody construct. Leukemia 2003, 17(5):900–909.

[99] Choi D, Kim T-G, Sung YC: The past, present, and future of adoptive T cell therapy. Immune Network 2012, 12(4):139–147.

[100] Rosenberg SA, Restifo NP, Yang JC, Morgan RA, Dudley ME: Adoptive cell transfer: a clinical path to effective cancer immunotherapy. Nature Reviews Cancer 2008, 8(4):299–308.

[101] Delorme EJ, Alexander P: Treatment of primary fibrosarcoma in the rat with immune lymphocytes. *Lancet* 1964, 2(7351):117–120.

[102] Dunn GP, Bruce AT, Ikeda H, Old LJ, Schreiber RD: Cancer immunoediting: from immunosurveillance to tumor escape. *Nature Immunology* 2002, 3(11):991–998.

[103] Swann JB, Smyth MJ: Immune surveillance of tumors. *Journal of Clinical Investigation* 2007, 117(5):1137–1146.

[104] Sallusto F, Lenig D, Forster R, Lipp M, Lanzavecchia A: Two subsets of memory T lymphocytes with distinct homing potentials and effector functions. *Nature* 1999, 401(6754):708–712.

[105] Darcy PK, Neeson P, Yong CSM, Kershaw MH: Manipulating immune cells for adoptive immunotherapy of cancer. *Current Opinion in Immunology* 2014, 27:46–52.

[106] Gattinoni L, Zhong XS, Palmer DC, Ji Y, Hinrichs CS, Yu Z, Wrzesinski C, Boni A, Cassard L, Garvin LM et al: Wnt signaling arrests effector T cell differentiation and generates CD8+ memory stem cells. *Nature Medicine* 2009, 15(7):808–813.

[107] Hacein-Bey-Abina S, Garrigue A, Wang GP, Soulier J, Lim A, Morillon E, Clappier E, Caccavelli L, Delabesse E, Beldjord K et al: Insertional oncogenesis in 4 patients after retrovirus-mediated gene therapy of SCID-X1. *Journal of Clinical Investigation* 2008, 118(9):3132–3142.

[108] Klebanoff CA, Gattinoni L, Torabi-Parizi P, Kerstann K, Cardones AR, Finkelstein SE, Palmer DC, Antony PA, Hwang ST, Rosenberg SA et al: Central memory self/tumor-reactive CD8+ T cells confer superior antitumor immunity compared with effector memory T cells. *Proceedings of the National Academy of Sciences of the United States of America* 2005, 102(27):9571–9576.

[109] Pule MA, Savoldo B, Myers GD, Rossig C, Russell HV, Dotti G, Huls MH, Liu E, Gee AP, Mei Z et al: Virus-specific T cells engineered to coexpress tumor-specific receptors: persistence and antitumor activity in individuals with neuroblastoma. *Nature Medicine* 2008, 14(11):1264–1270.

[110] Shook DR, Campana D: Natural killer cell engineering for cellular therapy of cancer. *Tissue Antigens* 2011, 78(6):409–415.

[111] Rosenberg SA, Lotze MT, Muul LM, Leitman S, Chang AE, Ettinghausen SE, Matory YL, Skibber JM, Shiloni E, Vetto JT et al: Observations on the systemic administration of autologous lymphokine-activated killer cells and recombinant interleukin-2 to patients with metastatic cancer. *New England Journal of Medicine* 1985, 313(23):1485–1492.

[112] Miller JS, Soignier Y, Panoskaltsis-Mortari A, McNearney SA, Yun GH, Fautsch SK, McKenna D, Le C, Defor TE, Burns LJ et al: Successful adoptive transfer and in vivo expansion of human haploidentical NK cells in patients with cancer. *Blood* 2005, 105(8): 3051–3057.

6

Circadian Regulation of Colon Cancer Stem Cells: Implications for Therapy

Sandra Ríos-Arrabal, José Antonio Muñoz-Gámez,
Sergio Manuel Jiménez-Ruíz, Jorge Casado-Ruíz,
Francisco Artacho-Cordón and Josefa León-López

Abstract

The presence of cancer stem cells (CSCs) in colorectal cancer (CRC) has been associated with tumor initiation, metastasis, relapse, and resistance to chemotherapy and radiotherapy. Therefore, a better knowledge of the molecular mechanisms involved in the regulation of CSCs is required to develop treatments that are more effective. Like normal cells, cancer cells contain molecular clocks that generate circadian rhythms in gene expression and metabolic activity. Disruption of circadian rhythms has been linked to increased cancer risk, chemoresistance, and progression in CRC. CSCs also generate rhythms, which could be exploited with a chronopharmacological approach. Although the regulation of the expression of circadian rhythm genes appears to be mediated mainly by transcription–translation feedback loops, the existence of forms of nontranscriptional regulation has been demonstrated. Particularly, microRNAs (miRNA) and SIRT1 are significant players in regulating various aspects of the circadian clock function. Furthermore, miRNA acts as a regulator of cancer progression by regulating the CSC characteristics through SIRT1. These findings led us to hypothesize that there is a circadian rhythm of CSC markers regulated by miRNAs in CRC with SIRT1 acting as a mediator of miRNA activity. The pharmacological regulation of SIRT1, and therefore of the circadian machinery, could result in antiproliferative effects and increased sensitivity to antitumor treatments in CRC.

Keywords: circadian rhythms, cancer stem cells, SIRT1, redox homeostasis, melatonin

1. Introduction

Cancer is a major health burden and one of the leading causes of death worldwide. There are more than 200 known types of cancer, being CRC one of the most common cancers. In men, CRC is the third most common, after lung and prostate cancer. In women, CRC is the second most common cancer behind breast cancer [1].

Cancer begins with the transformation of a normal cell into a tumor cell through a multistage process. In this process, the changes are the result of the interaction between the genetic factors of the patient and external agents, including physical, chemical, or biological agents. Aging is another fundamental factor in the development of cancer. The coming years will see an increase in the total number of cancer cases [2]. This will be caused by the dramatic increase in average life expectancy during the last century in the industrialized world and by the fact that about 5% of the population in the developed countries is predicted to have more than 85 years by 2050 [3].

CRC is an excellent example of the increased cell malignancy with age; according to the Centers for Control and Prevention of Diseases, the incidence rate of CRC increases progressively with age. In 2007, the Surveillance, Epidemiology, and End Results Program registry reported that CRC incidence was 74.5/100,000 in persons aged 50–64 years, 186.0/100,000 in persons aged 65–74 years, and 290.1/100,000 in persons aged ≥75 years [4].

Little is known about the precise biochemical mechanisms responsible for the rise in CRC rates with aging. Some authors have proposed cancer stem cells/stem-like cells (CSCs/CSLCs) as the main factor associated with age-related rise in CRCs [5]. CSCs are a small subpopulation of cells that might play a critical role in CRC progression and resistance to chemotherapy and radiotherapy. Because of these resistances, CSCs play an important role in the processes of tumor recurrence and metastasis [6–8]. Therefore, it is increasingly likely that therapies that specifically target CSCs will be needed for the complete eradication of the tumor [7] because these cells are responsible for the morbidity and mortality associated with this type of cancer [9].

2. CSCs and CRC

CSCs, also known as tumor-initiating cells, were first identified by John Dick in acute myeloid leukemia in the late 1990s. Since then, they have been an intense focus of cancer research. CSCs have recently been identified in several solid tumors, including breast [10], colon [11], head and neck [12], lung [13], pancreas [14], and central nervous system cancer [15]. CSCs are defined as cancer cells that possess characteristics associated with normal stem cells, specifically the ability to self-renew and differentiate into multiple cell types, in particular into all the heterogeneous cell types found in a particular cancer sample [16] (**Figure 1**).

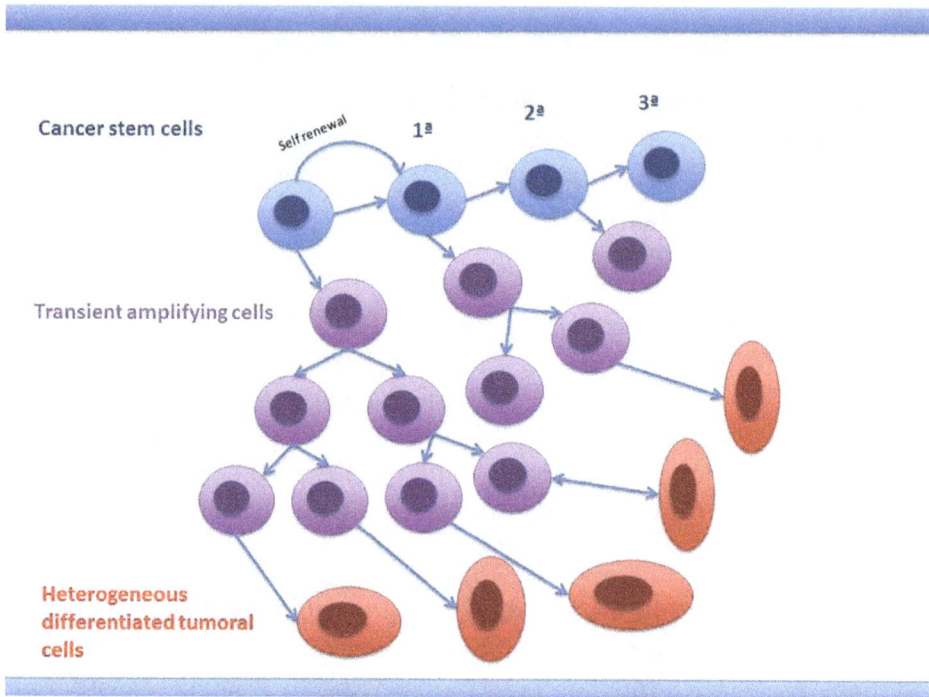

Figure 1. The cancer stem cells (CSCs) theory suggests that tumors grow like normal tissues of the body. In this way, the CSCs are able to both self-renew extensively, copying to them, and to produce the tissue grow (cancer tissue). In this process, the CSCs produce transit amplifying cells that have the capacity to divide a certain number of times, and then, they can differentiate into specialized heterogeneous tumor cells that do not have the skill to divide and therefore do not contribute to tumor growth.

Little is known about the origin of CSCs. Several proposals have been made regarding the origin of CSCs and probably several answers are possible depending on the tumor type and the tumor phenotype. In brief, CSC can arise if there are mutations in a developing stem or progenitor cells, in adult stem cells or adult progenitor cells, or in differentiated cells that acquire stem-like attributes [17]. Some data pointed to adult stem cells as origin of CSC in CRC. In this way, according to the most accepted model of CRC progression [18], four to five mutations in tumor suppressor genes or oncogenes are required and this takes about 8–12 years. As the colonic mucosa is a highly dynamic tissue, the mucosal cells are constantly replaced with cells derived from crypt stem cells. Therefore, only the long-lived cells (stem cells) may serve as reservoirs for accumulation of such mutations and epigenetic modifications.

In CRC, the presence of CSC has been correlated to tumor initiation, progression, metastasis, relapse, and resistance to chemotherapy and radiotherapy. [19]. CSCs have been isolated from CRC and are identified by the expression of specific surface markers and by their functional characteristics: CD44, CD166, CD133, ALDH1 (aldehyde dehydrogenase isoform 1), and ESA (epithelial-specific antigen, also known as EpCAM) [20]. Moreover, CSCs have been involved in the transition from adenoma to carcinoma, and this issue is age-dependent. In addition, an age-related rise in CSC has been observed in normal colonic mucosa and in premalignant adenomatous polyps. Moreover, the CSCs found showed an increased expression of CD44,

CD166, ALDH1, miR-21, and oncogenic miRNA, which suggests a predisposition of the organ to developing colorectal cancer [21]. Another characteristic of CSCs is that they can undergo epithelial–mesenchymal transition [22]. The fact that CSCs are resistant to conventional therapies has important implications in the development of novel strategies, such as CSCs-targeted treatments. It makes sense that eradication of CSCs or, alternatively, the attenuation of their malignant and stemness properties can lead us to achieve more effective therapeutic approaches. Therefore, development of specific CSCs-targeted therapies holds hope for improvement in the survival and quality of life of cancer patients, especially in patients with metastatic disease.

3. Epigenetic phenomena associated with CRC: miRNA regulatory network

Epigenetic processes are potentially reversible genetic modifications that lead to genomic instability and malfunction but that do not involve changes in DNA sequence. Epigenetic changes include (a) altered DNA methylation, (b) chromatin remodeling, and (c) small non-coding RNA (miRNAs). Notable changes in epigenetics have been reported for several age-related diseases, including CRC [23]. miRNAs are a small non-coding RNAs with 18–25 nucleotides found in plants, animals, and some viruses that are involved in RNA silencing and regulation of gene expression at the post-transcriptional level. miRNAs bind to the 3′-untranslated region (3′-UTR) of the protein-coding messenger RNAs (mRNAs). A single miRNA may regulate multiple mRNA targets and these small molecules are predicted to regulate approximately 60% of the human genes [24].

miRNAs are involved in different biological processes, including embryogenesis and the maintenance of stem cell characteristics, cell proliferation, metabolism, and transduction signals as in resistance to cancer treatments, including chemo- and radiotherapy [25, 26]. The presence of certain miRNAs has been associated with tumor development, tumor cell invasion, and cancer metastasis, and they may be of value as biomarkers for tumor detection and prognosis [27]. In addition, evidences show that miRNAs participate as oncogenic or tumor suppressors in the developmental and physiological processes of several human cancers, including CRC.

3.1. miRNA regulatory network in CRC

Approximately 450 unique miRNAs have been associated with CRC. In this disease, the aberrant expression of miRNAs has been associated with initiation and progression of CRC. Of special interest is miRNA involvement in the invasion, migration, and progression of disease through epithelial–mesenchymal transition into metastases. This event occurred due to IL6/STAT3 mediation and/or TP53 inactivation [28]. miRNAs are also involved in resistance to radio-chemotherapy [29].

Furthermore, miRNAs might regulate cell proliferation and apoptosis by targeting mitogen receptor tyrosine kinases and cell cycle regulators, such as cyclin-dependent kinases

(CDKs), reciprocal miRNA interactions with MYC (v-myc avian myelocytomatosis viral on-cogene homolog) and TP53, and by regulating the proapoptotic and antiapoptotic mRNAs [30].

Moreover, due to the altered expression of miRNAs in tumor development, they have been proposed as tissue and circulation biomarkers (blood derivates and feces). They might play a role in the prognostic and predictive diagnosis of CRC [31]. **Table 1** shows the potential roles of miRNA in CRC. Additionally, miRNA-related polymorphisms might disrupt their binding sites, miRNA processing, and expression. In this way, the single-nucleotide polymorphism (SNP) and other genetic abnormalities might be of utility in the study of the risk and prognosis of CRC.

	Role in CRC	**miRNA**
Oncogene	Proliferation	miR-21, miR-92a, miR-96, miR-135a, miR-135b
	Apoptosis	miR-21
	DNA damage response	miR-155
	Invasion	miR-21, miR-92a
	Epithelial–mesenchymal transition	miR-92a
	Metastasis	miR-224
	Inflammation	miR-224
Tumor suppressor	Proliferation	let-7, miR-7, miR-18a, miR-26b, miR-27b, miR-143, miR-144, miR-145, miR-194, miR-320a
	Apoptosis	miR-26b, miR-34a, miR-194, miR-195, miR-365, miR-491
	Angiogenesis	miR-27b, miR-145, miR-101, miR-126
	Invasion	miR-26b, miR-145, miR-194
	Migration	miR-26b, miR-145, miR-194
Circulatory biomarkers	Diagnosis	miR-21, miR-31, miR-34a, miR-92a, miR-143, miR-145, miR-601, miR-760
	Prognosis/survival	miR-21, miR-124-5p, miR-141, miR-155, miR-182, miR-200c
	Chemotherapy	miR-17-5p, miR-19a, miR-20a, miR-27b, miR-126, miR-130, miR-140, miR-145, miR-192, miR-216, miR-200c

Table 1. MiRNAs described in CRC

MiRNA has also been described with high potential as therapeutic target. According to Schetter et al., the two strategies for miRNA-based therapies are (a) to inhibit oncogenic miRNAs and (b) to restore tumor suppressor miRNAs. Some preclinical models have shown that both strategies might be effective in the treatment of CRC cancers [29].

3.2. miRNA regulation of CSC in CRC

Many studies have reported that miRNAs are key players in the regulation of CSCs [32]. Bitarte et al. [33] have described that miR-451 is involved in the self-renewal, tumorigenicity, and chemoresistance of CRC stem cells. Up-regulation of miR-451 resulted in reduction of colon sphere formation and growth, inhibition of tumorigenicity in vivo, and sensitization to the active metabolite of irinotecan, SN38. This metabolite might be related to miR-451–mediated down-regulation of cyclooxygenase-2 (COX-2) and WNT (Wingless-type MMTV integration site family) pathway, essential to maintain cell stemness. On the other hand, Bitarte et al. also described that the regulation of expression of ATP-binding cassette (ABCB1) by miR-451 could decrease SN38 resistance.

Moreover, it has been suggested that miR-215 and miR-140 could control the slow proliferation and the chemoresistance of CSCs in the colon. In this respect, Jones et al. [34] described miRNA-215 (miR-215) as a direct transcriptional target of CDX1 in CRC stem cell differentiation. Song et al. [35] suggested miR-215 as molecular modulator of chemoresistance in CSC in CRC. Moreover, Yu et al. [36] have reported that miR-93 suppresses proliferation and colony formation of human CRC stem cells.

4. Circadian rhythms and CSC in CRC

Circadian rhythms are daily rhythms that take the form of a sine wave with high or active and low or quiet periods over the 24-hour clock. Many biological processes are temporally coordinated so that groups of genes called "clock genes" and their products are expressed at different critical times of the day, being likewise coordinated in circadian time [37]. A master clock in the suprachiasmatic nucleus (SCN) of the hypothalamus organizes the circadian system in a hierarchical manner. The SCN receives photic input through direct retinal innervation that initiates gene expression in the SCN [38]. In this way, light exposure synchronizes the SCN clock to solar time, adapting the oscillator to exact 24-hour cycle. The master clock of the SCN communicates day-night information to the rest of the body. The SCN receives light input from the retina and then conveys the photic information into neural or humoral signals. This information is then sent to peripheral circadian clocks that exist in almost all cells of the body and synchronize them to the same phase [39]. Whereas light is the dominant rhythmic signal for the SCN oscillator, the peripheral clocks respond to other environmental signal, such as body temperature, hunger, and hormone secretion cycles, and modify their phase accordingly [40, 41].

4.1. Regulation of circadian rhythms in mammals

In mammals, these daily rhythms are maintained by autoregulatory transcriptional and translational feedback and feed-forward loops (TTFLs) [42]. The core clock genes are BMAL1 (brain and muscle aryl-hydrocarbon receptor nuclear translocator-like 1), CLOCK (circadian locomotor output cycles kaput), PER (period homolog), and CRY (cryptochrome) [41]. BMAL1 heterodimerizes with either CLOCK or NPAS2 (neuronal PAS domain protein 2) and binds to E-box elements in PER (PER1-3) and CRY (CRY1-2) promoter regions and activates their transcription. Upon accumulation in the cytoplasm, PER and CRY proteins translocate to the nucleus where they repress the BMAL1: CLOCK/NPAS2 regulatory complex, thereby shutting down their own transcription. The PER and CRY heterodimers are progressively degraded, allowing the circuit to start again. This negative feedback leads to a cycle in gene expression that takes approximately 24 hours to complete (**Figure 2**) [43].

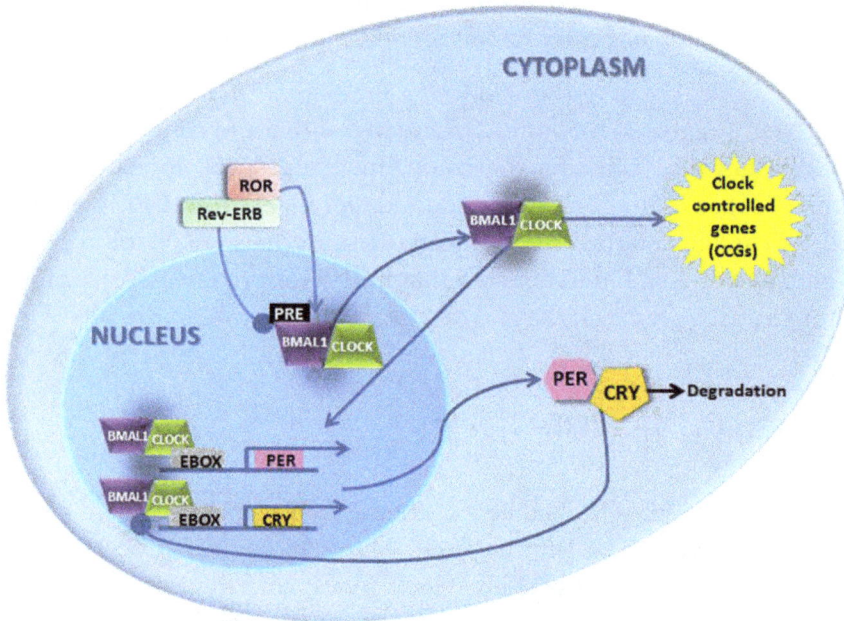

Figure 2. Schematic representation of the core circadian clock. (Adapted from Robinson and Reddy [52]. Copyright ©2014). BMAL1 and CLOCK transcription products translocate to the cytoplasm and dimerize. They then return to the nucleus and bind to E-box regions and promote Period (PER) and Cryptochrome (CRY) transcription. PER and CRY translocate to the cytoplasm, dimerize, and return to the nucleus and inhibit the binding of the CLOCK/BMAL complex. PER and CRY are subsequently degraded. REV-ERB inhibits the transcription of Bmal1, whereas ROR promotes BMAL1 expression. The clock-controlled genes REV-ERBα (REV-ERB) and RORα (ROR) generate additional circadian control by modulating the expression of BMAL1.

Post-transcriptional and post-translational modifications, such as phosphorylation, acetylation, methylation, sumoylation, and ubiquitination, are crucial to the clock molecular mechanism [44]. Post-translational modifications of the proteins of the circuit generate the essential time delay that maintains the period of the cycle at approximately 24 hours. Additional feedback pathways involving nuclear receptors, such as RORα (retinoid-related orphan receptor alpha), REV-ERBα (NR1D1, nuclear receptor subfamily 1, group D, member 1), PPARγ (peroxisome proliferator–activated receptor gamma), and PGC-1α (peroxisome proliferator–activated receptor gamma coactivator 1-alpha) provide further robustness to the circuit [45, 46]. Additionally, these clock genes control numerous target genes (termed clock controlled genes, CCGs) and they regulate the circadian rhythms of various biochemical and physiological processes [47].

4.2. Redox regulation of circadian rhythms

The possible relation between circadian rhythm and redox state has been long known but it was unclear whether redox oscillations are a driver of the clock or a biomarker of cellular time. The discovery that circadian redox oscillations appear to be conserved throughout evolution, and that circadian oscillations in redox parameters persist in the absence of transcriptional system, has consolidated the interplay between metabolic processes and the molecular clock [48]. In mammals, nearly 10,000 genes are known to be under circadian control [49]. Several studies have investigated circadian oscillations in gene expression in metabolic tissues, including brown fat, liver, and skeletal muscle [50]. Certain metabolic enzymes are rhythmically expressed in the liver, such as aconitase, aldolase 2, enolase 1, ketohexokinase, and succinate dehydrogenase 1 [51]. Since numerous metabolic diseases appear to have a circadian-related dysfunction, it follows that core cellular metabolism and the clock are intimately connected [52].

The redox state of a cell has been shown to be an integral component in the regulation of the molecular clock. DNA binding of NPAS2 and CLOCK is influenced by the redox state of NAD(H) and NHAP(H). NADP inhibits NPAS2:BMAL1 binding to DNA, but, on the other hand, DNA binding is promoted by NADPH. At a ratio of NADP:NADP(H) of over 75% NPAS2:BMAL1 DNA binding increases, whereas below 75% binding decreases [53].

Peroxiredoxins (PRDXs) are a family of antioxidants that help to prevent cellular damage resulting from the production of ROS and work by reducing H_2O_2 to water. Six PRDX isoforms are known (PRDX 1–6), and they are found in different cellular localizations: isoforms 1, 2, 5, and 6 in the cytosol, isoforms 3 and 5 in the mitochondria, isoform 5 in the peroxisome, and isoform 4 in the endoplasmic reticulum [54, 55]. PRDXs could have one or two redox active cysteine residues that bind H_2O_2 forming a sulfenic acid. In mammals, there are five two-Cysperoxiredoxins (PRDX 1–5) and a single one-Cysperoxiredoxin (PRDX 6) [56]. In most cases, a homodimer is formed by a resolving cysteine at the C terminus forming a disulphide bond with the cysteine sulfenic acid. This bond can then be 'resolved' by thioredoxin, enabling further catabolism of peroxide by PRDX [57].

The cycle of PRDX had been shown to follow a circadian rhythm, with two forms of PRDX6 oscillating in antiphase in the liver, emphasizing a role of post-translational modification in circadian rhythmicity [51]. While the core clockwork use TTFLs, many works suggest the redox state of PRDXs is driven by the metabolic state of the cell, but it is independent of transcription [58]. However, the reciprocal influence between the TTFL and the PRDX-based metabolic clock has not fully addressed yet.

4.3. Epigenetic regulation of circadian rhythms by miRNAs

Some miRNAs have regulatory functions contributing to the control over circadian protein expression [59]. The influences of the circadian clock function on miRNA expression or vice versa have been well established. Experimental evidence suggests that up to 30% of core clock genes are under the control of miRNA. Recently, miR-132 and miR-219 seem to be directly involved in the clock system and regulate light response [60].

Other studies examine the role of extracellular miRNAs in the regulation of molecular components and modulation of rhythmicity in peripheral cellular clocks. The studies revealed that exposure to miR-142-3p– and miR-494–enriched conditioned medium increases intracellular expression of these miRNAs and results in functional effects in recipient cells [59].

4.4. Circadian rhythms and CRC

In carcinogenesis, the levels of expression of many proteins may be dependent directly or indirectly on the circadian cycle. Investigations on the relation between the circadian clock and DNA damage response have revealed that DNA damage checkpoints, nucleotide excision repair, and apoptosis are appreciably influenced by the clock [61]. Changes in the circadian rhythm of cell division are considered important component in neoplastic transformation. The presence of DNA damage is usually associated with cell cycle arrest for attempted repairs or induction of apoptosis. The mechanism of repair happens before the S-phase of the cell cycle, and although there are post-replication mechanisms for induction of cell cycle arrest, the G1/S checkpoint is usually the most stringent cell cycle checkpoint and this event will take place at night for adjustment of the circadian rhythm [61]. On the other hand, disruptions of the circadian rhythm genes are associated with increased susceptibility to cancers [62].

Some experimental studies have showed the role of the disruption of the molecular clock work in colorectal carcinogenesis and CRC progression [63]. One example is seen in human cancer cells lines when PER1 is overexpressed. In this experiment, it was observed a reduced colony formation and clonogenic expansion, in sensitization to radiation-induced apoptosis, and in altered expression of transcriptional target genes, such as c-MYC and p21 [64]. In contrast, PER2-null mice showed an increase in hyperplasia and neoplasia in response to γ-radiation [65]. In line with this work, restoring CLOCK expression in a human colon adenocarcinoma cell line derived from a primary colon cancer, in response to ionizing radiation, conferred protection against ultraviolet (UV)-induced apoptosis and decreased G2/M arrest [66].

On the other hand, one study that used CRC tumor tissue from patients demonstrated that PER2 expression was higher in well-differentiated cancer cells when compared to poorly differentiated ones. Associations of decreased PER2 levels with patient age, histological grade, TNM (for tumors/nodes/metastases) stage, and expression of nuclear proliferation-related antigen Ki67 were also observed [67]. In addition, down-regulation of PER3 associated with various clinicopathological factors, including tumor location, differentiation, and stage, as well as poorer survival was seen in CRC tissues, thus suggesting an important role in CRC progression [68].

The efficacy of many drugs and the intensity of their effects depend on the time of day when they are administered (chronochemotherapy), and they are therefore associated with the circadian rhythm. The clock acts as a modulator of the pharmacokinetics and pharmacodynamics of chemotherapeutic drugs and of the activity of the DNA-repair enzymes that repair the DNA damage caused by anticancer drugs [61]. Some studies have demonstrated that chronomodulated chemotherapy has better tolerability and antitumor activity compared with conventional chemotherapy. A good example is the treatment of advanced stage CRC where oxaliplatin is administered in the afternoon and 5-FU and leucovorin are delivered late at night (chronoFLO4) [69]. Other authors have observed that 5-FU administration during the sleeping time before radiotherapy could have an advantage as a chronotherapy and also as a radiosensitizer [70].

4.5. Regulation of stemness by the circadian machinery

Numerous studies are demonstrating the importance of coherent circadian oscillations for a variety of homeostatic functions of tissues. One example is the timed activation and differentiation of stem and progenitor cells, and how perturbation of this temporal coordination leads to pathologies, including obesity and neurological diseases, aging, and cancer [71].

Like normal cells, cancer cells contain molecular clocks that generate circadian rhythms in gene expression and metabolic activity [72]. The circadian rhythms not only regulate the cell cycle in normal differentiated cells but there could also be a functional relation between circadian rhythm gene expression and the intrinsic control of the proliferation of CSCs and progenitor cells in different tissues [73]. In rodents and humans, all the hematopoietic stem and progenitor cells exhibit a predictable circadian variation [74, 75]. Some authors have shown that there is an increase in circadian rhythm gene expression of highly differentiated stem cell cultures. In both cancer and normal cells, a rhythmic nuclear translocation of PER2 and other critical clock proteins is an essential part of a clock timing mechanism based on transcriptional–translational feedback loops and rhythmic chromatin modification [73, 76].

The malignant phenotype depends not only on the characteristics of the cancer cell itself but also on the tumor microenvironment. CSCs have to survive for a long time in the body to generate the highly tumorigenic cells responsible for the clinical manifestations of cancer. During this period, the niche helps to shelter CSCs from different types of insults, such as the immune response and chemotherapy-induced genotoxic stress [77, 78]. This suggests that the niche may also play a protective role for CSCs, thus increasing the risk of cancer. In fact, BMAL1 suppresses cancer cell invasion by blocking the phosphoinositide 3-kinase-Akt-Matrix metalloproteinase-2 (MMP-2) signaling pathway [79]. Other authors have reported circadian oscillations in the levels of MMP-9 [80].

5. SIRT1 and the circadian regulation of CSCs by miRNAs

The silent information regulator (SIRT) 2 family of proteins, known as sirtuins, is a class III of histone deacetylases or NAD+−dependent deacetylases and is conserved from bacteria to humans. The requirement for NAD+ links the activity of sirtuins directly to the metabolic state of the cell, since the deacetylase activity of these proteins is controlled by the cellular NAD+/NADH ratio. There are seven sirtuins (SIRT1–7) in mammals. They have different specific substrates and biological functions and are found in various cell compartments [81].

The role of sirtuin activation in mammals is to regulate the progression of aging and age-associated disorders, including neurodegeneration, diabetes, cardiovascular diseases, and many types of cancer [82]. The best characterized and well-studied among the human sirtuins is SIRT1. It can be found in the nucleus and in the cytoplasm of the cells [83].

5.1. Sirt1 in cancer biology

SIRT1 is overexpressed in some types of human cancer tissues, such as ovary, liver, breast, stomach, pancreas and prostate, and down expressed in skin cancer. In CRC, SIRT1 is also overexpressed. However, other investigations have revealed pronounced SIRT1 expression in both normal colon and tumor tissues, although its expression is substantially reduced in higher grade CRC tumors [84].

SIRT1 has a dual role in tumorigenesis, where it can function as either a tumor promoter or a tumor suppressor. Its function in malignancy varies with concentration, cellular location, temporal and spatial distribution, and regulation by upstream and downstream factors [85].

The initial connection of sirtuins to cancer was made when SIRT1 was found to deacetylate and repress the activity of the tumor suppressor p53 [86, 87]. SIRT1-mediated deacetylation suppresses the functions of other tumor suppressors, including p73, hypermethylated in cancer 1 (HIC1), E2F transcription factor 1(E2F1, also known as retinoblastoma-associated protein 1), retinoblastoma protein (Rb), and phosphatase and tensin homologue deleted in chromosome 10 (PTEN), thus suggesting that SIRT1 acts as a promoter in tumor development and progression [88–93]. Other reports showed SIRT1 as a downstream of the oncoprotein BCR-ABL tyrosine kinase (Abelson murine leukemia viral oncogene homolog 1), implicated in the development of chronic myelogenous leukemia (CML)-like myeloproliferative disease [94].

Autophagy is a self-degradative process that plays a role by eliminating damaged organelles and misfolded or aggregated proteins through the lysosomal degradation pathway. Autophagy initially serves as a protective process to prevent cancer initiation; however, after neoplastic transformation, it can promote tumor cell survival and maintenance [95]. Autophagy can also affect chemotherapeutic and immunotherapeutic response in cancer cells making it an attractive target for development of anticancer drugs [96, 97]. SIRT1 forms a molecular complex with the genes related to autophagy and autophagosome formation, Atg5, Atg7, and Atg8. Loss of SIRT1 activity results in the acetylation of those factors thus leading to defects in the process of autophagy [98].

Consistent with a tumor-suppressor role, SIRT1 deacetylates and decreases the stability of the oncogene c-MYC [99]. In addition, the activity of SIRT1 can be increased by some tumor-suppressors, for example BRCA1 (breast cancer 1) [99]. SIRT1 exerts anticarcinogenic effects through multiple mechanisms [83]. SIRT1 can counteract various genotoxic insults, including oxidative DNA damage, thereby blocking initiation of carcinogenesis. SIRT1 deacetylates and inhibits proapoptotic p53 and PARP-1 (poly (ADP-ribose) polymerase 1) under stressful conditions, conferring cell survival [86, 100]. SIRT1 is also required for DNA repair processes to maintain genomic stability [101, 102].

SIRT1 inhibits the mediators involved in aberrantly amplified proinflammatory signaling during promotion and progression of carcinogenesis [103–105]. The anti-inflammatory effect of SIRT1 might be achieved by inhibition of several transcription factors related to inflammation, nuclear factor κB (NF-κB), signal transducer and activator of transcription 3 (STAT3), and the c-Jun and fos elements of transcription factor activator protein 1 (AP-1) [106–108]. Mainly through NF-κB and AP-1 pathways, SIRT1 was engaged in macrophage and T-cell activation [105, 109]. SIRT1 also regulates the differentiation and function of iTreg (induced Treg helper cells) [110]. Interestingly, SIRT1 translates metabolic cues during regulation of the immune responses, which would bring new insights into both pathogenesis and potential therapeutic strategies of a variety of immune-related diseases, such as cancer [111].

5.2. SIRT1 and stem cells

SIRT1 is considered an old multifaceted enzyme with an important role in the maintenance of pluripotency in various types of stem cells. Most of the in vivo data suggest that Sirt1 acts in early development as a modulatory molecule on basic developmental processes [112]. In cancer, SIRT1 has been implicated in the regulation of CSCs survival and differentiation. SIRT1 has been found to regulate the growth and survival of leukemia stem cells (LSCs) and confer resistance against chemotherapy [113], stimulate endometrial cell tumor growth through lipogenesis [114], maintain neural stem cells and promote oncogenic transformation [115], and foster hepatocellular carcinoma [116]. As a result, SIRT1 and agents that modulate SIRT1 activity may represent new therapeutic strategies against tumorigenesis.

One of the more intriguing hypotheses about aging and age-related disease is that age-associated phenotypic alterations derive from the inability of resident stem cells to maintain tissue structure and function [117]. This suggests that the aging process could arise from loss or malfunction of self-renewal and/or differentiation potential in adult stem cell populations. SIRT1 has a positive role in stemness by aiding in the silencing of differentiation genes, which suggests new potential explanations of its ability to extend lifespan and to avoid cell and organism senescence [112, 118].

5.3. SIRT1 and miRNAs

Expression of SIRT1 is controlled at multiple levels by transcriptional, post-transcriptional, and post-translational mechanisms under physiological and pathological conditions [119]. Deacetylation activity of SIRT1 can be modulated by multiple regulators. AROS (Active regulator of SIRT1) and DBC1 (deleted in breast cancer 1) are positive and negative regulators of SIRT1, respectively [120, 121].

Emerging evidence indicates that miRNAs are important regulators of SIRT1 expression and activity [119]. In cancer, SIRT1 mediates miR-34a activation of apoptosis by regulating p53 activity. In addition, p53 induces expression of miR-34a which suppresses SIRT1, increasing p53 activity [122]. In CRC, dysregulation of microRNA-34a expression causes drug-resistance to 5-FU in human colon cancer cells through the downregulation of Sirt1 and E2F3 [123, 124].

miRNAs play an important role in proper function and differentiation of human and mouse stem cells. Recently, it has been demonstrated that miR-34a is required for proper differentiation of mouse embryonic stem cells, mouse neural stem cell, and mouse embryonic fibroblasts and that it function in part by targeting SIRT1 and modulating p53 activity [125–127]. Also, the miR-29b-Sirt1 axis regulates self-renewal of mouse embryonic stem cells in response to reactive oxygen species [128]. miR-34a is also a critical regulator of cancer progression by the regulation of CSC characteristics, through SIRT1 as a mediator [129–133], and mainly, through up-regulation of p53/p21 [131].

5.4. SIRT1 as regulator of circadian rhythms

Two independent studies identified SIRT1 as a critical modulator of the circadian clock machinery. Asher et al. [134] observed oscillations in SIRT1 protein levels, and Nakahata et al. [135] demonstrated that SIRT1 activity, and not its protein levels, oscillates in a circadian manner. SIRT1 modulates circadian rhythms by deacetylating histone H3 Lys9 and Lys14 at promoters of rhythmic genes, BMAL1 and PER2. The CLOCK-BMAL1 complex interacts with SIRT1 and recruits it to the promoters of rhythmic genes. While BMAL1 acetylation acts as a signal for CRY recruitment, PER2 acetylation enhances its stability [134]. These findings led to the concept that SIRT1 operates as a rheostat of the circadian machinery, modulating the amplitude of CLOCK-mediated acetylation and consequent transcription cycles [135].

Circadian oscillation of SIRT1 activity suggested that cellular NAD+ levels may also oscillate. In fact, circadian clock controls the expression of NAMPT (nicotinamide phosphoribosyl-transferase), a key rate-limiting enzyme in the salvage pathway of NAD+ biosynthesis. The oscillatory expression of NAMPT is abolished in Clock/Clock mice, which results in drastically reduced levels of NAD+. These results imply the existence of an enzymatic/transcriptional feedback loop, wherein SIRT1 regulates the levels of its own cofactor [135]. These results also connect the circadian machinery to cell metabolism [134].

SIRT1 either directly or indirectly can influence the redox property of the cell [136]. In addition to reduce cellular oxidative stress burden, SIRT1 is also regulated by oxidative stress [137]. Since redox homeostasis influence circadian machinery, SIR1 could regulate circadian genes trough redox status of the cell. A recent report suggests that PRDX2 regulates the TTFL oscillation by decreasing the nuclear redox levels and increasing SIRT1 enzymatic activity, although neither a direct interaction between PRX and SIRT1 nor a modulation of SIRT1 intracellular levels by PRX was found [138].

5.5. SIRT1 regulators as new tools for cancer treatment

Recently, multiple research groups have pursued the identification and development of small molecule compounds that modulate sirtuins SIRT1 regulators as new tools for cancer treatment [139]. To date, SIRT1 inhibitors and activators have been described with different effects on cancer [140].

SIRT inhibitors require combined targeting of both SIRT1 and SIRT2 to induce p53 acetylation and cell death, like sirtinol and salermide [139]. Trichostatin A (TSA) and sirtinol induce p38MAPK- and AMPK-mediated downregulation of survivin and its functional correlation with decreased colon cancer cell viability in vitro [141]. Other salermide-related sirtuin inhibitors show antiproliferative effects in colon cancer cells in vitro, including CSCs [142]. Vorinostat activates p53, but does not require p53 for inducing its anticancer action in CRC [143]. The SIRT1 selective inhibitor Amurensin G may be effective in eliminating colon CSCs and may be applicable to potentiate the sensitivity of colon CSCs to TNF-related apoptosis-inducing ligand (TRAIL) [144].

Studies have shown that the sirtuin activator resveratrol, a polyphenol found in wines has chemopreventive activity against various cancers. In CRC, resveratrol induce apoptosis and suppressed the PI3K/Akt signaling pathway. The combination treatment with resveratrol and 5-FU induced a synergistic enhancement of growth inhibition and apoptosis in colon cancer DLD-1 cells. Interestingly, resveratrol increased the intracellular expression level of miR-34a, which down-regulated the target gene E2F3 and its downstream Sirt1, resulting in growth inhibition [145].

Melatonin is the main secretory product of the pineal gland and plays important roles in several biological functions, including circadian rhythms, sleep, mood, reproductive physiology, and aging diseases [146]. Numerous studies based on animal and clinical data have provided evidence that melatonin reduces the incidence of experimentally induced cancers and may significantly inhibit the growth of some human tumors [147]. Recently, melatonin was confirmed as a novel inhibitor of SIRT1. Melatonin inhibits prostate cancer and osteosarcoma cell growth through SIRT1 inhibition [148, 149]. Interestingly, it was recently reported that melatonin decreases CSCs and dysplastic injuries in colon tissue [150].

6. Concluding remarks

SIRT1 expression correlated with depth of invasion, lymph node metastasis, and TNM stage in CRC. Simultaneously, SIRT1 overexpression predicted a poor overall survival in CRC patients, and SIRT1 is a candidate negative prognostic biomarker for CRC patients [151]. SIRT1 has also been implicated in chemoresistance in CRC patients with [152] or without metastasis [124]. Further investigations aimed at targeting SIRT1 alone or in combination with chemotherapy deserve further attention and may ultimately increase response rates in the treatment of CRC. In this sense, melatonin can significantly amplify the cytostatic and the cytotoxic effects triggered by other compounds or conventional drugs. We are far from having a satisfactory understanding about how and when melatonin exerts its beneficial effects. Melatonin in the nanomolar range induces down-regulation of SIRT1. This finding is of great relevance because there is intense research ongoing to identify nontoxic feasible inhibitors of SIRT1. Melatonin should be evaluated for the management of those cancers where this protein is overexpressed and is functional.

Author details

Sandra Ríos-Arrabal[1], José Antonio Muñoz-Gámez[2], Sergio Manuel Jiménez-Ruíz[2], Jorge Casado-Ruíz[2], Francisco Artacho-Cordón[1] and Josefa León-López[3*]

*Address all correspondence to: pepileon@ugr.es

1 Department of Radiology and Physical Medicine, University of Granada, Granada, Spain, Biosanitary Research Institute, Granada, Spain

2 Clinical Management Unit of Digestive Disease and Research Support Unit, San Cecilio University Hospital Granada, Spain; Biosanitary Research Institute Granada, Spain

3 Clinical Management Unit of Digestive Disease and Research Support Unit, San Cecilio University Hospital Granada, Spain; Biosanitary Research Institute Granada, Spain; Ciber of Hepatic and Digestive Diseases (CIBERehd), Madrid, Spain

References

[1] Ferlay J, Soerjomataram I, Dikshit R, Eser S, Mathers C, Rebelo M, Parkin DM, Forman D, Bray F. Cancer incidence and mortality worldwide: sources, methods and major patterns in GLOBOCAN 2012. International Journal of Cancer. 2015;136(5):E359–86. DOI: 10.1002/ijc.29210

[2] Vaiopoulos AG, Kostakis ID, Koutsilieris M, Papavassiliou AG. Colorectal cancer stem cells. Stem Cells. 2012;30(3):363–71. DOI: 10.1002/stem.1031

[3] Todaro M, Francipane MG, Medema JP, Stassi G. Colon cancer stem cells: promise of targeted therapy. Gastroenterology. 2010;138(6):2151–62. DOI: 10.1053/j.gastro.2009.12.063

[4] Kemper K, Grandela C, Medema JP. Molecular identification and targeting of colorectal cancer stem cells. Oncotarget. 2010;1(6):387–95.

[5] Nangia-Makker P, Yu Y, Majumdar AP. Role of cancer stem cells in age-related rise in colorectal cancer. World Journal of Gastrointestinal Pathophysiology. 2015;6(4):86–9. DOI: 10.4291/wjgp.v6.i4.86

[6] Li X, Lewis MT, Huang J, Gutierrez C, Osborne CK, Wu MF, Hilsenbeck SG, Pavlick A, Zhang X, Chamness GC, Wong H, Rosen J, Chang JC. Intrinsic resistance of tumorigenic breast cancer cells to chemotherapy. Journal of the National Cancer Institute. 2008;100(9):672–9. DOI: 10.1093/jnci/djn123

[7] Ogawa K, Yoshioka Y, Isohashi F, Seo Y, Yoshida K, Yamazaki H. Radiotherapy targeting cancer stem cells: current views and future perspectives. Anticancer Research. 2013;33(3):747–54.

[8] Meirelles K, Benedict LA, Dombkowski D, Pepin D, Preffer FI, Teixeira J, Tanwar PS, Young RH, MacLaughlin DT, Donahoe PK, Wei X. Human ovarian cancer stem/ progenitor cells are stimulated by doxorubicin but inhibited by Mullerian inhibiting substance. Proceedings of the National Academy of Sciences of the United States of America. 2012;109(7):2358–63. DOI: 10.1073/pnas.1120733109

[9] Nigam A. Breast cancer stem cells, pathways and therapeutic perspectives 2011. The Indian Journal of surgery. 2013;75(3):170–80. DOI: 10.1007/s12262-012-0616-3

[10] Al-Hajj M, Wicha MS, Benito-Hernandez A, Morrison SJ, Clarke MF. Prospective identification of tumorigenic breast cancer cells. Proceedings of the National Academy of Sciences of the United States of America. 2003;100(7):3983–8. DOI: 10.1073/pnas. 0530291100

[11] Dalerba P, Dylla SJ, Park IK, Liu R, Wang X, Cho RW, Hoey T, Gurney A, Huang EH, Simeone DM, Shelton AA, Parmiani G, Castelli C, Clarke MF. Phenotypic characteri- zation of human colorectal cancer stem cells. Proceedings of the National Academy of Sciences of the United States of America. 2007;104(24):10158–63. DOI: 10.1073/pnas. 0703478104

[12] Prince ME, Sivanandan R, Kaczorowski A, Wolf GT, Kaplan MJ, Dalerba P, Weissman IL, Clarke MF, Ailles LE. Identification of a subpopulation of cells with cancer stem cell properties in head and neck squamous cell carcinoma. Proceedings of the National Academy of Sciences of the United States of America. 2007;104(3):973–8. DOI: 10.1073/ pnas.0610117104

[13] Ho MM, Ng AV, Lam S, Hung JY. Side population in human lung cancer cell lines and tumors is enriched with stem-like cancer cells. Cancer Research. 2007;67(10):4827–33. DOI: 10.1158/0008-5472.CAN-06-3557

[14] Li C, Lee CJ, Simeone DM. Identification of human pancreatic cancer stem cells. Methods in Molecular Biology. 2009;568:161–73. DOI: 10.1007/978-1-59745-280-9_10

[15] Singh SK, Hawkins C, Clarke ID, Squire JA, Bayani J, Hide T, Henkelman RM, Cusi- mano MD, Dirks PB. Identification of human brain tumour initiating cells. Nature. 2004;432(7015):396–401. DOI: 10.1038/nature03128

[16] Clarke MF, Dick JE, Dirks PB, Eaves CJ, Jamieson CH, Jones DL, Visvader J, Weissman IL, Wahl GM. Cancer stem cells--perspectives on current status and future directions: AACR Workshop on cancer stem cells. Cancer Research. 2006;66(19):9339–44. DOI: 10.1158/0008-5472.CAN-06-3126

[17] Rapp UR, Ceteci F, Schreck R. Oncogene-induced plasticity and cancer stem cells. Cell Cycle. 2008;7(1):45–51.

[18] Fearon ER, Vogelstein B. A genetic model for colorectal tumorigenesis. Cell. 1990;61(5): 759–67.

[19] Roy S, Majumdar AP. Cancer stem cells in colorectal cancer: genetic and epigenetic changes. Journal of Stem Cell Research & Therapy. 2012;Suppl 7(6). DOI: 31 10.4172/2157-7633.S7-006

[20] Rassouli FB, Matin MM, Saeinasab M. Cancer stem cells in human digestive tract malignancies. Tumour Biology: The Journal of the International Society for Oncodevelopmental Biology and Medicine. 2015. DOI: 10.1007/s13277-015-4155-y. [Epub ahead of print].

[21] Nautiyal J, Du J, Yu Y, Kanwar SS, Levi E, Majumdar AP. EGFR regulation of colon cancer stem-like cells during aging and in response to the colonic carcinogen dimethylhydrazine American Journal of Physiology. Gastrointestinal and Liver Physiology. 2012;302(7):G655-63. DOI: 10.1152/ajpgi.00323.2011

[22] Kanwar SS, Yu Y, Nautiyal J, Patel BB, Majumdar AP. The Wnt/beta-catenin pathway regulates growth and maintenance of colonospheres. Molecular Cancer. 2010;9:212. DOI: 10.1186/1476-4598-9-212

[23] Liu L, Wylie RC, Andrews LG, Tollefsbol TO. Aging, cancer and nutrition: the DNA methylation connection. Mechanisms of Ageing and Development. 2003;124(10–12): 989–98.

[24] Friedman RC, Farh KK, Burge CB, Bartel DP. Most mammalian mRNAs are conserved targets of microRNAs. Genome Research. 2009;19(1):92–105. DOI: 10.1101/gr. 082701.108

[25] Nam EJ, Yoon H, Kim SW, Kim H, Kim YT, Kim JH, Kim JW, Kim S. MicroRNA expression profiles in serous ovarian carcinoma. Clinical Cancer Research: An Official Journal of the American Association for Cancer Research. 2008;14(9):2690–5. DOI: 10.1158/1078-0432.CRC-07-1731

[26] Pourrajab F, Babaei Zarch M, BaghiYazdi M, Hekmatimoghaddam S, Zare-Khormizi MR. MicroRNA-based system in stem cell reprogramming; differentiation/dedifferentiation. The International Journal of Biochemistry & Cell Biology. 2014;55:318–28. DOI: 10.1016/j.biocel.2014.08.008

[27] Malek E, Jagannathan S, Driscoll JJ. Correlation of long non-coding RNA expression with metastasis, drug resistance and clinical outcome in cancer. Oncotarget. 2014;5(18): 8027–38.

[28] Rokavec M, Oner MG, Li H, Jackstadt R, Jiang L, Lodygin D, Kaller M, Horst D, Ziegler PK, Schwitalla S, Slotta-Huspenina J, Bader FG, Greten FR, Hermeking H. IL-6R/ STAT3/miR-34a feedback loop promotes EMT-mediated colorectal cancer invasion and metastasis. The Journal of Clinical Investigation. 2014;124(4):1853–67. DOI: 10.1172/ JCI73531

[29]   Schetter AJ, Okayama H, Harris CC. The role of microRNAs in colorectal cancer. Cancer Journal. 2012;18(3):244–52. DOI: 10.1097/PPO.0b013e318258b78f

[30]   Cekaite L, Eide PW, Lind GE, Skotheim RI, Lothe RA. MicroRNAs as growth regulators, their function and biomarker status in colorectal cancer. Oncotarget. 2015. DOI: 10.18632/oncotarget.6390. [Epub ahead of print].

[31]   Meiri E, Mueller WC, Rosenwald S, Zepeniuk M, Klinke E, Edmonston TB, Werner M, Lass U, Barshack I, Feinmesser M, Huszar M, Fogt F, Ashkenazi K, Sanden M, Goren E, Dromi N, Zion O, Burnstein I, Chajut A, Spector Y, Aharonov R. A second-generation microRNA-based assay for diagnosing tumor tissue origin. The Oncologist. 2012;17(6): 801–12. DOI: 10.1634/theoncologist.2011-0466

[32]   Liu X, Fu Q, Du Y, Yang Y, Cho WC. MicroRNA as regulators of cancer stem cells and chemoresistance in colorectal cancer. Current Cancer Drug Targets. 2015. [Epub ahead of print].

[33]   Bitarte N, Bandres E, Boni V, Zarate R, Rodriguez J, Gonzalez-Huarriz M, Lopez I, Javier Sola J, Alonso MM, Fortes P, Garcia-Foncillas J. MicroRNA-451 is involved in the self-renewal, tumorigenicity, and chemoresistance of colorectal cancer stem cells. Stem Cells. 2011;29(11):1661–71. DOI: 10.1002/stem.741

[34]   Jones MF, Hara T, Francis P, Li XL, Bilke S, Zhu Y, Pineda M, Subramanian M, Bodmer WF, Lal A. The CDX1-microRNA-215 axis regulates colorectal cancer stem cell differentiation. Proceedings of the National Academy of Sciences of the United States of America. 2015;112(13):E1550-8. DOI: 10.1073/pnas.1503370112

[35]   Song B, Wang Y, Titmus MA, Botchkina G, Formentini A, Kornmann M, Ju J. Molecular mechanism of chemoresistance by miR-215 in osteosarcoma and colon cancer cells. Molecular Cancer. 2010;9:96. DOI: 10.1186/1476-4598-9-96

[36]   Yu XF, Zou J, Bao ZJ, Dong J. miR-93 suppresses proliferation and colony formation of human colon cancer stem cells. World Journal of Gastroenterology. 2011;17(42):4711–7. DOI: 10.3748/wjg.v17.i42.4711

[37]   Hrushesky W, Rich IN. Measuring stem cell circadian rhythm. Methods in Molecular Biology. 2015;1235:81-95. doi: 10.1007/978-1-4939-1785-3_8.

[38]   Hastings MH, Herzog ED. Clock genes, oscillators, and cellular networks in the suprachiasmatic nuclei. Journal of Biological Rhythms. 2004;19(5):400–13. DOI: 10.1177/0748730404268786

[39]   Mohawk JA, Green CB, Takahashi JS. Central and peripheral circadian clocks in mammals. Annual Review of Neuroscience. 2012;35:445. DOI: 10.1146/annurev-neuro-060909-153128

[40]   Kohsaka A, Waki H, Cui H, Gouraud SS, Maeda M. Integration of metabolic and cardiovascular diurnal rhythms by circadian clock. Endocrine Journal. 2012;59(6):447–56. DOI: 10.1507/endocrj

[41] Chen L, Yang G. Recent advances in circadian rhythms in cardiovascular system. Frontiers in Pharmacology. 2015;6. DOI: 10.3389/fphar.2015.00071

[42] Yang G, Paschos G, Curtis AM, Musiek ES, McLoughlin SC, FitzGerald GA. Knitting up the raveled sleave of care. Science Translational Medicine. 2013;5(212):212rv3. DOI: 10.1126/scitranslmed.3007225

[43] Ukai H, Ueda HR. Systems biology of mammalian circadian clocks. Annual Review of Physiology. 2010;72:579–603. DOI: 10.1146/annurev-physiol-073109-130051

[44] Cardone L, Hirayama J, Giordano F, Tamaru T, Palvimo JJ, Sassone-Corsi P. Circadian clock control by SUMOylation of BMAL1. Science. 2005;309(5739):1390–4. DOI: 10.1126/science.1110689

[45] Liu C, Li S, Liu T, Borjigin J, Lin JD. Transcriptional coactivator PGC-1 alpha integrates the mammalian clock and energy metabolism. Nature. 2007;447(7143):477–81. DOI: 10.1038/nature05767

[46] Yang G, Jia Z, Aoyagi T, McClain D, Mortensen RM, Yang T. Systemic PPAR gamma deletion impairs circadian rhythms of behavior and metabolism. Plos One. 2012;7(8):e38117 DOI:10.1177/1534735409352083

[47] Paschos G. Circadian clocks, feeding time and metabolic homeostasis. Name: Frontiers in Pharmacology. 2015;6:112. DOI: 10.3389/fphar.2015.00112

[48] Edgar RS, Green EW, Zhao Y, van Ooijen G, Olmedo M, Qin X, Xu Y, Pan M, Valekunja UK, Feeney KA. Peroxiredoxins are conserved markers of circadian rhythms. Nature. 2012;485(7399):459–64. DOI: 10.1038/nature11088

[49] Ueda HR, Chen W, Adachi A, Wakamatsu H, Hayashi S, Takasugi T, Nagano M, Nakahama K, Suzuki Y, Sugano S. A transcription factor response element for gene expression during circadian night. Nature. 2002;418(6897):534–9. DOI: 10.1038/nature00906

[50] Storch K-F, Lipan O, Leykin I, Viswanathan N, Davis FC, Wong WH, Weitz CJ. Extensive and divergent circadian gene expression in liver and heart. Nature. 2002;417(6884):78–83. DOI: 10.1038/nature744

[51] Reddy AB, Karp NA, Maywood ES, Sage EA, Deery M, O'Neill JS, Wong GK, Chesham J, Odell M, Lilley KS. Circadian orchestration of the hepatic proteome. Current Biology. 2006;16(11):1107–15. DOI: 10.1016/j.cub.2006.04.026

[52] Robinson I, Reddy A. Molecular mechanisms of the circadian clockwork in mammals. FEBS Letters. 2014;588(15):2477–83. DOI: 10.1016/j.febslet.2014.06.005

[53] Rutter J, Reick M, Wu LC, McKnight SL. Regulation of clock and NPAS2 DNA binding by the redox state of NAD cofactors. Science. 2001;293(5529):510–4. DOI: 10.1126/science.1060698

[54] Rhee SG, Woo HA. Multiple functions of peroxiredoxins: peroxidases, sensors and regulators of the intracellular messenger H2O2, and protein chaperones. Antioxidants & Redox Signaling. 2011;15(3):781–94. DOI: 10.1089/ars.2010.3393

[55] Rhee SG, Woo HA, Kil IS, Bae SH. Peroxiredoxin functions as a peroxidase and a regulator and sensor of local peroxides. Journal of Biological Chemistry. 2012;287(7): 4403–10. DOI: 10.1074/jbc.R111.283432

[56] Hall A, Karplus PA, Poole LB. Typical 2-Cys peroxiredoxins: structures, mechanisms and functions. FEBS Journal. 2009;276(9):2469–77. DOI: 10.1111/j. 1742-4658.2009.06985.x.

[57] Hoyle NP, O'Neill JS. Oxidation-reduction cycles of peroxiredoxin proteins and nontranscriptional aspects of timekeeping. Biochemistry. 2015;54(2):184–93. DOI: 10.1021/bi5008386

[58] Avitabile D, Ranieri D, Nicolussi A, D'Inzeo S, Capriotti AL, Genovese L, Proietti S, Cucina A, Coppa A, Samperi R. Peroxiredoxin 2 nuclear levels are regulated by circadian clock synchronization in human keratinocytes. The International Journal of Biochemistry & Cell Biology. 2014;53:24–34. DOI: 10.1016/j.biocel.2014.04.024

[59] Shende VR, Kim S-M, Neuendorff N, Earnest DJ. MicroRNAs function as cis-and trans-acting modulators of peripheral circadian clocks. FEBS Letters. 2014;588(17):3015–22. DOI: 10.1016/j.febslet.2014.05.058

[60] Cheng H-YM, Papp JW, Varlamova O, Dziema H, Russell B, Curfman JP, Nakazawa T, Shimizu K, Okamura H, Impey S. microRNA modulation of circadian-clock period and entrainment. Neuron. 2007;54(5):813–29. DOI: 10.1016/j.neuron.2007.05.017

[61] Sancar A, Lindsey-Boltz LA, Gaddameedhi S, Selby CP, Ye R, Chiou Y-Y, Kemp MG, Hu J, Lee JH, Ozturk N. Circadian clock, cancer, and chemotherapy. Biochemistry. 2015;54(2):110–23. DOI: 10.1021/bi5007354

[62] Kettner NM, Katchy CA, Fu L. Circadian gene variants in cancer. Annals of Medicine. 2014;46(4):208–20. DOI: 10.3109/07853890.2014.914808

[63] Mazzoccoli G, Vinciguerra M, Papa G, Piepoli A. Circadian clock circuitry in colorectal cancer. World Journal of Gastroenterology. 2014;20(15):4197. DOI: 10.1016/jbbrc. 2006.05.094

[64] Yang X, Wood PA, Ansell C, Hrushesky WJ. Circadian time-dependent tumor suppressor function of period genes. Integrative Cancer Therapies. 2009;8(4):309–16. DOI: 10.1177/1534735409352083

[65] Wood PA, Yang X, Hrushesky WJ. Clock genes and cancer. Integrative Cancer Therapies. 2009;8(4):303–8. DOI: 10.1177/1534735409355292

[66] Alhopuro P, Björklund M, Sammalkorpi H, Turunen M, Tuupanen S, Biström M, Niittymäki I, Lehtonen HJ, Kivioja T, Launonen V. Mutations in the circadian gene

CLOCK in colorectal cancer. Molecular Cancer Research. 2010;8(7):952–60. DOI: 10.1158/1541-7786.MCR-10-0086

[67] Wang Y, Hua L, Lu C, Chen Z. Expression of circadian clock gene human Period2 (hPer2) in human colorectal carcinoma. World Journal of Surgical Oncology. 2011;9(1): 166. DOI: 10.1186/1477-7819-9-166

[68] Wang X, Yan D, Teng M, Fan J, Zhou C, Li D, Qiu G, Sun X, Li T, Xing T. Reduced expression of PER3 is associated with incidence and development of colon cancer. Annals of Surgical Oncology. 2012;19(9):3081–8. DOI: 10.1245/s10434-012-2279-5

[69] Levi F, Schibler U. Circadian rhythms: mechanisms and therapeutic implications. Annual Review of Pharmacology and Toxicology. 2007;47:593–628. DOI: 10.1146/annurev.pharmtox.47.120505.105208

[70] Asao T, Sakurai H, Harashima K, Yamaguchi S, Tsutsumi S, Nonaka T, Shioya M, Nakano T, Kuwano H. The synchronization of chemotherapy to circadian rhythms and irradiation in pre-operative chemoradiation therapy with hyperthermia for local advanced rectal cancer. Abbreviations: 5-FU 5-fluorouracil LV Leucovorin APR abdomino-perineal resection. International Journal of Hyperthermia. 2006;22(5):399–406. DOI: 10.1080/02656730600799873

[71] Janich P, Meng QJ, Benitah SA. Circadian control of tissue homeostasis and adult stem cells. Current Opinion in Cell Biology. 2014;31:8–15. DOI: 10.1016/j.ceb.2014.06.010

[72] Fujioka A, Takashima N, Shigeyoshi Y. Circadian rhythm generation in a glioma cell line. Biochemical and Biophysical Research Communications. 2006;346(1):169–74. DOI: 10.1016/jbbrc.2006.05.094

[73] Sharma VP, Anderson NT, Geusz ME. Circadian properties of cancer stem cells in glioma cell cultures and tumorspheres. Cancer Letters. 2014;345(1):65–74. DOI: 10.1016/j.canlet.2013.11.009

[74] Laerum O. Hematopoiesis occurs in rhythms. Experimental Hematology. 1995;23(11): 1145–7. DOI: 10.1111/j.1600-0609.1997.tb01680.x

[75] Bourin P, Ledain AF, Beau J, Mille D, Lévi F. In-vitro circadian rhythm of murine bone marrow progenitor production. Chronobiology International. 2002;19(1):57–67. DOI: 10.1081/CBI-120002677

[76] Lowrey PL, Takahashi JS. Genetics of circadian rhythms in mammalian model organisms. Advances in Genetics. 2011;74:175. DOI: 10.1016/B978-0-12-387690-4.00006-4

[77] Li L, Xie T. Stem cell niche: structure and function. Annual Review of Cell and Developmental Biology. 2005;21:605–31. DOI: 10.1146/annurev.cellbio.21.012704.131525

[78] McAllister SS, Weinberg RA. Tumor-host interactions: a far-reaching relationship. Journal of Clinical Oncology: Official Journal of the American Society of Clinical Oncology. 2010;28(26):4022–8. DOI: 10.1200/JCO.2010.28.4257

[79] Jung CH, Kim EM, Park JK, Hwang SG, Moon SK, Kim WJ, Um HD. Bmal1 suppresses cancer cell invasion by blocking the phosphoinositide 3-kinase-Akt-MMP-2 signaling pathway. Oncology Reports. 2013;29(6):2109–13. DOI: 10.3892/or.2013.2381

[80] Markoulli M, Papas E, Cole N, Holden BA. The diurnal variation of matrix metallo-proteinase-9 and its associated factors in human tears. Investigative Ophthalmology & Visual Science. 2012;53(3):1479–84. DOI: 10.1167/iovs.11-8365

[81] Carafa V, Nebbioso A, Altucci L. Sirtuins and disease: the road ahead. Frontiers in Pharmacology. 2012;3:4. DOI: 10.3389/fphar.2012.00004

[82] Guarente L. Franklin H. Epstein lecture: sirtuins, aging, and medicine. The New England Journal of Medicine. 2011;364(23):2235–44. DOI: 10.1056/NEJMra1100831

[83] Chalkiadaki A, Guarente L. The multifaceted functions of sirtuins in cancer. Nature Reviews Cancer. 2015;15(10):608–24. DOI: 10.1038/nrc3985

[84] Yang H, Bi Y, Xue L, Wang J, Lu Y, Zhang Z, Chen X, Chu Y, Yang R, Wang R, Liu G. Multifaceted modulation of SIRT1 in cancer and inflammation. Critical Reviews in Oncogenesis. 2015;20(1–2):49–64.

[85] Fang Y, Nicholl MB. A dual role for sirtuin 1 in tumorigenesis. Current Pharmaceutical Design. 2014;20(15):2634–6.

[86] Luo J, Nikolaev AY, Imai S, Chen D, Su F, Shiloh A, Guarente L, Gu W. Negative control of p53 by Sir2alpha promotes cell survival under stress. Cell. 2001;107(2):137–48.

[87] Vaziri H, Dessain SK, Ng Eaton E, Imai SI, Frye RA, Pandita TK, Guarente L, Weinberg RA. hSIR2(SIRT1) functions as an NAD-dependent p53 deacetylase. Cell. 2001;107(2):149–59.

[88] Dai JM, Wang ZY, Sun DC, Lin RX, Wang SQ. SIRT1 interacts with p73 and suppresses p73-dependent transcriptional activity. Journal of Cellular Physiology. 2007;210(1):161–6. DOI: 10.1002/jcp.20831

[89] Pediconi N, Guerrieri F, Vossio S, Bruno T, Belloni L, Schinzari V, Sciciani C, Fanciulli M, Levrero M. hSirT1-dependent regulation of the PCAF-E2F1-p73 apoptotic pathway in response to DNA damage. Molecular and Cellular Biology. 2009;29(8):1989–98. DOI: 10.1128/MCB.00552-08

[90] Zhang Q, Wang SY, Fleuriel C, Leprince D, Rocheleau JV, Piston DW, Goodman RH. Metabolic regulation of SIRT1 transcription via a HIC1:CtBP corepressor complex. Proceedings of the National Academy of Sciences of the United States of America. 2007;104(3):829–33. DOI: 10.1073/pnas.0610590104

[91] Wang C, Chen L, Hou X, Li Z, Kabra N, Ma Y, Nemoto S, Finkel T, Gu W, Cress WD, Chen J. Interactions between E2F1 and SirT1 regulate apoptotic response to DNA damage. Nature Cell Biology. 2006;8(9):1025–31. DOI: 10.1038/ncb1468

[92] Wong S, Weber JD. Deacetylation of the retinoblastoma tumour suppressor protein by SIRT1. The Biochemical Journal. 2007;407(3):451–60. DOI: 10.1042/BJ20070151

[93] Ikenoue T, Inoki K, Zhao B, Guan KL. PTEN acetylation modulates its interaction with PDZ domain. Cancer Research. 2008;68(17):6908–12. DOI: 10.1158/0008-5472.CAN-08-1107

[94] Yuan H, Wang Z, Li L, Zhang H, Modi H, Horne D, Bhatia R, Chen W. Activation of stress response gene SIRT1 by BCR-ABL promotes leukemogenesis. Blood. 2012;119(8): 1904–14. DOI: 10.1182/blood-2011-06-361691

[95] Guo JY, Xia B, White E. Autophagy-mediated tumor promotion. Cell. 2013;155(6):1216–9. DOI: 10.1016/j.cell.2013.11.019

[96] Wei Y, Zou Z, Becker N, Anderson M, Sumpter R, Xiao G, Kinch L, Koduru P, Christudass CS, Veltri RW, Grishin NV, Peyton M, Minna J, Bhagat G, Levine B. EGFR-mediated Beclin 1 phosphorylation in autophagy suppression, tumor progression, and tumor chemoresistance. Cell. 2013;154(6):1269–84. DOI: 10.1016/j.cell.2013.08.015

[97] Galluzzi L, Pietrocola F, Levine B, Kroemer G. Metabolic control of autophagy. Cell. 2014;159(6):1263–76. DOI: 10.1016/j.cell.2014.11.006

[98] Lee IH, Cao L, Mostoslavsky R, Lombard DB, Liu J, Bruns NE, Tsokos M, Alt FW, Finkel T. A role for the NAD-dependent deacetylase Sirt1 in the regulation of autophagy. Proceedings of the National Academy of Sciences of the United States of America. 2008;105(9):3374–9. DOI: 10.1073/pnas.0712145105

[99] Yuan J, Minter-Dykhouse K, Lou Z. A c-Myc-SIRT1 feedback loop regulates cell growth and transformation. The Journal of Cell Biology. 2009;185(2):203–11. DOI: 10.1083/jcb.200809167

[100] Rajamohan SB, Pillai VB, Gupta M, Sundaresan NR, Birukov KG, Samant S, Hottiger MO, Gupta MP. SIRT1 promotes cell survival under stress by deacetylation-dependent deactivation of poly(ADP-ribose) polymerase 1. Molecular and Cellular Biology. 2009;29(15):4116–29. DOI: 10.1128/MCB.00121-09

[101] Ming M, Shea CR, Guo X, Li X, Soltani K, Han W, He YY. Regulation of global genome nucleotide excision repair by SIRT1 through xeroderma pigmentosum C. Proceedings of the National Academy of Sciences of the United States of America. 2010;107(52): 22623–8. DOI: 10.1073/pnas.1010377108

[102] Oberdoerffer P, Michan S, McVay M, Mostoslavsky R, Vann J, Park SK, Hartlerode A, Stegmuller J, Hafner A, Loerch P, Wright SM, Mills KD, Bonni A, Yankner BA, Scully R, Prolla TA, Alt FW, Sinclair DA. SIRT1 redistribution on chromatin promotes genomic stability but alters gene expression during aging. Cell. 2008;135(5):907–18. DOI: 10.1016/j.cell.2008.10.025

[103] Zhu X, Liu Q, Wang M, Liang M, Yang X, Xu X, Zou H, Qiu J. Activation of Sirt1 by resveratrol inhibits TNF-alpha induced inflammation in fibroblasts. PLoS One. 2011;6(11):e27081. DOI: 10.1371/journal.pone.0027081

[104] Zhang Z, Lowry SF, Guarente L, Haimovich B. Roles of SIRT1 in the acute and restorative phases following induction of inflammation. The Journal of Biological Chemistry. 2010;285(53):41391–401. DOI: 10.1074/jbc.M110.174482

[105] Yoshizaki T, Schenk S, Imamura T, Babendure JL, Sonoda N, Bae EJ, Oh DY, Lu M, Milne JC, Westphal C, Bandyopadhyay G, Olefsky JM. SIRT1 inhibits inflammatory pathways in macrophages and modulates insulin sensitivity. American Journal of Physiology: Endocrinology and Metabolism. 2010;298(3):E419-28. DOI: 10.1152/ajpendo.00417.2009

[106] Yeung F, Hoberg JE, Ramsey CS, Keller MD, Jones DR, Frye RA, Mayo MW. Modulation of NF-kappaB-dependent transcription and cell survival by the SIRT1 deacetylase. The EMBO Journal. 2004;23(12):2369–80. DOI: 10.1038/sj.emboj.7600244

[107] Nie Y, Erion DM, Yuan Z, Dietrich M, Shulman GI, Horvath TL, Gao Q. STAT3 inhibition of gluconeogenesis is downregulated by SirT1. Nature Cell Biology. 2009;11(4):492–500. DOI: 10.1038/ncb1857

[108] Zhang R, Chen HZ, Liu JJ, Jia YY, Zhang ZQ, Yang RF, Zhang Y, Xu J, Wei YS, Liu DP, Liang CC. SIRT1 suppresses activator protein-1 transcriptional activity and cyclooxygenase-2 expression in macrophages. The Journal of Biological Chemistry. 2010;285(10): 7097–110. DOI: 10.1074/jbc.M109.038604

[109] Zhang J, Lee SM, Shannon S, Gao B, Chen W, Chen A, Divekar R, McBurney MW, Braley-Mullen H, Zaghouani H, Fang D. The type III histone deacetylase Sirt1 is essential for maintenance of T cell tolerance in mice. The Journal of Clinical Investigation. 2009;119(10):3048–58. DOI: 10.1172/JCI38902

[110] Beier UH, Wang L, Bhatti TR, Liu Y, Han R, Ge G, Hancock WW. Sirtuin-1 targeting promotes Foxp3+ T-regulatory cell function and prolongs allograft survival. Molecular and Cellular Biology. 2011;31(5):1022–9. DOI: 10.1128/MCB.01206-10

[111] Chen X, Lu Y, Zhang Z, Wang J, Yang H, Liu G. Intercellular interplay between Sirt1 signalling and cell metabolism in immune cell biology. Immunology. 2015;145(4):455–67. DOI: 10.1111/imm.12473

[112] Calvanese V, Lara E, Suarez-Alvarez B, Abu Dawud R, Vazquez-Chantada M, Martinez-Chantar ML, Embade N, Lopez-Nieva P, Horrillo A, Hmadcha A, Soria B, Piazzolla D, Herranz D, Serrano M, Mato JM, Andrews PW, Lopez-Larrea C, Esteller M, Fraga MF. Sirtuin 1 regulation of developmental genes during differentiation of stem cells. Proceedings of the National Academy of Sciences of the United States of America. 2010;107(31):13736–41. DOI: 10.1073/pnas.1001399107

[113] Li L, Osdal T, Ho Y, Chun S, McDonald T, Agarwal P, Lin A, Chu S, Qi J, Hsieh YT, Dos Santos C, Yuan H, Ha TQ, Popa M, Hovland R, Bruserud O, Gjertsen BT, Kuo YH,

Chen W, Lain S, Mc Cormack E, Bhatia R. SIRT1 activation by a c-MYC oncogenic network promotes the maintenance and drug resistance of human FLT3-ITD acute myeloid leukemia stem cells. Cell Stem Cell. 2014;15(4):431–46. DOI: 10.1016/j.stem.2014.08.001

[114] Lin L, Zheng X, Qiu C, Dongol S, Lv Q, Jiang J, Kong B, Wang C. SIRT1 promotes endometrial tumor growth by targeting SREBP1 and lipogenesis. Oncology Reports. 2014;32(6):2831–5. DOI: 10.3892/or.2014.3521

[115] Lee JS, Park JR, Kwon OS, Lee TH, Nakano I, Miyoshi H, Chun KH, Park MJ, Lee HJ, Kim SU, Cha HJ. SIRT1 is required for oncogenic transformation of neural stem cells and for the survival of "cancer cells with neural stemness" in a p53-dependent manner. Neuro-oncology. 2015;17(1):95–106. DOI: 10.1093/neuonc/nou145

[116] Mao B, Hu F, Cheng J, Wang P, Xu M, Yuan F, Meng S, Wang Y, Yuan Z, Bi W. SIRT1 regulates YAP2-mediated cell proliferation and chemoresistance in hepatocellular carcinoma. Oncogene. 2014;33(11):1468–74. DOI: 10.1038/onc.2013.88

[117] Rando TA. Stem cells, ageing and the quest for immortality. Nature. 2006;441(7097):1080–6. DOI: 10.1038/nature04958

[118] Calvanese V, Fraga MF. SirT1 brings stemness closer to cancer and aging. Aging. 2011;3(2):162–7.

[119] Choi SE, Kemper JK. Regulation of SIRT1 by microRNAs. Molecules and Cells. 2013;36(5):385–92. DOI: 10.1007/s10059-013-0297-1

[120] Kim EJ, Kho JH, Kang MR, Um SJ. Active regulator of SIRT1 cooperates with SIRT1 and facilitates suppression of p53 activity. Molecular Cell. 2007;28(2):277–90. DOI: 10.1016/j.molcel.2007.08.030

[121] Kim JE, Chen J, Lou Z. DBC1 is a negative regulator of SIRT1. Nature. 2008;451(7178):583–6. DOI: 10.1038/nature06500

[122] Yamakuchi M, Lowenstein CJ. MiR-34, SIRT1 and p53: the feedback loop. Cell Cycle. 2009;8(5):712–5.

[123] Akao Y, Noguchi S, Iio A, Kojima K, Takagi T, Naoe T. Dysregulation of microRNA-34a expression causes drug-resistance to 5-FU in human colon cancer DLD-1 cells. Cancer Letters. 2011;300(2):197–204. DOI: 10.1016/j.canlet.2010.10.006

[124] Amirkhah R, Farazmand A, Irfan-Maqsood M, Wolkenhauer O, Schmitz U. The role of microRNAs in the resistance to colorectal cancer treatments. Cell and Molecular Biology (Noisy-le-grand). 2015;61(6):17–23.

[125] Tarantino C, Paolella G, Cozzuto L, Minopoli G, Pastore L, Parisi S, Russo T. miRNA 34a, 100, and 137 modulate differentiation of mouse embryonic stem cells. FASEB Journal: Official Publication of the Federation of American Societies for Experimental Biology. 2010;24(9):3255–63. DOI: 10.1096/fj.09-152207

[126] Aranha MM, Santos DM, Sola S, Steer CJ, Rodrigues CM. miR-34a regulates mouse neural stem cell differentiation. PLoS One. 2011;6(8):e21396. DOI: 10.1371/journal.pone.0021396

[127] Lee YL, Peng Q, Fong SW, Chen AC, Lee KF, Ng EH, Nagy A, Yeung WS. Sirtuin 1 facilitates generation of induced pluripotent stem cells from mouse embryonic fibroblasts through the miR-34a and p53 pathways. PLoS One. 2012;7(9):e45633. DOI: 10.1371/journal.pone.0045633

[128] Xu Z, Zhang L, Fei X, Yi X, Li W, Wang Q. The miR-29b-Sirt1 axis regulates self-renewal of mouse embryonic stem cells in response to reactive oxygen species. Cellular Signalling. 2014;26(7):1500–5. DOI: 10.1016/j.cellsig.2014.03.010

[129] Nalls D, Tang SN, Rodova M, Srivastava RK, Shankar S. Targeting epigenetic regulation of miR-34a for treatment of pancreatic cancer by inhibition of pancreatic cancer stem cells. PLoS One. 2011;6(8):e24099. DOI: 10.1371/journal.pone.0024099

[130] Duan K, Ge YC, Zhang XP, Wu SY, Feng JS, Chen SL, Zhang LI, Yuan ZH, Fu CH. miR-34a inhibits cell proliferation in prostate cancer by downregulation of SIRT1 expression. Oncology Letters. 2015;10(5):3223–7. DOI: 10.3892/ol.2015.3645

[131] Ye Z, Fang J, Dai S, Wang Y, Fu Z, Feng W, Wei Q, Huang P. MicroRNA-34a induces a senescence-like change via the down-regulation of SIRT1 and up-regulation of p53 protein in human esophageal squamous cancer cells with a wild-type p53 gene background. Cancer Letters. 2016;370(2):216–21. DOI: 10.1016/j.canlet.2015.10.023

[132] Ma W, Xiao GG, Mao J, Lu Y, Song B, Wang L, Fan S, Fan P, Hou Z, Li J, Yu X, Wang B, Wang H, Xu F, Li Y, Liu Q, Li L. Dysregulation of the miR-34a-SIRT1 axis inhibits breast cancer stemness. Oncotarget. 2015;6(12):10432–44. DOI: 10.18632/oncotarget.3394

[133] Wang Z, Chen CC, Chen W. CD150 Side Population Defines Leukemia Stem Cells in a BALB/c Mouse Model of CML and Is Depleted by Genetic Loss of SIRT1. Stem Cells. 2015. DOI: 10.1002/stem.2218

[134] Asher G, Gatfield D, Stratmann M, Reinke H, Dibner C, Kreppel F, Mostoslavsky R, Alt FW, Schibler U. SIRT1 regulates circadian clock gene expression through PER2 deacetylation. Cell. 2008;134(2):317–28. DOI: 10.1016/j.cell.2008.06.050

[135] Nakahata Y, Kaluzova M, Grimaldi B, Sahar S, Hirayama J, Chen D, Guarente LP, Sassone-Corsi P. The NAD+–dependent deacetylase SIRT1 modulates CLOCK-mediated chromatin remodeling and circadian control. Cell. 2008;134(2):329–40. DOI: 10.1016/j.cell.2008.07.002

[136] Chung S, Yao H, Caito S, Hwang JW, Arunachalam G, Rahman I. Regulation of SIRT1 in cellular functions: role of polyphenols. Archives of Biochemistry and Biophysics. 2010;501(1):79–90. DOI: 10.1016/j.abb.2010.05.003

[137] Volonte D, Zou H, Bartholomew JN, Liu Z, Morel PA, Galbiati F. Oxidative stress-induced inhibition of Sirt1 by caveolin-1 promotes p53-dependent premature senes-

cence and stimulates the secretion of interleukin 6 (IL-6). The Journal of Biological Chemistry. 2015;290(7):4202–14. DOI: 10.1074/jbc.M114.598268

[138] Ranieri D, Avitabile D, Shiota M, Yokomizo A, Naito S, Bizzarri M, Torrisi MR. Nuclear redox imbalance affects circadian oscillation in HaCaT keratinocytes. The International Journal of Biochemistry & Cell Biology. 2015;65:113–24. DOI: 10.1016/j.biocel. 2015.05.018

[139] Villalba JM, Alcain FJ. Sirtuin activators and inhibitors. Biofactors. 2012;38(5):349–59. DOI: 10.1002/biof.1032

[140] Kozako T, Suzuki T, Yoshimitsu M, Arima N, Honda S, Soeda S. Anticancer agents targeted to sirtuins. Molecules. 2014;19(12):20295–313. DOI: 10.3390/molecules191220295

[141] Hsu YF, Sheu JR, Lin CH, Yang DS, Hsiao G, Ou G, Chiu PT, Huang YH, Kuo WH, Hsu MJ. Trichostatin A and sirtinol suppressed survivin expression through AMPK and p38MAPK in HT29 colon cancer cells. Biochimica et biophysica acta. 2012;1820(2):104– 15. DOI: 10.1016/j.bbagen.2011.11.011

[142] Rotili D, Tarantino D, Nebbioso A, Paolini C, Huidobro C, Lara E, Mellini P, Lenoci A, Pezzi R, Botta G, Lahtela-Kakkonen M, Poso A, Steinkuhler C, Gallinari P, De Maria R, Fraga M, Esteller M, Altucci L, Mai A. Discovery of salermide-related sirtuin inhibitors: binding mode studies and antiproliferative effects in cancer cells including cancer stem cells. Journal of Medicinal Chemistry. 2012;55(24):10937–47. DOI: 10.1021/jm3011614

[143] Sonnemann J, Marx C, Becker S, Wittig S, Palani CD, Kramer OH, Beck JF. p53-dependent and p53-independent anticancer effects of different histone deacetylase inhibitors. British Journal of Cancer. 2014;110(3):656–67. DOI: 10.1038/bjc.2013.742

[144] Lee SH, Kim MJ, Kim DW, Kang CD, Kim SH. Amurensin G enhances the susceptibility to tumor necrosis factor-related apoptosis-inducing ligand-mediated cytotoxicity of cancer stem-like cells of HCT-15 cells. Cancer Science. 2013;104(12):1632–9. DOI: 10.1111/cas.12299

[145] Kumazaki M, Noguchi S, Yasui Y, Iwasaki J, Shinohara H, Yamada N, Akao Y. Anticancer effects of naturally occurring compounds through modulation of signal transduction and miRNA expression in human colon cancer cells. The Journal of Nutritional Biochemistry. 2013;24(11):1849–58. DOI: 10.1016/j.jnutbio.2013.04.006

[146] Reiter RJ, Tan DX, Galano A. Melatonin: exceeding expectations. Physiology (Bethesda). 2014;29(5):325–33. DOI: 10.1152/physiol.00011.2014

[147] Zamfir Chiru AA, Popescu CR, Gheorghe DC. Melatonin and cancer. Journal of Medicine and Life. 2014;7(3):373–4.

[148] Jung-Hynes B, Schmit TL, Reagan-Shaw SR, Siddiqui IA, Mukhtar H, Ahmad N. Melatonin, a novel Sirt1 inhibitor, imparts antiproliferative effects against prostate

cancer in vitro in culture and in vivo in TRAMP model. Journal of Pineal Research. 2011;50(2):140–9. DOI: 10.1111/j.1600-079X.2010.00823.x

[149] Cheng Y, Cai L, Jiang P, Wang J, Gao C, Feng H, Wang C, Pan H, Yang Y. SIRT1 inhibition by melatonin exerts antitumor activity in human osteosarcoma cells. European Journal of Pharmacology. 2013;715(1–3):219–29. DOI: 10.1016/j.ejphar. 2013.05.017

[150] Kannen V, Marini T, Zanette DL, Frajacomo FT, Silva GE, Silva WAJr., Garcia SB. The melatonin action on stromal stem cells within pericryptal area in colon cancer model under constant light. Biochemical and Biophysical Research Communications. 2011;405(4):593–8. DOI: 10.1016/j.bbrc.2011.01.074

[151] Zu G, Ji A, Zhou T, Che N. Clinicopathological significance of SIRT1 expression in colorectal cancer: A systematic review and meta analysis. The International Journal of Surgery. 2016;26:32–7. DOI: 10.1016/j.ijsu.2016.01.002

[152] Vellinga TT, Borovski T, de Boer VC, Fatrai S, van Schelven S, Trumpi K, Verheem A, Snoeren N, Emmink BL, Koster J, Rinkes IH, Kranenburg O. SIRT1/PGC1alpha-dependent increase in oxidative phosphorylation supports chemotherapy resistance of colon cancer. Clinical Cancer Research: An Official Journal of the American Association for Cancer Research. 2015;21(12):2870–9. DOI: 10.1158/1078-0432.CRC-14-2290

7

Colorectal Cancer Prevention and Risk Counseling

Serife Koc, Melek Nihal Esin and Aysun Ardic

Abstract

Colorectal cancer (CRC) is one of the leading causes of cancer death in the world. Many risk factors have been identified in the development of colorectal cancer. It is necessary to carry out activities related to risk factors in order to implement effective CRC early diagnosis and screening programs and achieve positive outcomes. International screening guidelines have been created and these are being implemented by individual countries according to their own health policies. Colorectal cancer prevention and early training in terms of disease identification, counseling against negative disease perceptions, and changing false beliefs will reduce the fear of CRC and ensure the development of positive health behaviors and acceptance of screening. Among recent developments in cancer prevention, "cancer risk counseling" has become quite prominent. Individual-specific colorectal cancer risk counseling programs are developed through the assessment of individual risk factors by focusing on a genetic assessment and the development of a risk management plan. This chapter will examine and define colorectal cancer prevention and risk counseling strategies in relation with the relative literature.

Keywords: Colorectal cancer, prevention, cancer risk counseling, screening, clinical guidelines

1. Introduction

Colorectal cancer (CRC) is one of the leading causes of cancer death in the world. Colorectal cancer is a significant public health problem in many countries considering its incidence, mortality rate, and treatment costs [1]. Among all cancer deaths, mortality due to CRC ranks second in the world and accounts for 9–10% of all cancers deaths [2–4]. Colorectal cancer is the second most common cancer worldwide [5]. The incidence of CRC in North America and highly industrialized areas such as northwestern Europe and Australia is high, but is low in less developed regions such as Asia, Africa, and South America [2, 5, 6]. Lifetime risk of developing CRC varies between 2.4 and 6%. Risk factors possessed by individuals may increase this rate [2, 3]. It is necessary to carry out activities related to risk factors in order to implement effective CRC early diagnosis and screening programs and achieve positive outcomes. Moreover, implementing cost-effective screening programs decreases costs and increases the effectiveness of CRC screening [7, 8]. Many people do not know the risk factors for CRC; it is reported that those who do know them should be encouraged and supported by professionals to apply safeguard measures and effective interventions. More than half of CRC incidents can be prevented by implementing protection strategies in accordance with risk factors [9, 10]. However, to achieve this, negative behaviors must be changed to positive, and individuals should be directed toward early diagnosis in accordance with their risk conditions and monitored [11, 12]. In the realization of primary and secondary prevention strategies, bespoke colon cancer risk counseling is important for reducing morbidity and mortality [11–13].

2. Colorectal cancer prevention and risk counseling

2.1. Colorectal cancer prevention

2.1.1. Colorectal cancer risk factors

Advancing age, familial and genetic factors, environmental factors, and lifestyle/behavioral factors affect the development of CRC [2, 6–8]. Colorectal cancer risk factors are divided into two groups, those that can be changed and those that cannot [1, 6, 10].

Nonchangeable risk factors: These factors cannot be taken under control by the individual. These include age, sex, genetics (personal or family history of CRC), chronic colon diseases such as ulcerative colitis, inflammatory bowel disease or Crohn's disease, and a history of adenomatous polyps [6, 8, 10, 13].

Changeable risk factors: These are behavioral factors that can be altered or managed to help reduce the risk of CRC. It is reported that more than half of all cancers are linked to risky health behaviors. Changeable factors include but are not limited to smoking, moderate-to-heavy levels of alcohol consumption, being overweight and obesity, unbalanced diet, excessive consumption of red meat and/or processed meat products, physical inactivity, and/or sedentary lifestyle [3, 4, 6, 8–10, 13–19]. Risk factors and their relative risk for CRC are shown in **Table 1**. Colorectal cancer risk with relative risk above 1 indicates high risk, and less than 1 indicates low risk [10].

2.1.2. Colorectal cancer prevention strategies

The aim is to prevent cancer, precancerous lesions, and reduce the incidence of cancer-related morbidity and mortality and cancer spread, or at least diagnose it at earlier stages. Cancer prevention research, and the reduction of cancer morbidity and mortality, requires a three-dimensional approach: primary, secondary, and tertiary prevention [4, 6, 11, 20].

Factors increasing the risk	Relative risk
Family history and genetics	
One first-degree relative	2.2
More than one relative	4.0
Relative diagnosed before 45	3.9
Individual history	
Crohn's disease	2.6
Ulcerative colitis	2.8
Colon	1.9
Rectum	
Diabetes	1.2
Behavioral risk factors	
Excessive alcohol consumption	1.6
Obesity	1,.2
Red meat consumption	1.2
Processed meat consumption	1.2
Smoking cigarette	1.2
Risk reducing factors	
Physical activity (colon)	0.7
Consumption of dairy products	0.8
Fruit consumption	0.9
Vegetable consumption	0.9
Total dietary fiber consumption (10 g/day)	0.9

Table 1. Colorectal cancer risk factors and relative risk.

2.1.2.1. Primary prevention strategies

Primary prevention includes reducing the effects of carcinogens by using chemopreventive agents or removing environmental carcinogens. The goal of primary prevention is to prevent cancer from starting by reducing individual risk. Primary prevention focuses on lifestyle changes and risk factors related to chemoprevention. Primary prevention measures focus on two areas: making lifestyle changes toward changing primary risk factors and chemoprevention (chemical protection) strategies [20, 21].

2.1.2.1.1. Lifestyle changes

Healthy body weight: Being overweight obesity increases the risk of CRC, independent of physical activity. It is noted that abdominal obesity as measured by waist diameter is a more important risk factor than general obesity for both women and men [8, 10]. Patient education about ways to gain and maintain a healthy body weight is an important health professional task. Most people know its importance but there is a need for the encouragement and support of health professionals to implement effective interventions for individuals. Excess body fat can be reduced by reducing caloric intake and increasing physical activity. Reducing daily calorie intake by 50–100 calories can prevent gradual weight gain in adults, 500 calories/day or more weight loss program is the first joint reduction target. Research has shown that up to 60 minutes a day of moderate to vigorous physical activity may be necessary to prevent weight gain. For overweight people, daily physical activity up to 90 minutes of moderate intensity can help in losing weight [21].

Healthy nutrition and diet: Positive dietary factors that reduce the risk of cancer include low-fat diet (less than 24% of dietary fat content), high in fiber, high in omega 3, high fruits and vegetables, citrus fruits, cruciferous vegetables, carotene and lycopene-rich foods, plant-based diet, calcium, selenium, vitamin D, folic acid, omega 3 nutritional factors, and fatty acids. Dietary factors that increase the risk of cancer include animal fat, saturated fat, red meat, burnt/charred meat, trans fatty acids, and excessive alcohol consumption. Animal fats and consumption of excessive red meat and processed meat products increase the risk of high-calorie diet and consumptionless fiber-rich foods [2, 6, 8, 15, 16]. An oil-poor fiber-rich diet, 20–35 g of fiber daily for adults, and reducing total daily calories from fat by about 30%, with limited consumption of red meat is said to help reduce the risk of CRC. Also, regular consumption of fruits, vegetables, and calcium are recommended to reduce the risk for CRC for women and men. Nutritional advice for cancer prevention includes plant-derived diet containing at least five servings of fruits and vegetables every day, choosing whole grains instead of refined carbohydrates, eating saturated fat, and restricting alcohol and excessive calorie intake [11, 17, 19, 21].

Physical activity: Physical inactivity is one of the behavioral risk factors most often associated with CRC. Risk of CRC is lower for physically active people. Risk of CRC for very physically active people is 25% lower than in most physically inactive people [10]. Being physically active during both work and leisure time also reduces the risk. The American Cancer Society recommends a minimum of 150 minutes of moderate intensity every week, and preferably spread over the week, or 75 minutes of vigorous physical activity (or combination thereof) [10].

Avoidance of tobacco and alcohol: Smoking is more related to lung cancer but it also has quite harmful effects on the colon and rectum. Cigarette smoking increases the risk of colorectal adenoma [2, 6, 10, 17] and long-term use is associated with large polyps in the colon/rectum. The numbers of polyps have been reported to increase in patients even after they quit smoking 10 years previously [8, 17]. It is stated that the relative risk of CRC development is 1.64 in current smokers relative to nonsmokers [2], and 12% of all CRC deaths are related to tobacco use [8, 17]. Age of smoking initiation, duration of smoking, and the amount of cigarettes consumed per day increase the risk of CRC [18]. The difference in life risk of developing CRC in individuals who consume —two to four alcoholic beverages per day is greater than 23% compared with those who consume less than one alcoholic beverage per day. Alcohol consumption as a factor that plays a role in CRC is seen at an earlier age. The relative risk is 1.08 for alcohol intake of 25 g/day. Smoking together with alcohol consumption doubles the risk of CRC [10, 17, 19].

2.1.2.1.2. Chemopreventive measures

The administration of drugs or natural compounds to prevent the development of CRC is called chemoprevention. Colorectal cancer chemoprevention can be considered for advanced adenomas greater than 1 cm with villous histology, and more than two adenomas independent of the size of the adenoma and histology. Also, patients with a family history of cancer or cancer in first-degree relatives benefit from chemoprevention. Some 10% of all CRC groups can benefit from chemoprevention [22]. Research into chemoprevention of CRC is very active and chemical measures are recommended to more people in the high-risk group [6, 18, 21, 22]. Results of studies on chemical measures vary. Nonsteroidal anti-inflammatory drugs (NSAIDs) and aspirin have been determined to inhibit the enzyme cyclo-oxygenase (COX-1 and COX-2), which is involved in development of CRC. Regular aspirin or other NSAID use in humans reduces CRC development by 30–50%. In the recent past, these agents were not recommended for the general population (average risk), but today aspirin and other NSAIDs are recommended for the average-risk group. However, aspirin and other NSAIDs have adverse effects such as gastrointestinal bleeding and stroke, thus the benefit/risk balance of these drugs has restricted their use. In addition, calcium, vitamin D, folic acid, hormone replacement therapy, and the protection provided by statins need to be evaluated in further studies [6, 18, 21, 22].

2.1.2.2. Secondary prevention strategies

Secondary prevention, which enables slow-growing lesions to be diagnosed at early stages, includes early diagnosis and screening methods. Screening achieves better results because it avoids the onset of new cases and enables treatment of tumors at an early stage, which provides a better prognosis. Screening methods such as colonoscopy can identify abnormal cancerous changes so cancer can be prevented from fully developing. Secondary prevention is often associated with the removal of precancerous lesions or intraepithelial neoplasia (e.g., ductal carcinoma in situ, adenoma, or hyperplasia). In this way, disease is caught at an early stage, and the incidence of patients with advanced stage disease and mortality decreases [20, 23]. Polyps, especially adenomatous-type polyps, are known to be the precursor of CRC. The estimated 5-year survival rate of localized tumor (limited to the bowel wall) is 90%, it is 68% when the regional lymph node is involved, and 10% in the presence of distant metastases. CRC screening is recommended for the entire population; some people have a higher risk of developing CRC than others. The most important step is to assess the correct risk of developing CRC, screening is most effective test for individuals [6, 21, 23–27].

Colorectal cancer screening tests are divided into two groups:

- Stool tests: guaiac-based fecal occult blood test (gFOBT), fecal immunochemical test, stool DNA test.

- Structural analysis: flexible sigmoidoscopy (FS), colonoscopy, double barium contrast radiography, computed tomographic (CT) colonography, virtual colonoscopy, capsule endoscopy.

Each test has different advantages and disadvantages and can be used alone or in combination according to the request and the status of the individual [6]. Secondary prevention measures "Who should be screened and how?" The answer to the questions of who and which test brings clarity to the issue of how and how much will be applied at intervals, which is why CRC screening recommendations/guidelines have been established in many countries [6, 11, 21].

2.1.2.3. Clinical guidelines on colorectal cancer prevention

The aim of screening is to detect a precancer condition in the healthy population, as well as very early-stage malignancies that can be treated with a clearly curative intervention. In this context, international clinical guidelines have been created by the following organizations:

- American Cancer Society (ACS), The US Multi-Society Task Force on Colorectal Cancer (USMSTF), and American College of Radiology

- U.S. Preventive Services Task Force (USPSTF)

- National Comprehensive Cancer Network (NCCN)

- European Society for Medical Oncology (ESMO)

Screening tests and follow-up intervals are implemented and updated frequently by these organizations, depending on study results and technical improvements. The recommendations are not applied in the same way for the whole population; there are variations between countries and appropriate tests are recommended based on individual risk situations [6, 11, 16, 21, 24–28]. Although all guidelines recommend starting routine screening for CRC and adenomatous polyps in asymptomatic adults at age 50, there is less agreement as to the screening method, frequency of screening, and at which age screening may be safely discontinued. The recommendations differ for the method, frequency, and age of screening commencement in high-risk patients.

American Cancer Society, the US Multi-Society Task Force on Colorectal Cancer, and American College of Radiology (ACR) guidelines were published in 2008 [6, 21, 24]. These guidelines recommend starting screening in asymptomatic men and women at age 50 years. Any test that can detect adenomatous polyps can be used for screening adults at average risk. **Table 2** lists the tests and their recommended frequency of use. Individuals with family history of CRC, polyps, or one of the hereditary CRC syndromes, or a personal history of CRC or chronic inflammatory bowel disease are recommended to undergo colonoscopy at younger ages and more frequently than individuals at average risk (**Tables 3** and 4) [24, 28].

Test	Interval recommendations	Training issues to facilitate decision-making advantage/disadvantage
Flexible sigmoidoscopy	Every 5 years[1,2] Every 10 years[3] The optimal interval should not be <10 years and may even be extended to 20 years[3]	• Full or partial bowel preparation is required • Sedation is not generally used, so there may be some difficulties during the process • The protective effect is limited to the examined column section • If results are positive, people are generally directed to colonoscopy • Low risk of bleeding, infection, and perforation
Colonoscopy	Every 10 years[1,2,3] The optimal interval should not be <10 years and may even be extended up to 20 years[3]	• Full bowel preparation is required • Awareness under sedation used in most centers • A business day may be needed for resting before the preparation and after the process • Transportation (car cannot be used after sedation) and travel companion is required • Biopsy can be taken during the procedure, polyps can be removed • Rare but potentially serious risk of perforation and hemorrhage; risk increases with polypectomy
Double-contrast colonography	Every 5 years[1,2] Uncertain[3]	• Full bowel preparation is required • The biopsy cannot be done during the procedure • If one or more polyps >6 mm, colonoscopy will be recommended; follow-up colonoscopy will require full bowel preparation • Sedation is generally not used, so there may be some difficulties during the process • Low-risk, rare perforations have been reported
Virtual colonoscopy/ CT colonography	Every 5 years[1] Uncertain[2,3]	• Full bowel preparation is required • If one or more polyps > 6 mm, colonoscopy will be recommended; if colonoscopy is not possible on the same day, full bowel preparation is needed before the colonoscopy • Sedation is not used, so there may be some difficulties during the process

Test	Interval recommendations	Training issues to facilitate decision-making advantage/disadvantage
		• Low-risk, rare perforations have been reported
		• Extracolonic abnormalities can be identified and require further evaluation

[1]American Cancer Society, USMSTF, American College of Radiology screening guide.
[2]National Comprehensive Cancer Network (NCCN).
[3]ESMO guidelines and European guidelines for quality assurance in colorectal cancer screening and diagnosis [6, 13, 21, 24–27].

Table 2. Average risk for colorectal cancer, tips for individuals in the group, follow-up frequency, and advantages and disadvantages.

Test	Recommendations interval	Training issues to facilitate decision-making advantage/disadvantage
Guiac-based FOBT	Annually[1, 2] Annually[3] The test interval should not exceed 2 years[3]	• Depending on the manufacturer's recommendation, 2–3 stool samples collected at home are required to complete the test; stool sample collected during a single examination at the clinic, touching stool test is not acceptable and should not be used • No risk of perforation of the intestine • Can be done at home, increase the protection of privacy • It is relatively cheap compared with other tests • If results are positive, further evaluation with colonoscopy is needed • Avoid consumption aspirin, NSAIDs, vitamin C, red meat, poultry, fish, and raw vegetables for 48 hours before the test
Fecal immuno-chemical test	Annually[1] Uncertain[2] The test interval should not exceed 3 years[3]	• If results are positive, further evaluation with colonoscopy I needed • Single tests are often ineffective • The transportation of the material to the laboratory requires specific instructions and appropriate protective material • No risk of perforation • Protection of privacy as can be done at home
Stool DNA test	Uncertain[1,2,3]	• A test sample should be sufficient and should be packaged in suitable preservative for transportation to the laboratory • More expensive than other stool tests • If the test result is positive, further evaluation with colonoscopy is needed. If the test is negative, it is not clear, the test should be

Test	Recommendations interval	Training issues to facilitate decision-making advantage/disadvantage
		repeated at appropriate intervals
		• No dietary restrictions
		• Protection of privacy increased as can be done at home
		• No risk of perforation

[1]American Cancer Society, USMSTF, American College of Radiology screening guide.
[2]National Comprehensive Cancer Network (NCCN).
[3]ESMO guidelines and European guidelines for quality assurance in colorectal cancer screening and diagnosis [6, 13, 21, 24–27].

Table 2. Moderate risk for colorectal cancer, tips for individuals in the group, follow-up frequency, advantages and disadvantages (continued).

Risk category	Starting year	Recommendations/interval	Comment
CRC or adenomatous polyps in the first 60 years of first-degree relative or two or more first-degree relatives at any age	40 years, or 10 years younger than the age of the CRC diagnosis in the youngest relative CRC diagnosis[1,2] 40 years, or 5 years younger than the age of cancer onset in first-degree relatives[3]	Colonoscopy[1,2] FOBT and colonoscopy[3] Every 5 years[1,2,3]	
Two adenomatous/CRC polyps in first- or second-degree relatives aged over 60 years	40 years[1,2] or 5 years younger than the age of disease onset in first-degree relatives[3]	Screening frequency and recommendations for moderate risk individuals are applied[1,2] Screening/follow-up procedure will be determined by clinical follow-up of patients[3]	Individuals can now scan any screening test but should begin at an early age

[1]American Cancer Society, USMSTF, American College of Radiology screening guide.
[2]National Comprehensive Cancer Network (NCCN).
[3]ESMO guidelines and European guidelines for quality assurance in colorectal cancer screening and diagnosis [6, 13, 21, 24–27].

Table 3. Recommendations and colorectal cancer screening tests for individuals in the increased-risk group.

Risk category	Starting year	Recommendations/interval	Comment
Genetically diagnosed with FAP or without evidence of	10 or 12 years old[1,2] Starting at age 12–14 years and continued lifelong in mutation carriers[3]	Individual genetic anomaly that carries genetic tests to determine the annual FSA and consulting requirements[1,2] Sigmoidoscopy every 2 years[3]	If genetic testing is positive, colectomy should be considered Screening and monitoring procedures following clinical cases will be determined[3]

Risk category	Starting year	Recommendations/interval	Comment
genetic testing and those suspected in FAP			Once adenomas are detected, annual colonoscopy should be carried out until colectomy is planned[3]
For AFAP	Starting at age 18–20 years and continued lifelong in mutation carriers.[3]	Colonoscopy every 2 years[3]	After adenomas are detected, colonoscopy should be carried out annually[3]
Genetically or clinically diagnosed with HNPCC individuals, or high-risk individuals for HNPCC	20–25 years of age or their immediate family members or 10 years younger than the age of the CRC diagnosis in the youngest relative[1,2] Starting at age 20–25 or 5 years before the youngest case in the family[3]	Colonoscopy every 1–2 years and counseling on whether the genetic testing is necessary[1,2]Colonoscopy every 1–2 years.[3] Upper limit is not established.[3]	First-degree relatives of people with known hereditary MMR gene mutations should be offered genetic testing for HNPCC. Family mutation as yet unknown, but also those having one of the first three criteria of modified Bethesda should be recommended Screening and monitoring procedures following clinical cases will be determined[3]

[1]American Cancer Society, USMSTF, American College of Radiology screening guide.
[2]National Comprehensive Cancer Network (NCCN).
[3]ESMO guidelines and European guidelines for quality assurance in colorectal cancer screening and diagnosis [6, 13, 21, 24–27].

Table 4. Recommendations and colorectal cancer screening tests for individuals in the high-risk group.

US Preventive Services Task Force (USPSTF):

The US Preventive Services Task Force (USPSTF) recommends using high-sensitivity fecal occult blood testing, sigmoidoscopy, or colonoscopy from the age 50 years and to continue until the age of 75 years [28]. Higher risk individuals should begin screening at a younger age, and likely more frequently. Whether individuals need to be screened beyond the age of 75 years must be decided on an individual basis. Recommended screening tests and intervals are as follows:

- High-sensitivity fecal occult blood test (FOBT)—annual

- Flexible sigmoidoscopy—5 yearly (every 3 years with FOBT)

- Colonoscopy—every 10 years

Colonoscopy can be used for screening or as a follow-up diagnostic tool in symptomatic patients, or when the results of another CRC screening test are unclear or abnormal [28].

The National Comprehensive Cancer Network (NCCN):

The National Comprehensive Cancer Network (NCCN) has released separate guidelines for average- (**Table 2**), increased- (**Table 3**), and high-risk individuals (**Table 4**). For average individuals, the NNCN's guidance is almost identical to that of the ACS, USMSTF, and ACR. These guidelines make recommendations for each risk factor for individuals at high risk [27, 28].

European Society for Medical Oncology (ESMO):

According to all international guidelines, screening tests are stratified according to the personal risk of disease. The CRC screening guidelines of ESMO are in parallel with the guiding principles of the European guidelines. The ESMO recommendations for average-, increased-, and high-risk individuals are shown in **Tables 2–4**, respectively. Guaiac (g) FOBT reduced CRC mortality in average-risk populations by 15% in different age groups. To date, only FOBT has been recommended for men and women aged 50–74 years. Fecal immunochemical testing appears to be superior to gFOBT with respect to detection rates and positive predictive values for adenomas and cancer. Flexible sigmoidoscopy has been demonstrated to reduce CRC and mortality rates when conducted in organized screening programs. FS screening should be discontinued in patients of average risk aged more than 74 years because of the increased number of comorbidities in this population. There is no current evidence to support adding in a one-off sigmoidoscopy to FOBT screening. There is limited efficacy of colonoscopy in reducing CRC incidence and mortality. The optimal age for a single colonoscopy is circa 55 years but the age range for this test is 50–74 years. Newer screening techniques such as computed tomography colonography, stool DNA testing, and capsule endoscopy are still under evaluation and as such should not yet be relied upon to screen the average-risk population [29, 30].

Colorectal cancer screening remains a subject of debate regarding to whom, with which method, and at what frequency; however, its cost-effectiveness has been demonstrated and this is key in influencing the decision to implement CRC screening programs [7, 31]. Policy-makers and health professionals who decide on which CRC screening strategy to recommend or implement must be well informed. It is vital that resources are used efficiently when planning or implementing nationwide CRC screening programs, and that a cost-effective option for CRC screening is selected. According to the results of recent review studies, there is a complexity which screening test is the most cost-effective and which screening test should be chosen [7, 31].

Individuals are divided into categories according to their risk of CRC, and the type and frequency of screening methods varies depending on the risk category [6, 21, 23–27]. The risk of developing CRC for an individual is classified into three categories: moderate risk, increased risk, and high risk; screening is recommended in accordance with the risk group of individuals [6, 13]. Persons with known gene mutation or those with suspected gene mutations have a very high risk of contracting the disease [6, 13, 21, 24–27].

2.1.2.3.1. Moderate/average-risk group

Everyone is under the lowest risk for CRC [21]. Personal and family history of colorectal polyps or ulcerative colitis without CRC, chronic inflammatory bowel disease such as Crohn's disease without CRC, and all individuals aged 50 years and over are at average risk [6, 21, 24–27].

Individuals at average risk are recommended for screening; the frequency of follow-up is shown in **Table 2**.

2.1.2.3.2. Increased risk group

In this group, risk of CRC is growing twice according to the individuals in average risk. Individuals with a history of adenomatous polyps are at significantly higher risk. A family history of CRC or adenoma increases a person's risk of developing CRC. If there is a family history CRC or adenomas including first-degree relatives (mother, father, sibling, or child) before the age of 60, the risk of developing CRC at any age (−three to four times the average risk) significantly increases. Screening recommendations for high-risk individuals are shown in **Table 3**.

2.1.2.3.3. High-risk group

The risk of CRC in individuals with a known genetic mutation is high. The most common hereditary CRC syndrome, HNPCC, also known as Lynch syndrome, is an autosomal dominant syndrome and accounts for 3–5% of all CRCs. Familial adenomatous polyposis, which is characterized by multiple adenomatous colonic polyps, is an autosomal dominant syndrome comprising 1% of all CRC cases. For the FAP, the average age of cancer diagnosed is 39 years for FAP, but in the individuals with FAP 75% of adenomas occurred in 20 years. Recommended screening and surveillance programs for high-risk individuals are shown in **Table 4** [6, 21, 24, 30].

2.1.2.4. Tertiary prevention strategies

Tertiary prevention is used in the treatment of specified diseases or prevention of complications associated with the disease, is often used to treat one type of cancer and metastasis, or involves treating patients at risk for development of a secondary primary cancer [20]. The target of tertiary prevention in cancer patients is to reduce morbidity and mortality with the optimal treatment. Primary and secondary prevention practices are recommended in developing or less developed countries due to the fact that greater economic burden of tertiary prevention [20].

2.2. Colon cancer risk counseling

Today, although advances in treatment and screening standards established successful tests for CRC, it is not perceived as a curable and preventable disease. Many people do not know that even simple measures can prevent CRC. Cancer can be prevented in some individual cases, and it is very important to develop the perception in the community and belief that cancer can be prevented and is curable. Determining the level of risk and interpretation, encouraging preventive behaviors, and improving the early diagnosis and screening behaviors are important parts of early detection and screening programs. Prevention of colon cancer will be successful with the health efforts of professionals to increase awareness of the disease, risk assessments, counseling programs with appropriate recommendations, and diagnose the patients in an early stage [32, 33]. In studies conducted in recent years in the prevention of cancer, "cancer risk counseling" concept stands out [32, 34]. Physicians and nurses who work in primary healthcare services and oncology units have an important role and responsibilities in implementing programs and changing behavior that encourages early screening and diagnosis of cancer. Cancer risk counseling focuses on genetic assessment, assessment of individual risk factors, and the development of a risk management plan [35]. At this point, health professionals trained in CRC counseling can take control of their risk by reaching the individuals at an early stage [11, 12, 32, 36, 37]. Cancer risk counseling should be done in a second step in primary care with asymptomatic individuals at moderate risk and members of the increased-risk and high-risk groups. For example, risk counseling to individuals who have registered in family medicine and family health centers in the moderate-risk group is given by public health nurses. Family of individuals with hereditary CRC and of patients are counseled by doctors and nurses in clinical oncology for as long as treatment continues, or by clinical staff of family cancer clinics/genetic private surveillance programs or outpatient clinics, for those with chronic bowel disease if they are under follow-up [32, 36–38]. To conduct CRC risk counseling, physicians and nurses must have the authority and knowledge on this subject.

This risk counseling process encompasses a comprehensive cancer risk assessment, and determining genetic predisposition, information, guidance training and screening, genetic counseling, and creation of a risk management plan that includes the monitoring and evaluation plan. To achieve effective results in risk counseling, giving individual-specific messages, making an assessment of risk status together with the individual, and supporting the individual in the decision-making process is essential. In addition, it is aimed to follow-up screening participation of the individuals, and guide individuals who receive abnormal test results. Thus, CRC risk counseling aims to reduce morbidity and mortality with an increase in screening rates and to detect disease at an early stage [33, 35, 38].

Risk advisor staff who conduct risk counseling and risk assessments must have certain characteristics. CRC staff have to have adequate current information about hardware, communication techniques, good training, and counseling skills. Also, a counseling room should have adequate ventilation and lighting systems suitable for training and counseling. Colorectal cancer risk counseling identifies risk factors for an individual that can and cannot be changed (hazard identification/risk assessment); screening for risk factors proposition includes monitoring of behavior change initiatives and behavioral changes [38].

2.2.1. Stages of colorectal cancer risk counseling

Colorectal cancer risk counseling includes individual education and counseling and is implemented in three stages [32, 38]:

Stage 1: Application phase

Stage 2: Follow-up phase

Stage 3: Evaluation phase

2.2.1.1. Application phase

The creation of awareness through risk assessment and transfer of disease-specific information/education consist of three parts. Before making giving detailed information, disease awareness should be created for the individual, the individual's attention should be directed toward the subject and they should be allowed to ask questions [38]. At this stage, awareness about factors that increase the risk of disease must be created, and behavioral changes must be implemented in order to ensure appropriate counseling skills and evidence-based interventions [14]. A wide range of communication media have been used in studies aiming to increase awareness of CRC screening ranging from personal letters to TV advertisements. While facilitating effective participation in CRC screening initiatives, such as reminders, mass media and the media, group training, personal training, and assessments, are taken by reducing structural barriers to healthcare professionals and include initiatives such as feedback. The effectiveness of personal reminders, personal training, and counseling in improving CRC screening has been proven [10, 25, 39–44].

Sections	Initiatives/methods	Tools
Application phase		
Creating awareness	**Initiative:** CRC risk factors, prevention, information about early diagnosis **Method:** Face-to-face interviews, telephone interviews, video/slide show, introduce role models, motivational interviewing, send letters	Banners, posters, models, TV and newspaper advertisements, letters, mail/invitation via e-mail, phone messages, calendars, giveaway/inducers such as promotion, promotional stands
Risk assessment	**Initiative:** Determine the risk rating of the individual **Method:** Face-to-face interviews, computer-aided risk assessment models	Risk assessment tables, pedigree charts, graphs, histograms, electronic health records
Disease-specific information	**Initiative:** Provide adequate and appropriate information about the disease **Method:** Face to face interviews	Slides, posters, pamphlets, educational videos, health beliefs scales, written materials
Follow-up phase		
	Initiative: Maintain awareness, support positive behavior, follow-up/surveillance of screening behavior **Method:** Interview	Phone calls, text messages, e-mail, reminders, call center awards
Evaluation phase		
	Initiative: Preventive screening behavior and participation in evaluation, assessment test results **Method:** Face-to-face interviews	Automated phone calls Web-based assessment

Table 5. Colorectal cancer risk counseling can be applied in all stages of evidence-based initiatives.

Creating awareness: Various implications may be used in order to create awareness in the individuals about the importance of their protective behaviors in the prevention of CRC and their health. Evidence-based interventions recommended in the recent relevant studies are shown in **Table 5** [10, 25, 39–44]. Due to purpose of encouraging individuals take action to protective behaviors, it is important to give positive messages in materials (e.g., posters, banners) that it is possible to protect against CRC [11, 36, 37]. Risk assessment is required for each individual in order to determine the screening interval and proper test [21, 33].

Risk assessment: It is important to be able to receive adequate health history. The scope of individual members in the counseling process assessment includes the following:

- demographic, socioeconomic, cultural characteristics, and medical history (previous/ existing diseases, especially chronic bowel disease, polyps),

- a detailed family history (especially first- and second-degree relatives),

- cognitive and psychosocial (cognitive capacity, CRC knowledge, risk perception, CRC-related health beliefs and attitudes, perceptions, motivation, concerns, barriers, CRC relevant experience, anxiety and fears, coping mechanisms and social support status, decision-making and decision support systems),

- lifestyle behaviors (habits that increase the risk of CRC, dietary behaviors, physical activity status, smoking and alcohol use, stress level, given the importance of such a negative attitude and a healthy lifestyle),

- do not collect data on exposure to environmental risk factors and other characteristics.

Risk assessment tools for practical risk assessment (risk calculation tool, pedigram) can be made using electronic health records [10, 25, 33, 35, 39, 45]. According to the data obtained, a risk rating of the risk assessment is performed. The risk rating is how to determine whether an individual is at risk and making orientation relative to the risk. The degree of risk of cancer is important in guiding the individual screening tests [6, 11, 21]. In this regard, national/ international guidelines should be considered. Risk assessment, web-based tools, and mathematical models of interpretation of risk may make it easier to use directed individual protection proposals. Graphical presentation of risk status (bar, pie, histogram) makes it easier to explain and to understand the risk [6, 21, 33, 45]. Health behavior models have been developed for people to understand why there are different health behaviors or practices they are going to implement. While counseling individuals, health behavior models act as a "black box" to determine factors that affect preventive behaviors and to change negative behaviors to positive. These models are Health Belief Model, Transtheoretic Model, Health Promotion, and Preventive Health Model [11, 12, 14, 38, 39].

The risk status of the individual is described in a way that can be understood. Words, tone of voice, body images, and facial expressions of health personnel can affect the understanding individual risk information. The level of education of the individual, age, cultural, and linguistic differences should be taken into account. In addition, the cost of diagnosis and treatment, transportation requirements, communication, and cultural characteristics are important for the care of the patient's decision. Particular circumstances of the individual (e.g., affected my social and personal values, and economic and environmental conditions) should be considered. Individuals are given information regarding their assessment and risk diagnostics; when interpreting cancer risks, results that will disrupt the motivation for the individual's protection behavior or descriptions that will cause anxiety/fear should be avoided [33, 45].

Sufficient disease-specific information: The aim is to address the lack of knowledge about the disease and the individual CRC screening tests (fecal occult blood test, colonoscopy, double-contrast bowel X-ray, sigmoidoscopy). Patients training sessions should include information on colon and rectal anatomy of the digestive system, CRC generation, CRC signs and symptoms, risk factors, the importance of disease prevention, prevention, healthy lifestyle behaviors, early diagnosis and screening tests, the advantages and disadvantages of each test, and information about CRC protection behavior information [11, 21, 32, 35, 38, 39, 45]. Taking appropriate initiatives to scan an individual's risk rating should be provided and monitored (see **Table 5**). Encouragement of positive behavior aimed at reducing CRC risk and altering health beliefs associated with the disease are very important. Therefore, the individual's health beliefs during counseling, motivation, and barriers to education in this direction may be determined by a variety of scales [11, 21, 38]. Video display and printed materials in the education department, presentations, and motivational interviewing techniques such as active listening are available. There are no studies on the use of individual incentives that promote screening (a small amount of money, coupons, gift certificates); therefore, there is insufficient evidence to support this initiative alone. After the training, short appropriate tests should be conducted in order to evaluate the effectiveness of the training; individuals who then wish to undergo screening should be referred to the relevant departments and clinics [38].

2.2.1.2. Follow-up phase

Maintainance of awareness of the individual is intended to support the CRC protection behavior. It will increase the importance of the disease and practical initiatives to ensure the consistency of behavior covered in the training. The next follow-up face-to-face meeting in the implementation phase can be done through methods such as e-mail or telephone (**Table 5**). During these initiatives, any information that was given during training that was not clear can be questioned. For example, healthy lifestyle behaviors and screening recommendations for prevention of CRC can be repeated/reviewed, and information can be discussed about where to go in the event of receiving negative test results. At this stage, the behavior of individuals regarding disease protection is expected to show increased enthusiasm. All associated individuals (family, friends, healthcare professionals) are encouraged to support positive and protective behavior [11, 12, 21, 25, 35, 38].

2.2.1.3. Evaluation phase

At this stage, CRC protection behavior exhibited by the individual is evaluated. Changing an individual's behavior is not a goal that can be realized in a short time, it requires long-term follow-up. In order to ensure continuity, to maintain positive behaviors and enable behavior changes to occur, regular implementation of risk counseling (e.g., 3, 6, 12, 24 months) should be carried out [34, 35, 39]. The evaluation phase, which allows for obtaining feedback from individuals, is usually advised to be face to face. Reasons for an individual wishing to end the program should be taken to identify obstacles and need to reschedule procedures overcome these barriers [11, 12, 21, 32, 35, 38, 41, 45].

3. Conclusions

Primary and secondary prevention practices in the management of CRC are to be carried out together. Applying primary measures alone will not be enough, only having screening tests will not prevent the disease occurrence. Primary healthcare physicians and nurses have an important role in the implementation of risk counseling. Colorectal cancer risk counsellers are required to have special knowledge and skills. Therefore, the staff who undertake counseling are required to have received appropriate training. Colorectal cancer risk counseling is a process that applies to all stages of implementation, including monitoring, evaluation stages, and health services. Many initiatives and recommended methods for each stage of the process have been demonstrated in research. Adequate training in CRC risk counseling practice of health professionals, all relevant employees in surgery, oncology, and public health has been estimated to reduce the incidence of CRC.

Author details

Serife Koc[1*], Melek Nihal Esin[2] and Aysun Ardic[2]

*Address all correspondence to: serife.koc@istanbul.edu.tr

1 Karamanoglu Mehmetbey University, Karaman School of Health, Karaman, Turkey

2 Istanbul University, Florence Nightingale Faculty of Nursing, Istanbul, Turkey

References

[1] Chan AD, Giovannucci ED. Primary prevention of colorectal cancer. Gastroenterology. 2010; 138: 2029–2043.

[2] Wilkes GM. Colon, rectal, and anal cancers. In: Yarbro CH, Wujcik D, Gobel BH, editors. Cancer Nursing Principles and Practice. 7th ed. Sudbury, MA: Jones and Barlett Publishers; 2011. pp. 1205–1257.

[3] Johnson CM, Wei C, Ensor JE, Smolenski DJ, Amos CI, Levin B. et al. Meta-analyses of colorectal cancer risk factors. Cancer Causes Control. 2013; 24: 1207–1222.

[4] Tarraga LPJ, Albero JS, Rodriguez-Montes JA. Primary and secondary prevention of colorectal cancer. Clinical Medicine Insights: Gastroenterology. 2014; 7: 33–46.

[5] Ferlay J, Soerjomataram I, Ervik M, Dikshit R, Eser S, Mathers C, Rebelo M, Parkin DM, Forman D, Bray F. GLOBOCAN 2012 v1.0, Cancer Incidence and Mortality Worldwide: IARC CancerBase No. 11 [Internet]. Lyon, France: International Agency for Research on Cancer; 2013. Available from: http://globocan.iarc.fr [Accesssed: 2014/08/30].

[6] Erturk S. Colorectal cancers: Epidemiology, factors that play a role in the etiology, screening and chemoprevention. In: Baykan A, Zorluoglu A, Gecim E, Terzi C, editors. Colon and Rectum Cancers. Istanbul: Turkish Society of Colon and Rectal Surgery, Secil Offset Printing and Packaging Industry Co.Ltd.; 2010. pp. 15-30. [in Turkish]

[7] Patel SS, Kilgore ML. Cost effectiveness of colorectal cancer screening strategies. Cancer Control: Journal of the Moffitt Cancer Center. 2015; 22(2): 248–258.

[8] Oxentenko AS, Wei EK, Limburg PJ, Giovanucci E. Risk factors and prevention. In: Couric K, editor. American Cancer Society's Complete Guide to Colorectal Cancer. Atlanta: American Cancer Society; 2006. pp. 11–34.

[9] Glasper A. Can nurses help to promote earlier diagnosis of bowel cancer? British Journal of Nursing. 2012; 21(1): 50–51.

[10] American Cancer Society (ACS). Colorectal Cancer Facts and Figures 2014-2016. Atlanta: American Cancer Society, Inc.; 2014. Available from: http://www.cancer.org/acs/groups/content/documents/document/acspc-042280.pdf [Accesssed: 2015/10/30].

[11] Price AS. Primary and secondary prevention of colorectal cancer. Gastroenterology Nursing. 2003; 26(2): 73–81.

[12] Myers ER. Decision counseling in cancer prevention and control. Health Psychology. 2005; 24(4): 71–77.

[13] Cavdar I. Colon Rectum and Anal Cancers. In: Can G, editor. Oncology Nursing. Istanbul: Nobel Medical Publishers; 2015. pp. 707–717. [in Turkish]

[14] Simons VA, Flynn SP, Flocke SA. Practical behavior change counseling in primary care. Primary Care: Clinics in Office Practice. 2007; 34(3): 611–622.

[15] Thomson CA, Chen Z. The role of diet, physical activity and body composition in cancer prevention. In: Alberts DS, Hess LM, editors. Fundamentals of Cancer Prevention. 2nd ed. Tucson: Springer; 2010. pp. 31–78. DOI: 10.1007/978-3-540-68986-7.

[16] James, WPT. The role of nutrition in cancer prevention. In: Miller AB, editor. Epidemiologic studies in cancer prevention and screening. New York: Springer; 2013; pp. 121–140.

[17] Bazensky I, Shoobridge-Moran C, Yoder LH. Colorectal cancer: an overview of the epidemiology, risk factors, symptoms, and screening guidelines. Medsurg Nursing. 2007; 16(1): 46–51.

[18] Kahler CJ, Rex D, Imperiale TF. Screening for Colorectal Cancer, Social Follow-up and Primary Prevention: An Overview of Current Literature. Gastroenterology Turkish pressure. 2008; 3 (4): 193–217. [in Turkish]

[19] Keith JN, Jackson SC. Environmental factors and colorectal cancer. In: Kim KE, editor. Early Detection and Prevention of Colorectal Cancer. New Jersey: Slack Incorporated; 2009. pp. 49–71.

[20] Alberts DS, Hess LM. Introduction to cancer prevention. In: Alberts DS, Hess LM, editors. Fundamentals of Cancer Prevention. 2nd ed. Tucson: Springer; 2010. pp. 1–12. DOI: 10.1007/978-3-540-68986-7.

[21] Mahon SM. Prevention and screening of gastrointestinal cancers. Seminars in Oncology Nursing. 2009; 25(1): 15–31.

[22] Lance P. Chemical prevention for colorectal cancer: There is a long way to go although some progress. Gastroenterology Turkish pressure. 2008; 3(2): 98–106. [in Turkish]

[23] Patel SG, Ahnen DJ. Screening for colon polyps and cancer. In: Miller AB, editor. Epidemiologic Studies in Cancer Prevention and Screening. New York: Springer; 2013; pp. 169–182.

[24] Levin B, Lieberman BA, McFarland B, Andrews KS, Brooks D, Bond J. et al. Screening and surveillance for the early detection of colorectal cancer and adenomatous polyps, 2008: a joint guideline from the American Cancer Society, the US Multi-Society Task Force on Colorectal Cancer, and the American College of Radiology. Gastroenterology. 2008; 134(5): 1570–1595.

[25] European Commission. European guidelines for quality assurance in colorectal cancer screening and diagnosis. [Internet]. First ed., Luxemburg: Publication Office of the European Union; 2010. DOI: 10.2772/15379. Available from: http://www.kolorektum.cz/file/guidelines [Accessed: 2016/01/03].

[26] Lionis C, Petelos E. Early detection of colorectal cancer and population screening tests. In: Ettarh R, editor. Colorectal Cancer—From Prevention to Patient Care. Rijeka: InTech; 2012. pp. 45–66. Available from: http://www.intechopen.com/books/colorectal-cancer-from-prevention-to-patientcare/early-detection-of-colorectal-cancer-and-population-screening-tests [Accessed: 2015/12/30].

[27] NCCN Guidelines Version 2.2014, Colorectal Cancer Screening. Available from: http://www.nccn.org [Accessed: 2015/10/04].

[28] Cabebe EC. Colorectal cancer guidelines: colorectal cancer screening. In: Espat NJ, editor. [Internet]. 2015. Available from: http://emedicine.medscape.com/article/2500006-overview#a1 [Accessed: 2016/02/25].

[29] Labianca R, Nordlinger B, Beretta GD, Mosconi S, Mandalà M, Cervantes A, Arnold D. Early colon cancer: ESMO clinical practice guidelines for diagnosis, treatment and follow up. Annals of Oncology. 2013; 24(6): 64–72.

[30] Balmaña J, Balaguer F, Cervantes A, Arnold D. Familial risk-colorectal cancer: ESMO Clinical Practice Guidelines. Annals of Oncology. 2013; 24(6): 73–80.

[31] Lansdorp-Vogelaar I, Knudsen AB, Brenner H. Cost-effectiveness of colorectal cancer screening. Epidemiologic Reviews. 2011; 33(1): 88–100.

[32] Koc S, Esin MN. Screening behaviors, health beliefs, and related factors of first-degree relatives of colorectal cancer patients with ongoing treatment in Turkey. Cancer Nursing. 2014; 37(6): E51–60.

[33] Mahon SM. Screening and detection for asymptomatic individuals. In: Yarbro CH, Wujcik D, Gobel BH, editors. Cancer Nursing Principles and Practice. 7th ed. Sudbury, MA: Jones and Barlett Publishers; 2011. pp. 115–134.

[34] Glanz K, Steffen AD, Taglialatela LA. Effects of colon cancer risk counseling for first degree relatives. Cancer Epidemiology, Biomarkers and Prevention. 2007; 16(7): 1485–1491.

[35] MacDonald DJ. The oncology nurse's role in cancer risk assessment and counseling. Seminars in Oncology Nursing. 1997; 13(2): 123–128.

[36] Greenwald B. Health fairs: an avenue for colon health promotion in the community. Gastroenterology Nursing. 2003; 26(5): 191–194.

[37] Greenwald B. How to market colorectal cancer screening awareness and colonoscopy services. Gastroenterology Nursing. 2005; 28(5): 435–437.

[38] Koc S. The effect of colorectal cancer risk counseling on the promoting of primary and secondary preventive behaviors of the individuals at risk. [thesis] Istanbul: Istanbul University; 2014. [in Turkish]

[39] Gimeno Garcia AZ, Hernandez Alvarez Buylla N, Nicolas-Perez D, Quintero E. Public awareness of colorectal cancer screening: knowledge, attitudes, and interventions for increasing screening uptake. ISRN Oncology. 2014; 2014: 1–19.

[40] Rawl SM, Menon U, Burness A, Breslau ES. Interventions to promote colorectal cancer 26 screening: an integrative review. Nursing Outlook. 2012; 60(4): 172–181.

[41] Sabatino SA, Lawrence B, Elder R, Mercer SL, Wilson KM, DeVinney B, et al. Effectiveness of interventions to increase screening for breast, cervical, and colorectal cancers: nine updated systematic reviews for the guide to community preventive services. American Journal of Preventive Medicine. 2012; 43(1): 97–118.

[42] Brouwers CM, Vito C, Bahirathan L, Carol A, Carroll JC, Cotterchio M, et al. Effective interventions to facilitate the uptake of breast, cervical and colorectal cancer screening: an implementation guideline. Implementation Science. 2011a; 6(112): 1–8.

[43] Brouwers CM, Vito C, Bahirathan L, Carol A, Carroll JC, Cotterchio M, et al. What implementation interventions increase cancer screening rates? A systematic review. Implementation Science. 2011b; 6(111): 1–17.

[44] Holden DJ, Jonas DE, Porterfield DS, Reuland D, Harris R. Systematic review: enhancing the use and quality of colorectal cancer screening. Annals of Internal Medicine. 2010; 152(10): 668–676.

[45] National Cancer Institute. Cancer Genetics Risk Assessment and Counseling-for health professionals. [Internet]. Bethesda, MD: National Cancer Institute; 2015. Available from: http://www.cancer.gov/about-cancer/causes-prevention/genetics/risk-assessment-pdq#link/_323_toc [Accessed: 2015/12/30].

8

Immunotherapy in Colorectal Cancer

Gabriel Mak, Michele Moschetta and
Hendrik-Tobias Arkenau

Abstract

Colorectal cancer (CRC) remains one of the most common malignancies and the second leading cause of cancer-related death worldwide; treatment algorithms include surgery, chemotherapy and targeted therapies. Immunotherapy has recently emerged as an effective treatment approach in several types of cancer, including non–small cell lung cancer, melanoma and kidney cancer. In CRC, novel immune-checkpoint inhibitors such as anti-CTLA4 and PD1/PDL1 monoclonal antibodies have shown limited efficacy, although ongoing trials in mismatch repair-deficient CRC have shown significant and promising results. Here, we review the role of immune-microenvironment in colorectal cancer and current clinical data about therapeutic activity of immunotherapy in the treatment of CRC.

Keywords: colorectal cancer, immunotherapy, drug development, checkpoint inhibition, mismatch repair

1. Introduction

Colorectal cancer (CRC) is the fourth most common cancer and the second leading cause of cancer-related death worldwide. Surgery, chemotherapy, radiation therapy and targeted agents including anti-angiogenic and anti-epidermal growth factor receptor (EGFR) therapies form the backbone of treatment for CRC in various stages. Unfortunately, when diagnosed at advanced stage, CRC is still inevitably fatal. More than 50% of patients diagnosed with CRC eventually develop metastases, and almost 90% of these patients have unresectable disease [1–3]. In some patients with metastatic disease, metastectomy is still possible and can result in a cure in appropriately selected patients [2, 3]. The almost totality of metastatic CRC patients eventually develops resistance to all available standard therapies leading to cancer progression and death [4].

As we will discuss here, immunotherapy and immunomodulatory drugs may represent future therapeutic options to be included in the therapeutic armamentarium in the treatment of CRC. The importance of inflammation in CRC is partially supported by the evidence that patients with inflammatory bowel diseases, i.e., patients with ulcerative colitis and Crohn's disease are at increased risk for developing CRC [5]. It is assumed that chronic inflammation is a significant contributor to cancer development. This is supported by the fact that colon cancer risk increases with longer duration of colitis, greater anatomic extent of colitis, the concomitant presence of other inflammatory manifestations like primary sclerosing cholangitis [6] and the fact that certain drugs used to treat inflammation, such as 5-aminosalicylates and steroids, may prevent the development of CRC in this clinical setting [7]. It may be thus possible that by shaping the immune composition of the CRC microenvironment through novel immunotherapies, this may ultimately lead to a therapeutic effect in CRC.

2. The immune-cell microenvironment in colorectal cancer

An important step in tumour progression is the evasion and suppression of the host immune system [8, 9], as shown in **Figure 1**. In the normal microenvironment, the effector cells, including the natural killer (NK) cells and cytotoxic T lymphocytes (CTLs), are capable of driving potent anti-tumour suppressive activities. Tumour cells are often able to induce an

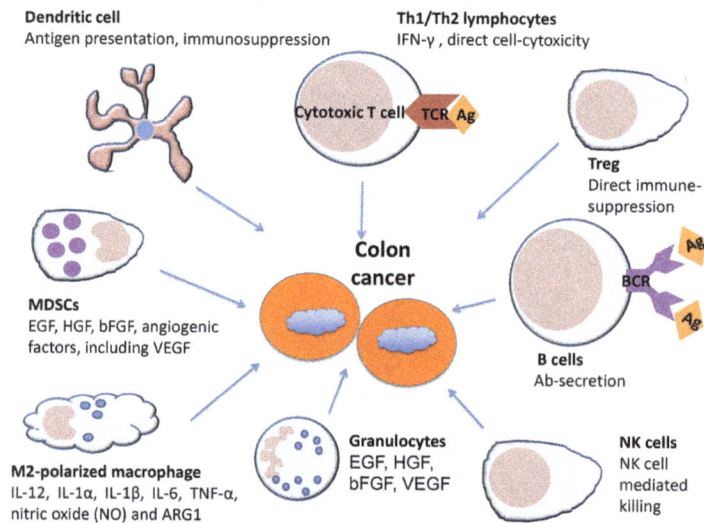

Figure 1. Immune-cell microenvironment in colorectal cancer. The evasion and suppression of the host immune system is an important step of colorectal cancer (CRC) progression. In physiologic conditions, effector cells, including the natural killer (NK) cells and cytotoxic T lymphocytes (CTLs), exert tumour surveillance and tumour suppressive activities. Tumour cells are able to induce an immunosuppressive microenvironment that protects them from the host immune system through the expansion of regulatory immune cells (i.e., myeloid-derived suppressor cells (MDSCs) and regulatory T cells (Tregs)) and alternative activation of other immune cells, including macrophages, granulocytes and dendritic cells.

immunosuppressive microenvironment that protects them from the host immune system. Overall, tumour cells are able to shape the host microenvironment, which is rich of immune cell populations, in a suitable way for them to survive to the host immune system recognition [10, 11]. The two major immunosuppressive mechanisms in cancer are (1) expansion of regulatory immune cells (i.e., myeloid-derived suppressor cells (MDSCs) and regulatory T cells (Tregs)) and (2) activation of the inhibitory T-cell pathways—programmed cell death-1/ programmed cell death-ligand 1 pathways (PD-1/PD-L1 pathways).

3. Myeloid-derived suppressor cells

Myeloid-derived suppressor cells are a heterogeneous and immature subset of circulating cells of myeloid derivation that can differentiate into, macrophages, granulocytes or dendritic cells (DCs) under physiologic conditions. However, under pathological conditions such as cancer or inflammation, the differentiation of these immature myeloid cells is inhibited resulting in accumulation of MDSCs in the tumour microenvironment or in the sites of inflammation [12]. For example, in cancer patients and tumour models, MDSCs accumulate in the tumour microenvironment because of the release of soluble factors by tumour cells or by other cells of the microenvironment, i.e., granulocyte macrophage colony stimulating factor (GM-CSF), interleukin-1 β and stromal-derived growth factor 1-α [13, 14]. MDSCs can then suppress T-cell proliferation through expression of several immune suppressive factors, including arginase, reactive oxygen species (ROS) and nitric oxide (NO). MDSCs can also promote the development of Treg cells *in vivo*, which are anergic and immune-suppressive [15]. Several studies have consistently shown that cancer patients with higher MDSC levels have shorter survival compared to patients with lower MDSC levels [16, 17]. Moreover, depletion of MDSCs in tumour-bearing mice using anti Gr-1 antibody [18, 19] or MDSC-targeting specific peptides have shown anti-tumour activities [20] suggesting that MDSCs can be a good target for future anti-tumour treatments. Two main subsets of MDSCs have been described, namely, granulo-cytic MDSC (G-MDSC) or polymorphonuclear (PMN)-MDSCs and monocytic MDSC (Mo-MDSC). G-MDSCs have granulocyte-like morphology characterised by increased levels of ROS and low levels of NO, whereas Mo-MDSCs have monocyte-like morphology with increased level of NO, but low levels of ROS. Human G-MDSCs and Mo-MDSCs are classically defined as $CD11b^+ CD33^+ HLA-DR^{-/low}CD14^-$ and $CD11b^+ CD33^+ HLA-DR^{-/low} CD14^+$, respectively. In tumour-bearing mice, G-MDSCs are the major MDSC subset that expands in the peripheral lymphoid organs after tumour engraftment pointing to a different biology of these cells in human and mice [21].

MDSCs promote metastasis development and primary tumour growth both in CRC patients and CRC murine models [22]. Importantly, MDSCs have also been implicated in the resistance to anti-angiogenic therapies used for the treatment CRC [23] via their ability to stimulate the expression of genes, whose products promote leukocyte recruitment, alternative angiogenic mechanisms, tumour migration, wound healing and formation of premetastatic niches in distal metastatic organs [23].

4. Regulatory T cells (Tregs)

Treg cells are a subset of CD4$^+$ T lymphocytes characterised by the expression of Forkhead Box P3 (FOXP3) transcription factor [24]. Tregs are able to suppress the function of antigen presenting cells (APCs), i.e., dendritic cells, and effector T cells by direct contact or by release of anti-inflammatory cytokines (IL-10 and TGF-β). Tregs are major players in the development of tumour immunosuppressive microenvironment; these cells accumulate both in the tumour microenvironment and the peripheral blood of patients with cancer [25, 26]. The increased frequency of Tregs both in the peripheral blood and especially in the sites of tumour growth has generally been considered a marker of poor prognosis due to Treg-mediated suppression of anti-tumour immunity [27, 28]. In transgenic mouse models, it has been shown in mice that Treg depletion induces regression of solid tumours and lymphomas, following increased intratumoural accumulation of activated CD8$^+$ cytotoxic T cells [29–31]. These data indicate that targeting Tregs can represent a potential anti-tumour strategy; however, the development of autoimmune diseases following administration of Treg cells has been described in these preclinical studies and may represent a limitation in the pursue of novel anti-Treg treatments in patients. In CRC, several studies have shown that Treg density in tumour specimens represents an independent negative prognostic factor [32–34]. Low-dose cyclophosphamide has been shown to reduce the numbers and function of Tregs and to induce anti-tumour, immune-mediated effects [35, 36]; this has been shown to be true in preclinical models of CRC [37], but no studies have been carried out in CRC patients so far.

5. Dendritic cells

Dendritic cells are cells of bone marrow origin defined as professional antigen presenting cells, which have the ability to present self and non-self antigens to T cells, thus promoting immunity or immune-tolerance [38]. Antigen presentation by DCs is able to induce naive T cells differentiation into effector and memory T cells; however, it can also lead to different forms of T-cell tolerance, depending on the local microenvironment stimuli and the functional status of the DCs. Myeloid-DCs (mDCs) and plasmacytoid-DCs (pDCs) are two major DC subsets that have been identified based on their origin, immune-phenotype and functional status [39]. In human, mDCs are usually defined as Lin$^-$HLADR$^+$CD11c$^+$CD123^{dim} cells, whereas pDCs are Lin$^-$CD11c$^-$CD4$^+$CD45RA$^+$CD123$^+$ILT3$^+$. Several studies have documented accumulation of DCs in tumour sites, which often correlated with poor prognosis [40–42]. The loss of tumour-derived antigen presentation ability by tumour-infiltrating DCs has been shown to be the consequence of the suppressive effects of the tumour microenvironment mediated by various cytokines [43]. For example, it has been demonstrated that tumour-infiltrating pDCs from solid tumours express high levels of inducible T-cell co-stimulator ligand (ICOS-L), which explains their ability to induce Tregs proliferation [44, 45], thus leading to local immunosuppression. Moreover, TGF-β secreted by DCs from breast cancer patients is able to induce Treg-cell proliferation and accumulation, thus leading to tumour growth [46]. The role of DCs in CRC has been controversial mostly due to the technical difficulties associated with their quantification and identification. For these reasons, it is difficult to draw a conclusion about the role of DCs and performance of DCs as a predictor of outcome for CRC [47, 48].

6. Natural killer cells

NK cells represent a heterogeneous lymphocyte population with direct-cytotoxic anti-tumour capacity and multiple immunoregulatory properties. Natural killer group 2D (NKG2D) is one of the NK cell activating receptors that recognises various proteins expressed on the surface of target cells in response to several forms of cellular stress. One of the ligand of NKG2D is the MHC class I polypeptide-related sequence A (MICA); target tumour cells that express MICA are efficiently killed via NKG2D despite the expression of MHC class I molecules, describing a pathway of anti-tumour activity mediated by NK cells [49]. Several preclinical studies have shown the susceptibility of CRC cells to the NK cell–mediated killing [50–52], which can be enhanced by the contemporary treatment with anti-CRC drugs like anti-EGFR inhibitors [53].

Interestingly Gharagozloo et al. [54] have recently shown that metastatic CRC patients present a significant reduction in the percentage of circulating NKG2D+NK cells as well as NKG2D mRNA expression in peripheral blood as compared to healthy controls, suggesting a specific defect of NK cell–mediated natural immunity in CRC patients.

7. Macrophage in colorectal cancer

Cells of the monocyte–macrophage lineage are one of the major components of the leukocyte infiltration in tumours; there is strong evidence that these cells promote inflammatory circuits that ultimately lead to tumour progression, tumour cell invasion and metastasis [55].

Macrophages recruited to the tumour-associated microenvironment may exist both in a classically activated inflammatory phenotypes (M1) with anti-tumour capacity or an alternatively activated, immunosuppressive (M2) phenotype with tumour supporting ability [56]; M1-polarised macrophage secretes a large amount of IL-12, IL-1α, IL-1β, IL-6, TNF-α, nitric oxide (NO) and ARG1, and stimulate secretion of IFN-γ by Th1 lymphocytes, thus activating Th1 immune response which in turn stimulate the tumour specific-CTL cytotoxicity. However, during tumour progression, macrophages shift towards a M2-polarised phenotype induced by the exposure of these cells to IL-4, IL-13, M-CSF/CSF-1, IL-10 and TGF-β1, among other factors present in the tumour microenvironment. In this state, macrophages are defined as tumour-associated macrophages (TAMs) and are able to support tumour growth, survival and metastasis. TAMs mostly derived by circulating monocyte which are recruited to the tumour bed by the secretion from tumour cells and the other cells of the tumour microenvironment of inflammatory cytokines such as M-CSF/CSF-1, SDF-1/CCL12 and MCP-1/CCL2. M2 macrophages then are able to secrete large amount of growth factors, such as EGF, HGF, bFGF, inflammatory factors (such as COX2) and angiogenic factors, including VEGF and angiogenic chemokines, which in turn all together promote progression of tumours (reviewed in [55, 57]).

In general, higher densities of TAMs in tumours and overexpression of key stimulators of M2 differentiation are considered markers of poor prognosis in a number of cancers [55, 57]. TAMs are associated with tumour progression and poor survival in CRC patients [58, 59], in line with *in vitro* and *in vivo* studies showing that macrophages are able to promote survival and induce proliferation of CRC cells via activation of Wnt pathway in CRC cells [60–62]. However, some other studies have shown that macrophages actually exert a tumour-suppressive activity in CRC via direct inhibition of tumour cell proliferation and via production of chemokines that attract T cells, stimulate proliferation of allogeneic T cells and activate type-1 T cells associated with anti-tumour immune responses [63]. In CRC, the role of macrophages may be ultimately context and stage dependent with implications for the design of future therapies aiming to target these cells.

8. Immune therapy in CRC

Given the complexity of the immune microenviroment and immune-cell composition of CRC, targeting this type of cancer via novel immunotherapies has been proved challenging. However, as described in the following paragraphs, recent advanced in the immunotherapy drug-development together with a better understanding of the genetic basis of immune stimulation have finally lead to the proof of concept demonstration that immunotherapy may represent an important therapeutic tool in the treatment of CRC.

9. Immune-cytokine therapy in CRC

Non-specific immunotherapy utilising cytokines such as interferon (IFN), interleukins and granulocyte macrophage colony-stimulating factor (GM-CSF) have been studied because of the potential ability to modulate and promote host immunity against tumour antigens. A Phase II trial of 29 patients with metastatic CRC using gemcitabine, oxaliplatin and 5-fluorouracil (GOLF) in combination with IL-2 and GM-CSF immune adjuvant regimen (GOLFIG) yielded promising results, with an overall response rate of 56.5%, disease control rate of 96% and median time to progression of 12.5 months [64]. A Phase III study comparing the GOLFIG regimen against the control arm of FOLFOX-4 in first line treatment of metastatic CRC was terminated early due to poor recruitment into the control arm. However, the experimental arm did show superiority in Progression Free Survival and Overall Response Rate with a trend towards improvement of overall survival; this trial does provide proof-of-concept that GOLFIG chemoimmunotherapy may represent a novel reliable option for first-line treatment of metastatic CRC [65].

10. Vaccines as therapeutic tools in CRC

Vaccine-based therapy can be delivered as whole-tumour-cell vaccines, peptide vaccines, viral vector vaccines or dendritic call vaccines, each with its inherent advantages and disadvantages (reviewed in [66, 67]). Overall in the treatment of CRC, there have been only small Phase I and Phase II studies with suggestions that vaccines may have a role in the adjuvant setting, and limited efficacy in metastatic disease. [68].

11. Rationale of checkpoint receptor pathway as a target in colorectal cancer

Immune checkpoints refer to a very complex and articulated series of inhibitory pathways that intricate into the immune system and that are crucial for regulating self-tolerance and modulating the duration and extent of physiological immune responses in peripheral tissues in order to avoid excessive immune-activation and subsequent collateral tissue damage (**Figure 2**) [69]. It is now well established that tumour cells can co-opt certain immune-checkpoint pathways; this represents a novel and important mechanism of immune resistance, particularly against T cells that are specific for tumour antigens. Consequently, the blockade of immune checkpoints is able to unleash T-cell–mediated anti-tumour immune response in a potent and sometime curative way [69].

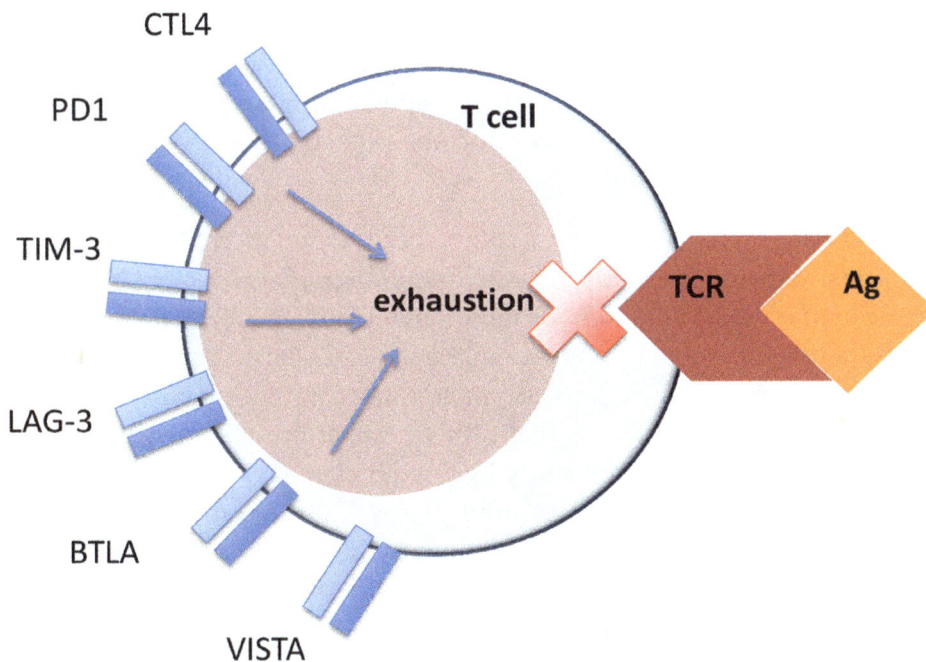

Figure 2. **Immune checkpoint and immunosuppression in CRC.** Immune checkpoints activate inhibitory pathways in T cell that ultimately lead to T-cell–mediated immunity suppression. Tumour cells can co-opt these immune-checkpoint pathways thus leading to T-cell exhaustion and tumour immunotolerance.CTLA4: cytotoxic T-lymphocyte-associated antigen 4; PD1: programmed cell death protein 1; TIM3: T-cell membrane protein 3; LAG3: lymphocyte activation gene 3; BTLA: B- and T-lymphocyte attenuator; VISTA: V-domain Ig suppressor of T-cell activation.

The two immune-checkpoint receptors that have been most studied in the context of clinical cancer immunotherapy, cytotoxic T-lymphocyte-associated antigen 4 (CTLA4; also known as CD152) and programmed cell death protein 1 (PD1; also known as CD279) are both inhibitory receptors and have both shown to be appropriate targets (**Figure 2**). Importantly, several other checkpoint immune pathways have recently emerged to be additional targets for the development of new immunotherapy drugs mostly in preclinical studies (**Figure 2**); these include lymphocyte activation gene 3 (LAG3; also known as CD223), 2B4 (also known as CD244), B- and T-lymphocyte attenuator (BTLA; also known as CD272), T-cell membrane protein 3 (TIM3; also known as HAVcr2), adenosine A2a receptor (A2aR) to name a few [70].

Programmed cell death 1 is a Type I transmembrane protein, which belongs to the CD28 family [71]. PD-1 is expressed on activated and exhausted T and B cells and has two ligands PD-L1 and PD-L2. Importantly, PD-L1 is not expressed on normal epithelial tissues, but can aberrantly be expressed on a variety of solid tumours [72]. On the other hand, PD-L2 is more broadly expressed on normal healthy tissues. Binding of PD-L1 to PD-1 reduces cytokine production and activation of the target T cells, leading to an immunosuppressive microenvironment.

Clinical trials targeting PD-1/PD-L1 pathway to overcome tumour-associated immune suppression have shown promising results for a variety of solid tumours. Checkpoint inhibitor immunotherapy is currently FDA-approved for the treatment of melanoma, kidney cancer and NSCLC. However, it has been shown active in many other types of solid, including gastric, ovarian cancer, and bladder cancer, and hematologic cancers, particularly Hodgkin lymphoma [73–76]. It is currently unclear what determines response to this type of treatment and this is an area of active research giving the costs and the potential toxicity associated with these treatments.

The accumulation of somatic mutations accompanies the initiation and progression of most cancers conferring to the tumour cells unrestricted proliferative capacity [77]. The analysis of cancer genomes has revealed that tumour mutational landscapes [78] are extremely variable among patients, among different tumours from the same patient and even among the different regions of a single tumour. Two separate papers have recently shown that response to checkpoint inhibitors, i.e., anti-CTL4 and anti-PDL1 Ab, critically depend on the mutational load of the specific tumours. The first study by Snyder et al. [79] found that mutational load associates with exceptional response to the anti-CTLA-4 Ab ipilimumab in melanoma patients. Using genome-wide somatic neoepitope analysis and patient-specific HLA-typing, they identified candidate tumour neoantigens for each patient predicted to be able to activate a T-cell response in anti-CTLA-4 treated patients.

Interestingly, the probability for a tumour to carry such neoantigens was dependent on the mutational load of the specific tumour, as it was the probability to respond to anti-CTLA-4 Ab. Similar results were obtained in NSCLC patients treated with pembrolizumab, an antibody-targeting PD-1 [80]. A higher non-synonymous mutation burden in tumours was associated with improved objective response, durable clinical benefit and progression-free survival. Therapeutic benefit in these patients correlated with the molecular smoking signature, higher neoantigen burden and DNA repair pathway mutations. All these factors were associated with increased mutation burden [80].

Both studies suggest for the first time a genomic-based mechanism to the response to novel immunotherapy drugs that can potentially help with designing rational combination treatments, i.e., DNA-damaging agents plus immune-checkpoint inhibitors.

12. PD1/PDL1—immune-checkpoint inhibitors

In unselected colon cancer, the response to immune-checkpoint inhibitors has shown limited efficacy [73]. In tumours that have shown response, predictive markers to checkpoint inhibition are being evaluated—with microsatellite insufficiency (MSI) or mismatch-repair (MMR) status being the most promising thus far [81].

Pembrolizumab (MK-3475)—a highly selective humanised IgG4 monoclonal antibody that blocks the interaction of PD-1 with its ligands PD-L1 and PD-L2—has undergone extensive testing in multiple tumour types. In the KEYNOTE-028 study—a multicohort, Phase Ib trial of pembrolizumab for programmed death-ligand 1 (PD-L1) positive advanced solid tumours; there were 156 screened patients with advanced colorectal cancer, with 33 (21%) of these being PD-L1 positive and 23 went on to receive treatment. Although the safety profile was acceptable with only one patient experiencing a grade ≥3 treatment-related adverse events with elevated bilirubin; it was felt there was overall minimal anti-tumour activity. One patient who had microsatellite instability high disease experienced a partial response, with four patients (17%) having the best response of stable disease, and progressive disease in 16 patients (70%) [82].

The initial Phase I study of anti-PD-1 antibody nivolumab included 17 colorectal patients, who were heavily pre-treated; the majority of these patients had PD-L1 negative tumours and thus overall, this study showed limited clinical efficacy [83]. However, one patient with colorectal cancer treated with five doses in this study experienced a complete response at 6 months, which was ongoing after 3 years; it was noted that the patient's tumour was MSI-high, and evidence of PD-L1 expression by infiltrating macrophages and lymphocytes [84].

Based on the previous reports associating mutational load to response to checkpoint inhibitors, Le et al. hypothesised that mismatch repair–deficient tumours and mismatch repair (MMR)–deficient tumours are more responsive to PD-1 blockade than are MMR-proficient tumours. A Phase II study of 41 patients evaluating the clinical activity of pembrolizumab in metastatic carcinoma with or without MMR-deficiency showed hazard ratios for disease progression or death (0.10; 95% CI, 0.03–0.37; $P < 0.001$) and for death (0.22; 95% CI, 0.05–1.00; $P = 0.05$) that favoured patients with mismatch repair-deficient colorectal cancer [85]. Thus, ongoing studies are exploring this particular subset.

The KEYNOTE-164 study (NCT02460198) is a Phase II study currently recruiting patients with previously treated locally advanced unresectable or metastatic mismatched repair-deficient or MSI-high colorectal carcinoma to assess efficacy of pembrolizumab monotherapy [85]. In the same patient population of MSI-high colorectal cancers, the Phase III KEYNOTE-177 (NCT02563002) study will compare pembrolizumab monotherapy against standard of care chemotherapy in first line treatment of advanced CRC [86].

Regarding anti-PD-L1 compounds, atezolizumab (MPDL3280A) has shown activity in Phase I studies—with one of four patients with colorectal cancer having a durable partial response [87]. In the Phase Ib study of atezolizumab in combination with bevacizumab in refractory metastatic CRC, and that of atezolizumab and bevacizumab with FOLFOX in the oxaliplatin naïve population, this confirmed acceptable safety and clinical activity—unconfirmed ORR 8% (1/13) and 44% (8/18) in the two arms respectively [88]. However, the Phase I study of BMS936559, which included 18 colorectal patients showed no response in this tumour type [89]. There are ongoing studies with other anti-PD-L1 compounds including durvalumab/ MEDI4736 (NCT01693562) and avelumab (NCT01772004).

13. Anti-CTLA4 Therapy

Tremilimumab, a fully human immunoglobulin (Ig) G2 monoclonal antibody that blocks inhibitory signalling from CTLA4 was studied as monotherapy treatment in a Phase II single arm study, of 47 patients with refractory metastatic CRC. Tremelimumab was intended to be administered every 90 days. Clinical activity was unable to be demonstrated, with 43 of 45 evaluable patients unable to receive a second dose—with a median duration on study of 2.3 months [90]. However, a Phase I combination study of tremelimumab with durvalumab (NCT01975831) is ongoing; and ipilimumab is also being studied in combination with nivolumab (NCT02060188).

14. Other immune-checkpoint inhibitors

In MSI-high colon cancers, it has been shown that up-regulation of PD-1, PD-L1, CTLA-4, LAG-3 and IDO immune checkpoints enables evasion from Th1 response [91]. As described, PD-L1, PD-1, CTLA-4 have been and are being investigated in the treatment of CRC. Anti-LAG-3 monoclonal antibodies (BMS-986016), alone and in combination with nivolumab are also being evaluated (NCT01968109).

15. Other combined immunotherapy strategies

As there has been limited efficacy from current immunotherapy strategies, it has been proposed that combination of immunotherapy with conventional chemotherapy, radiotherapy and targeted agents should be trialled [92]. The use of DNA damaging agents may increase the mutation burden, thus increase the efficacy of checkpoint inhibition.

16. Conclusion

Advanced CRC remains inevitably lethal despite optimal management, thus novel therapeutic approaches are urgently needed. Immunotherapy, particularly novel immune-checkpoint inhibitors, is transforming the therapeutic landscape of many types of cancer. Although in CRC the clinical data have been disappointing so far, this is probably due to the lack of knowledge of biomarkers/clinical features that can allow us the optimal selection of patients likely to respond to the specific immunotherapies. This has been proved by the identification of MMR status as a specific marker of response to anti-PD1/PDL1 treatment in CRC. In the future, a deeper understanding of immunobiology of CRC together with the development of novel immunotherapeutic agents will surely lead to new successful treatments for advanced CRC patients. This will be followed by further studies of combination of novel immunotherapies together with the present standard of care, i.e., surgery, chemotherapy and target therapies that will additionally improve the prognosis of advanced metastatic CRC.

Author details

Gabriel Mak[1], Michele Moschetta[1] and Hendrik-Tobias Arkenau[1,2*]

*Address all correspondence to: Tobias.Arkenau@hcahealthcare.co.uk

1 Sarah Cannon Research Institute, London, UK

2 University College London, London, UK

References

[1] Lee WS, Yun SH, Chun HK, Lee WY, Yun HR, Kim J, et al. Pulmonary resection for metastases from colorectal cancer: prognostic factors and survival. Int J Colorectal Dis. 2007;22(6):699–704.

[2] Choti MA, Sitzmann JV, Tiburi MF, Sumetchotimetha W, Rangsin R, Schulick RD, et al. Trends in long-term survival following liver resection for hepatic colorectal metastases. Ann Surg. 2002;235(6):759–766.

[3] Kanas GP, Taylor A, Primrose JN, Langeberg WJ, Kelsh MA, Mowat FS, et al. Survival after liver resection in metastatic colorectal cancer: review and meta-analysis of prognostic factors. Clin Epidemiol. 2012;4:283–301.

[4] Bergers G, Hanahan D. Modes of resistance to anti-angiogenic therapy. Nat Rev Cancer. 2008;8(8):592–603.

[5] Itzkowitz SH, Yio X. Inflammation and cancer IV. Colorectal cancer in inflammatory bowel disease: the role of inflammation. Am J Physiol Gastrointest Liver Physiol. 2004;287(1):G7–G17.

[6] Kim ER, Chang DK. Colorectal cancer in inflammatory bowel disease: the risk, pathogenesis, prevention and diagnosis. World J Gastroenterol. 2014;20(29):9872–9881.

[7] Stolfi C, De Simone V, Pallone F, Monteleone G. Mechanisms of action of non-steroidal anti-inflammatory drugs (NSAIDs) and mesalazine in the chemoprevention of colorectal cancer. Int J Mol Sci. 2013;14(9):17972–17985.

[8] Quail DF, Joyce JA. Microenvironmental regulation of tumor progression and metastasis. Nat Med. 2013;19(11):1423–1437.

[9] Swann JB, Smyth MJ. Immune surveillance of tumors. J Clin Invest. 2007;117(5):1137–1146.

[10] Smyth MJ, Ngiow SF, Ribas A, Teng MW. Combination cancer immunotherapies tailored to the tumour microenvironment. Nat Rev Clin Oncol. 2016 Mar;13(3):143–58. doi: 10.1038/nrclinonc.2015.209. Epub 2015 Nov 24.

[11] Kawano Y, Moschetta M, Manier S, Glavey S, Gorgun GT, Roccaro AM, et al. Targeting the bone marrow microenvironment in multiple myeloma. Immunol Rev. 2015;263(1): 160–172.

[12] Gabrilovich DI, Nagaraj S. Myeloid-derived suppressor cells as regulators of the immune system. Nat Rev Immunol. 2009;9(3):162–174.

[13] Almand B, Clark JI, Nikitina E, van Beynen J, English NR, Knight SC, et al. Increased production of immature myeloid cells in cancer patients: a mechanism of immunosuppression in cancer. J Immunol. 2001;166(1):678–689.

[14] Diaz-Montero CM, Salem ML, Nishimura MI, Garrett-Mayer E, Cole DJ, Montero AJ. Increased circulating myeloid-derived suppressor cells correlate with clinical cancer stage, metastatic tumor burden, and doxorubicin-cyclophosphamide chemotherapy. Cancer Immunol Immunother. 2009;58(1):49–59.

[15] Huang B, Pan PY, Li Q, Sato AI, Levy DE, Bromberg J, et al. Gr-1+CD115+ immature myeloid suppressor cells mediate the development of tumor-induced T regulatory cells and T-cell anergy in tumor-bearing host. Cancer Res. 2006;66(2):1123–1131.

[16] Walter S, Weinschenk T, Stenzl A, Zdrojowy R, Pluzanska A, Szczylik C, et al. Multipeptide immune response to cancer vaccine IMA901 after single-dose cyclophosphamide associates with longer patient survival. Nat Med. 2012;18(8):1254–1261.

[17] Solito S, Falisi E, Diaz-Montero CM, Doni A, Pinton L, Rosato A, et al. A human promyelocytic-like population is responsible for the immune suppression mediated by myeloid-derived suppressor cells. Blood. 2011;118(8):2254–2265.

[18] Serafini P, Meckel K, Kelso M, Noonan K, Califano J, Koch W, et al. Phosphodiesterase-5 inhibition augments endogenous antitumor immunity by reducing myeloid-derived suppressor cell function. J Exp Med. 2006;203(12):2691–2702.

[19] Li H, Han Y, Guo Q, Zhang M, Cao X. Cancer-expanded myeloid-derived suppressor cells induce anergy of NK cells through membrane-bound TGF-beta 1. J Immunol. 2009;182(1):240–249.

[20] Qin H, Lerman B, Sakamaki I, Wei G, Cha SC, Rao SS, et al. Generation of a new therapeutic peptide that depletes myeloid-derived suppressor cells in tumor-bearing mice. Nat Med. 2014;20(6):676–681.

[21] Youn JI, Nagaraj S, Collazo M, Gabrilovich DI. Subsets of myeloid-derived suppressor cells in tumor-bearing mice. J Immunol. 2008;181(8):5791–5802.

[22] Inamoto S, Itatani Y, Yamamoto T, Minamiguchi S, Hirai H, Iwamoto M, et al. Loss of SMAD4 promotes colorectal cancer progression by accumulation of myeloid-derived suppressor cells through the CCL15-CCR1 chemokine axis. Clin Cancer Res. 2016;22(2): 492–501.

[23] Ichikawa M, Williams R, Wang L, Vogl T, Srikrishna G. S100A8/A9 activate key genes and pathways in colon tumor progression. Mol Cancer Res. 2011;9(2):133–148.

[24] Fontenot JD, Gavin MA, Rudensky AY. Foxp3 programs the development and function of CD4+CD25+ regulatory T cells. Nat Immunol. 2003;4(4):330–336.

[25] Nishikawa H, Sakaguchi S. Regulatory T cells in tumor immunity. Int J Cancer. 2010;127(4):759–767.

[26] Mougiakakos D, Choudhury A, Lladser A, Kiessling R, Johansson CC. Regulatory T cells in cancer. Adv Cancer Res. 2010;107:57–117.

[27] Curiel TJ, Coukos G, Zou L, Alvarez X, Cheng P, Mottram P, et al. Specific recruitment of regulatory T cells in ovarian carcinoma fosters immune privilege and predicts reduced survival. Nat Med. 2004;10(9):942–949.

[28] Bates GJ, Fox SB, Han C, Leek RD, Garcia JF, Harris AL, et al. Quantification of regulatory T cells enables the identification of high-risk breast cancer patients and those at risk of late relapse. J Clin Oncol. 2006;24(34):5373–5880.

[29] Lahl K, Loddenkemper C, Drouin C, Freyer J, Arnason J, Eberl G, et al. Selective depletion of Foxp3+ regulatory T cells induces a scurfy-like disease. J Exp Med. 2007;204(1):57–63.

[30] Klages K, Mayer CT, Lahl K, Loddenkemper C, Teng MW, Ngiow SF, et al. Selective depletion of Foxp3+ regulatory T cells improves effective therapeutic vaccination against established melanoma. Cancer Res. 2010;70(20):7788–7799.

[31] Teng MW, Ngiow SF, von Scheidt B, McLaughlin N, Sparwasser T, Smyth MJ. Conditional regulatory T-cell depletion releases adaptive immunity preventing carcinogenesis and suppressing established tumor growth. Cancer Res. 2010;70(20):7800–7809.

[32] Vlad C, Kubelac P, Fetica B, Vlad D, Irimie A, Achimas-Cadariu P. The prognostic value of FOXP3+ T regulatory cells in colorectal cancer. J BUON. 2015;20(1):114–119.

[33] Wang Q, Feng M, Yu T, Liu X, Zhang P. Intratumoral regulatory T cells are associated with suppression of colorectal carcinoma metastasis after resection through overcoming IL-17 producing T cells. Cell Immunol. 2014;287(2):100–105.

[34] Lin YC, Mahalingam J, Chiang JM, Su PJ, Chu YY, Lai HY, et al. Activated but not resting regulatory T cells accumulated in tumor microenvironment and correlated with tumor progression in patients with colorectal cancer. Int J Cancer. 2013;132(6):1341–1350.

[35] Lutsiak ME, Semnani RT, De Pascalis R, Kashmiri SV, Schlom J, Sabzevari H. Inhibition of CD4(+)25+ T regulatory cell function implicated in enhanced immune response by low-dose cyclophosphamide. Blood. 2005;105(7):2862–2868.

[36] Ghiringhelli F, Larmonier N, Schmitt E, Parcellier A, Cathelin D, Garrido C, et al. CD4+CD25+ regulatory T cells suppress tumor immunity but are sensitive to cyclophosphamide which allows immunotherapy of established tumors to be curative. Eur J Immunol. 2004;34(2):336–344.

[37] Son CH, Bae JH, Shin DY, Lee HR, Jo WS, Yang K, et al. Combination effect of regulatory T-cell depletion and ionizing radiation in mouse models of lung and colon cancer. Int J Radiat Oncol Biol Phys. 2015;92(2):390–398.

[38] Banchereau J, Steinman RM. Dendritic cells and the control of immunity. Nature. 1998;392(6673):245–252.

[39] O'Doherty U, Peng M, Gezelter S, Swiggard WJ, Betjes M, Bhardwaj N, et al. Human blood contains two subsets of dendritic cells, one immunologically mature and the other immature. Immunology. 1994;82(3):487–493.

[40] Bell D, Chomarat P, Broyles D, Netto G, Harb GM, Lebecque S, et al. In breast carcinoma tissue, immature dendritic cells reside within the tumor, whereas mature dendritic cells are located in peritumoral areas. J Exp Med. 1999;190(10):1417–1426.

[41] Treilleux I, Blay JY, Bendriss-Vermare N, Ray-Coquard I, Bachelot T, Guastalla JP, et al. Dendritic cell infiltration and prognosis of early stage breast cancer. Clin Cancer Res. 2004;10(22):7466–7474.

[42] Sandel MH, Dadabayev AR, Menon AG, Morreau H, Melief CJ, Offringa R, et al. Prognostic value of tumor-infiltrating dendritic cells in colorectal cancer: role of maturation status and intratumoral localization. Clin Cancer Res. 2005;11(7):2576–2582.

[43] Zou W. Immunosuppressive networks in the tumour environment and their therapeutic relevance. Nat Rev Cancer. 2005;5(4):263–274.

[44] Conrad C, Gregorio J, Wang YH, Ito T, Meller S, Hanabuchi S, et al. Plasmacytoid dendritic cells promote immunosuppression in ovarian cancer via ICOS costimulation of Foxp3(+) T-regulatory cells. Cancer Res. 2012;72(20):5240–5249.

[45] Faget J, Bendriss-Vermare N, Gobert M, Durand I, Olive D, Biota C, et al. ICOS-ligand expression on plasmacytoid dendritic cells supports breast cancer progression by

promoting the accumulation of immunosuppressive CD4+ T cells. Cancer Res. 2012;72(23):6130–6141.

[46] Ramos RN, Chin LS, Dos Santos AP, Bergami-Santos PC, Laginha F, Barbuto JA. Monocyte-derived dendritic cells from breast cancer patients are biased to induce CD4+CD25+Foxp3+ regulatory T cells. J Leukoc Biol. 2012;92(3):673–682.

[47] Malietzis G, Lee GH, Jenkins JT, Bernardo D, Moorghen M, Knight SC, et al. Prognostic value of the tumour-infiltrating dendritic cells in colorectal cancer: a systematic review. Cell Commun Adhes. 2015;22(1):9–14.

[48] Legitimo A, Consolini R, Failli A, Orsini G, Spisni R. Dendritic cell defects in the colorectal cancer. Hum Vaccin Immunother. 2014;10(11):3224–3235.

[49] Groh V, Rhinehart R, Secrist H, Bauer S, Grabstein KH, Spies T. Broad tumor-associated expression and recognition by tumor-derived gamma delta T cells of MICA and MICB. Proc Natl Acad Sci USA. 1999;96(12):6879–6884.

[50] Kim GR, Ha GH, Bae JH, Oh SO, Kim SH, Kang CD. Metastatic colon cancer cell populations contain more cancer stem-like cells with a higher susceptibility to natural killer cell-mediated lysis compared with primary colon cancer cells. Oncol Lett. 2015;9(4):1641–1646.

[51] Taglia L, Matusiak D, Benya RV. GRP-induced up-regulation of Hsp72 promotes CD16+/94+ natural killer cell binding to colon cancer cells causing tumor cell cytolysis. Clin Exp Metastasis. 2008;25(4):451–463.

[52] Helms RA, Bull DM. Natural killer activity of human lymphocytes against colon cancer cells. Gastroenterology. 1980;78(4):738–744.

[53] Bae JH, Kim SJ, Kim MJ, Oh SO, Chung JS, Kim SH, et al. Susceptibility to natural killer cell-mediated lysis of colon cancer cells is enhanced by treatment with epidermal growth factor receptor inhibitors through UL16-binding protein-1 induction. Cancer Sci. 2012;103(1):7–16.

[54] Gharagozloo M, Kalantari H, Rezaei A, Maracy MR, Salehi M, Bahador A, et al. The decrease in NKG2D+ natural killer cells in peripheral blood of patients with metastatic colorectal cancer. Bratisl Lek Listy. 2015;116(5):296–301.

[55] Cook J, Hagemann T. Tumour-associated macrophages and cancer. Curr Opin Pharmacol. 2013;13(4):595–601.

[56] Sica A, Schioppa T, Mantovani A, Allavena P. Tumour-associated macrophages are a distinct M2 polarised population promoting tumour progression: potential targets of anti-cancer therapy. Eur J Cancer. 2006;42(6):717–727.

[57] Pollard JW. Tumour-educated macrophages promote tumour progression and metastasis. Nat Rev Cancer. 2004;4(1):71–78.

[58] Nagorsen D, Voigt S, Berg E, Stein H, Thiel E, Loddenkemper C. Tumor-infiltrating macrophages and dendritic cells in human colorectal cancer: relation to local regulatory

T cells, systemic T-cell response against tumor-associated antigens and survival. J Transl Med. 2007;5:62.

[59] Ohnishi K, Komohara Y, Saito Y, Miyamoto Y, Watanabe M, Baba H, et al. CD169-positive macrophages in regional lymph nodes are associated with a favorable prognosis in patients with colorectal carcinoma. Cancer Sci. 2013;104(9):1237–1244.

[60] Kaler P, Galea V, Augenlicht L, Klampfer L. Tumor associated macrophages protect colon cancer cells from TRAIL-induced apoptosis through IL-1beta-dependent stabilization of Snail in tumor cells. PLoS One. 2010;5(7):e11700.

[61] Kaler P, Augenlicht L, Klampfer L. Macrophage-derived IL-1beta stimulates Wnt signaling and growth of colon cancer cells: a crosstalk interrupted by vitamin D3. Oncogene. 2009;28(44):3892–902.

[62] Kaler P, Godasi BN, Augenlicht L, Klampfer L. The NF-kappaB/AKT-dependent induction of Wnt signaling in colon cancer cells by macrophages and IL-1beta. Cancer Microenviron. 2009;2(1):69–80.

[63] Ong SM, Tan YC, Beretta O, Jiang D, Yeap WH, Tai JJ, et al. Macrophages in human colorectal cancer are pro-inflammatory and prime T cells towards an anti-tumour type-1 inflammatory response. Eur J Immunol. 2012;42(1):89–100.

[64] Correale P, Cusi MG, Tsang KY, Del Vecchio MT, Marsili S, Placa ML, et al. Chemo-immunotherapy of metastatic colorectal carcinoma with gemcitabine plus FOLFOX 4 followed by subcutaneous granulocyte macrophage colony-stimulating factor and interleukin-2 induces strong immunologic and antitumor activity in metastatic colon cancer patients. J Clin Oncol. 2005;23(35):8950–8958.

[65] Correale P, Botta C, Rotundo MS, Guglielmo A, Conca R, Licchetta A, et al. Gemcitabine, oxaliplatin, levofolinate, 5-fluorouracil, granulocyte-macrophage colony-stimulating factor, and interleukin-2 (GOLFIG) versus FOLFOX chemotherapy in metastatic colorectal cancer patients: the GOLFIG-2 multicentric open-label randomized phase III trial. J Immunother. 2014;37(1):26–35.

[66] Halama N, Zoernig I, Jaeger D. Advanced malignant melanoma: immunologic and multimodal therapeutic strategies. J Oncol. 2010;2010:8.

[67] Singh PP, Sharma PK, Krishnan G, Lockhart AC. Immune checkpoints and immunotherapy for colorectal cancer. Gastroenterol Rep. 2015;3(4):289–297.

[68] Nagorsen D, Thiel E. Clinical and immunologic responses to active specific cancer vaccines in human colorectal cancer. Clin Cancer Res. 2006;12(10):3064–3069.

[69] Pardoll DM. The blockade of immune checkpoints in cancer immunotherapy. Nat Rev Cancer. 2012;12(4):252–264.

[70] Dong ZY, Wu SP, Liao RQ, Huang SM, Wu YL. Potential biomarker for checkpoint blockade immunotherapy and treatment strategy. Tumour Biol. 2016 Apr;37(4):4251–61. doi: 10.1007/s13277-016-4812-9. Epub 2016 Jan 16.

[71] Ishida Y, Agata Y, Shibahara K, Honjo T. Induced expression of PD-1, a novel member of the immunoglobulin gene superfamily, upon programmed cell death. EMBO J. 1992;11(11):3887–3895.

[72] Dong H, Strome SE, Salomao DR, Tamura H, Hirano F, Flies DB, et al. Tumor-associated B7-H1 promotes T-cell apoptosis: a potential mechanism of immune evasion. Nat Med. 2002;8(8):793–800.

[73] Topalian SL, Hodi FS, Brahmer JR, Gettinger SN, Smith DC, McDermott DF, et al. Safety, activity, and immune correlates of anti-PD-1 antibody in cancer. N Engl J Med. 2012;366(26):2443–2454.

[74] Brahmer JR, Tykodi SS, Chow LQ, Hwu WJ, Topalian SL, Hwu P, et al. Safety and activity of anti-PD-L1 antibody in patients with advanced cancer. N Engl J Med. 2012;366(26):2455–2465.

[75] Powles T, Eder JP, Fine GD, Braiteh FS, Loriot Y, Cruz C, et al. MPDL3280A (anti-PD-L1) treatment leads to clinical activity in metastatic bladder cancer. Nature. 2014;515(7528):558–562.

[76] Ansell SM, Lesokhin AM, Borrello I, Halwani A, Scott EC, Gutierrez M, et al. PD-1 blockade with nivolumab in relapsed or refractory Hodgkin's lymphoma. N Engl J Med. 2015;372(4):311–319.

[77] Hanahan D, Weinberg RA. Hallmarks of cancer: the next generation. Cell. 2011;144(5): 646–674.

[78] Kandoth C, McLellan MD, Vandin F, Ye K, Niu B, Lu C, et al. Mutational landscape and significance across 12 major cancer types. Nature. 2013;502(7471):333–339.

[79] Snyder A, Makarov V, Merghoub T, Yuan J, Zaretsky JM, Desrichard A, et al. Genetic basis for clinical response to CTLA-4 blockade in melanoma. N Engl J Med. 2014;371(23):2189–2199.

[80] Rizvi NA, Hellmann MD, Snyder A, Kvistborg P, Makarov V, Havel JJ, et al. Cancer immunology. Mutational landscape determines sensitivity to PD-1 blockade in non-small cell lung cancer. Science. 2015;348(6230):124–128.

[81] Ciombor KK, Wu C, Goldberg RM. Recent therapeutic advances in the treatment of colorectal cancer. Annu Rev Med. 2015;66:83–95.

[82] B.H. O'Neil JW, D. Lorente, E. Elez, J. Raimbourg, C. Gomez-Roca, S. Ejadi, S.A. Piha-Paul, R.A. Moss, L.L. Siu, K. Dotti, A. Santoro, M. Gould, S.S. Yuan, M. Koshiji, S.W. Han. Pembrolizumab (MK-3475) for patients (pts) with advanced colorectal carcinoma (CRC): preliminary results from KEYNOTE-028. Eur J Cancer. 2015;51:S3–S103.

[83] Brahmer JR, Drake CG, Wollner I, Powderly JD, Picus J, Sharfman WH, et al. Phase I study of single-agent anti–programmed death-1 (MDX-1106) in refractory solid tumors: safety, clinical activity, pharmacodynamics, and immunologic correlates. J Clin Oncol. 2010;28(19):3167–3175.

[84] Lipson EJ, Sharfman WH, Drake CG, Wollner I, Taube JM, Anders RA, et al. Durable cancer regression off-treatment and effective reinduction therapy with an anti-PD-1 antibody. Clin Cancer Res. 2013;19(2):462–468.

[85] Dung T, Le NSA, Laheru D, Browner IS, Wang H, Uram JN, Kemberling H, Zheng L, Iannone R, Friedman E, Meister A, Donehower RC, De Jesus-Acosta A, Diaz LA. Phase 2 study of programmed death-1 antibody (anti-PD-1, MK-3475) in patients with microsatellite unstable (MSI) tumors. J Clin Oncol 2014;32:5s:(suppl; abstr TPS3128).

[86] Luis A, Diaz DTL, Yoshino T, Andre T, Bendell JC, Zhang Y, Lam B, Koshiji M, Jäge D. KEYNOTE-177: first-line, open-label, randomized, phase III study of pembrolizumab (MK-3475) versus investigator-choice chemotherapy for mismatch repair deficient or microsatellite instability-high metastatic colorectal carcinoma. J Clin Oncol. 2016;34: (suppl 4S; abstr TPS789).

[87] Herbst R, Gordon MS, Fine G, Sosman J, Soria J, Hamid O, et al. A study of MPDL3280A, an engineered PD-L1 antibody in patients with locally advanced or metastatic tumors. J Clin Oncol (Meeting Abstracts) May 2013;31(15_suppl 3000).

[88] Bendell J, Powderly JD, Lieu C, Eckhardt SG, Hurwitz H, Hochster H, et al. Safety and efficacy of MPDL3280A (anti-PDL1) in combination with bevacizumab (bev) and/or FOLFOX in patients (pts) with metastatic colorectal cancer (mCRC). Journal of Clinical Oncology, 2015 Gastrointestinal Cancers Symposium (January 15-17, 2015);33(3_suppl) (January 20 Supplement), 2015: 704.

[89] Brahmer JR, Tykodi SS, Chow LQM, Hwu W-J, Topalian SL, Hwu P, et al. Safety and activity of anti–PD-L1 antibody in patients with advanced cancer. N Engl J Med. 2012;366(26):2455–2465.

[90] Chung KY, Gore I, Fong L, Venook A, Beck SB, Dorazio P, et al. Phase II study of the anti-cytotoxic T-lymphocyte-associated antigen 4 monoclonal antibody, tremelimumab, in patients with refractory metastatic colorectal cancer. J Clin Oncol. 2010;28(21): 3485.

[91] Llosa NJ, Cruise M, Tam A, Wicks EC, Hechenbleikner EM, Taube JM, et al. The vigorous immune microenvironment of microsatellite instable colon cancer is balanced by multiple counter-inhibitory checkpoints. Cancer Discov. 2015;5(1):43–51.

[92] Markman JL, Shiao SL. Impact of the immune system and immunotherapy in colorectal cancer. J Gastrointestinal Oncol. 2014;6(2):208–223.

9

Endoscopic Submucosal Dissection for Early Colon Cancer

Valentin Ignatov, Anton Tonev, Nikola Kolev,
Aleksandar Zlatarov, Shteryu Shterev,
Tanya Kirilova and Krasimir Ivanov

Abstract

Endoscopic submucosal dissection (ESD) was first implemented in early gastric cancer allowing for en-bloc resection of the lesions. With the experience came the expertise to introduce ESD for early colon cancer (ECC). ESD demonstrates several advantages in comparison with the endoscopic mucosa resection. It allows accurate histological assessment of the depth of invasion, minimizes the risk of local recurrence and helps in the determination of additional therapy. Indications for ESD are placed only after adequate endoscopic morphological classification of the lesions excluding higher risk of nodal metastases. This chapter provides an overview of the application of ESD techniques in ESD for ECC and provides assessment on its technical aspects and complications. In order to decrease the rate of complications a standard protocol for the ESD should be adopted. The protocol includes recommendations for patient selection, bowel and patient preparation, appropriate equipment (knives, endoscopes, and power devices). The chapter will review the current ESD techniques and oncological results. ESD could have great impact on the treatment of early colon cancer. Its role is already proven in rectal localizations and despite the challenges it should be adopted for the colon. Safe strategy for ESD is the cornerstone in decreasing complications, which includes suitable resection of specialized ESD devices.

Keywords: Early colon cancer, endoscopic submucosal dissection, minimally invasive treatment

1. Introduction

The endoscopic treatment method for gastrointestinal neoplastic lesion has developed in recent years. Another modality to the existing techniques is the endoscopic submucosal dissection which is a novel method which broadens the possibilities for endoscopic treatment of neoplastic lesion. First introduced in Japan for early gastric cancer, now the method has advanced and is also applied for early colon cancer. After gaining initial experience the ESD can be used safely on condition that the indications are strictly followed and the technical issues and associated complications are recognized. The chapter will review the current ESD techniques and oncological results. ESD could have great impact on the treatment of early colon cancer. Its role is already proven in rectal localizations and despite the challenges it should be adopted for the colon. Safe strategy for ESD is the cornerstone in decreasing complications, which includes suitable resection of specialized ESD devices.

2. Indications for colonic ESD

The indications for ESD are object of debate. The Colon ESD standardization Implementation Working Group has proposed a draft of "Criteria of Indications for Colorectal ESD). They include large-sized (more than 20 mm in diameter) lesion, which are unsuitable for snare endoscopic mucosal resection, non-granular types of laterally spreading tumours, lesion with type VI pit pattern, cancer with less than 1000 μm submucosal infiltration, large depressed-type lesions, large elevated lesion, suspected of cancer [1]. Additional indications for ESD include sporadic tumours in IBD, local residual carcinoma after endoscopic piecemeal resection, mucosal lesion with fibrosis, adenoma with non-lifting sign.

The diagnostic process includes chromo-endoscopy, magnified endoscopy, NBI-enhanced magnified endoscopy or EUS. The histological confirmation of diagnosis is not required because the adequate chromo-endoscopic evaluation is confirmed to be sufficient. Biopsy is not always required. The occurring submucosal fibrosis may increases the difficulty of the procedure and the associated risk [2].

3. Muscle retracting sign

Other useful criteria which may help the selection of patients suitable for ESD is the muscle retracting (MR) sign. The MR sign is described as retraction of muscularis propria with submucosal fibrosis. ESD of lesions with positive MR sign is more difficult, which poses as a threat for a safe procedure [2]. Usually in such cases ESD is aborted. The sign is not universally exhibited by all larger lesions with protruding areas, despite the morphological similarities. The conclusion is that MR sign may serve as indication for difficult ESD with risk of resection failure. Therefore it may indicate patients for surgical resection to avoid adverse events and complications of the ESD.

4. CO2 insufflation

The ESD is performed after insufflation of the colon lumen with CO_2, which has been proven to be effective [3]. It decreases the risk of pneumoperitoneum in cases of perforation and further complications, related to the ESD.

5. Treatment devices

ESD is technically dependent method and various devices have been introduced. Most of them have been developed in Japan [1, 4–21] (**Figure 1**). The devices can be divided in two more general categories: needle-knife type and grasping type.

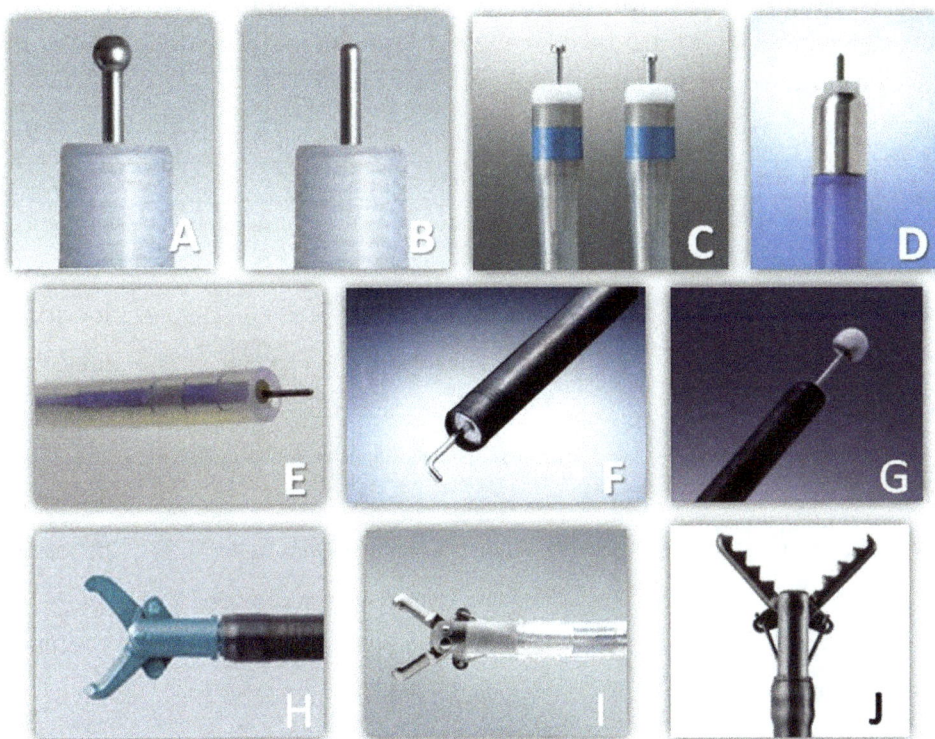

Figure 1. Devices used for colonic endoscopic submucosal dssection: A: Flush Knife (Fujifilm Medical, Tokyo, Japan); B: Flush Knife Ball Tip (Fujifilm Medical, Tokyo, Japan); C: DualKnife (Olympus Medical Systems Co., Tokyo, Japan); D: B-Knife (Zeon Medical, Tokyo, Japan); E: Splash needle (Pentax Co., Tokyo, Japan); F: Hook Knife (Olympus Medical Systems Co., Tokyo, Japan); G: IT Knife 2 (Olympus Medical Systems Co., Tokyo, Japan); H: Clutch Cutter (Fujifilm, Tokyo, Japan); I: SB knife Jr (Sumitomo Bakelite); J: Hemostat-Y forceps (PENTAX MEDICAL, Germany).

The needle-type knife device has two modifications – uncovered and covered type. The Flush Knife (Fujifilm Medical, Tokyo, Japan), the DualKnife (OlympusMedical Systems Co., Tokyo, Japan), the B-Knife (Zeon Medical, Tokyo, Japan), and the Splash needle (Pentax Co., Tokyo, Japan) belong to the obtuse, short tipped types [22–24]. As suggested by their name, the Flush Knife and the Splash needle also have the capability to inject substances in the submucosa.

This option is very helpful, because it obviates the need to change the injection and the cutting device during the procedure [23, 25]. Having a ball-disk at the tip, the Dual Knife is able to hook the submucosa, separate it from the muscularis propria. In contrast to the monopolar devices, the BKnife is a bipolar knife and therefore it may reduce the risk of complications. The HookKnife is usually used in cases of poor submucosal elevation [26]. Because of the special tip, the submucosa can be hooked and separated from muscularis propria and be safely cut [30]. On the other hand, the DualKnife and the Flush Knife are short tipped and may cause perforation of the thin wall of the colon in the presence of folds. The Flush Knife has two modifications – with needle tip and ball tip. Another product of Olympus Medical Systems Co. is the insulated-tipped knife 2 (IT Knife 2). Its efficacy is reported to be high when used for gastric lesion [27]. The procedure time is reported to be shortened because of the faster dissection time due to the longer blade. It also enables coagulation of small vessels. However, it is difficult to manipulate with this device and the long blade may also cause long perforations. A new device was later introduced, called IT knife nano. Its blade is smaller than of the IT Knife 2 and is targeted for submucosal dissection of the colon.

Author	Year	Country	Number of cases	Main device	Generator
Tamegai et al.	2007	Japan	71	Hook Knife	
Hurlstone et al.	2007	UK	42	Flex knife, IT knife	–
Fujishiro et al.	2007	Japan	200	Flex knife, Hook Knife, electrosurgical knife	ICC-2(X) or VI0300D
Zhou et al.	2009	China	74	Needle-knife, IT knife, Hook Knife	ICC-200
Isomoto et al.	2009	Japan	292	Flex knife, Hash knife, Hook Knife	ICC-200 or VI0300D
Saito et al.	2009	Japan	405	Bipolar needle knife (B-knife), IT knife	–
Iizuka et al.	2009	Japan	38	Flex knife	ICC-200 or VI0300D
Hotta et al.	2010	Japan	120	Flex knife, Flush Knife, Hook Knife	ICC-200 or VI0300D
Niimi et al.	2010	Japan	310	Flex knife, Hook Knife, electrosurgical knife	ICC-200 or VI0300D
Yoshida et al.	2010	Japan	250	Flush Knife	VI0300D
Toyonaga et al.	2010	Japan	512	Flex knife, Flush Knife	–
Matsumoto et al.	2010	Japan	203	Flex knife, Hook Knife, Dual Knife	–
Uraoka et al.	2011	Japan	202	B-Knife, Dual Knife, IT knife, mucoscctome	–
Shono et al.	2011	Japan	137	Flush Knife, Hook Knife, precutting knife	–
Kim et al.	2011	Korea	108	Flex knife, Hook Knife	VI0300D
Lee et al.	2011	Korea	499	Flex knife, Hook Knife	VI0300D
Probst et al.	2012	Germany	76	Hook Knife, IT knife, triangle knife	VI0300D
Okamoto et al.	2013	Japan	30	Dual Knife, mucosectome-2	VI0300D
Nawata et al.	2014	Japan	150	SB knife Jr, IT knife nano	–

Table 1. List of most commonly used devices and generators.

The grasping type devices have two major representatives – Clutch Cutter device (Fujifilm, Tokyo, Japan) and SB knife Jr (Sumitomo Bakelite) [21, 28]. The cutting method involves use of grasping type scissor forceps. It avoids fixing the knife to the target, although their use is associated with higher risk of perforation and bleeding after unexpected bowel movement [28]. Another useful device is the Hemostat-Y forceps (H-S2518; Pentax Co., Tokyo, Japan), which is used in bipolar mode to control visible bleeding and minimize the risk of any burning effect on the muscle layer. Some authors describe the use of double-balloon colonoscope in cases of difficult lesion location or to avoid paradoxical movement [29]. The procedure requires electrosurgical device. On **Table 1** are presented the most commonly used generators.

6. Practical aspects of the ESD

The bowel preparation is essential for a successful ESD. Any feces and liquid should be cleared from the colon. If any still remains in the lumen, ESD should not be initiated. The feces do not only prevent adequate dissection, but also pose as a serious treat in case of perforation.

A single channel general lower gastrointestinal endoscope is used for the procedure. Some centres have adopted the use of upper gastrointestinal endoscope. It is slimmer and can be used in retroflexed position [4]. The tip of the endoscope can be fitted with a transparent cap (Olympus Medical Systems Co., Tokyo, Japan).

ESD starts with submucosal injection. It is crucial to maintain adequate elevation during the procedure. Different solutions have been used. Some centres use in their practice two solutions: Glyceol (10% glycerin and 5% fructose; Chugai Pharmaceutical Co., Ltd., Tokyo, Japan) mixed with a small amount of Indigo Carmine and epinephrine, and 0.4% sodium hyaluronate solution (MucoUp; Seikagaku Corp, Tokyo, Japan) [30]. First, small amount of Glyceol is injected in the submucosal layer to confirm the appropriate localization and then MucoUp is injected until proper elevation is achieved. The final step is to inject small amout of Glyceol to flush the residual MucoUp [31]. Repeated submucosal injections are required during the procedure to maintain adequate submucosal elevation [29].

7. Sedation

ESD is usually a long procedure and can continue for more than 2.5 hours. Additionally, the abdominal discomfort caused by gas insufflation causes restlessness. Restlessness due to abdominal fullness and pain occurs frequently in cases with an operation time exceeding 2.5 h. Several medicaments are used for sedation. Some authors report use of midazolam and pentazocine with monitoring by automatic blood pressure monitor. They observed restlessness in 15 out of these 22 cases (68.1%) despite conscious sedation when the procedure lasted more than 2.5 hours. When the procedure lasted less than 2.5 h, restlessness was observed in only 10 out of 83 cases (12.0%) [32]. Carbon dioxide insufflations have also been reported to be effective for the prevention of abdominal fullness [33]. Another option is the use of propofol for conscious sedation which could be used for longer procedure without restlessness and discomfort [10].

8. Technique of ESD

The process of ESD is divided in several consecutive steps which are presented on **Figure 2**. After adequate elevation of the mucosa has been achieved, the process is initiated. The first step is mucosal incision and simultaneous incision to the deep submucosa layer. The lifting solution is injected at the proximal end of the lesion and mucosal incision is made. Sometimes the insertion of the endoscopic tip into the submucosal layer may become difficult and in these cases trimming of the mucosa is performed. To clear space for dissection after the trimming the submucosal layer near the mucosa is precisely cut. One of the practices for the mucosal incision is to circumvent the tumour. In cases where partial circumferential incision is performed the proximal side of the lesion is incised after the submucosal injection. Various endocut modes are recommended for the incision, which depend on the generator used. The described techniques for incision have their advantages and disadvantages. The circumferential incision may lead to undesired leakage of lifting liquid and loss of submucosal elevation. When injected at the distal side the tumour takes perpendicular to the endoscope position, which may hamper the dissection. The remaining uncut mucosa at the distal side pulls the tumour upward and also changes the position of the tumour. These situations are observed for tumours larger than 50 mm. When the incision is partially circumferential the elevation of the mucosa is easily maintained, because the uncut residual mucosa prevents liquid leakage. On the other hand after the partial resection of the tumour, the residual mucosa may become difficult for resection. Therefore each approach has its advantages and disadvantages. The specific type of incision should be chosen according to the tumour characteristics such as size,

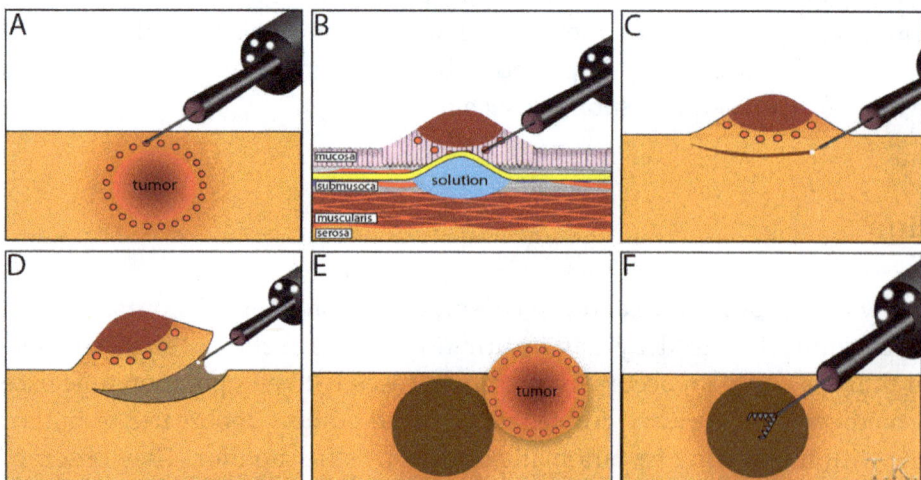

Figure 2. Steps of endoscopic submucosal dissection for early stage colon cancer: A: electrocautery marking around the lesion; B: injection of solution underneath the lesion; C: incision around the lesion; D: lifting and removal of the lesion; E: extraction of the tumor; F: meticulous hemostasis.

location, types of knives. During the submucosal dissection, the endoscopist can easily recognize the advantages of ESD. Structures such as vessels, fibrosis, etc. are clearly visible. Hemorrhage is controlled by precoagulation of the blood vessels. The thinner vessels are coagulated by cutting devices. The thicker ones can be dealt with forceps. Unlike for adenomatous lesion, in cases of early colon cancer the cutting line should be near the mucosal layer in order to achieve R0 resection. This step should be carried out with precision due to the higher perforation risk. The ESD is only finalized after careful inspection for any bleeding vessels. If any are found these are coagulated.

9. Complications

ESD in the colon is technically challenging procedure due to the anatomical characteristic of the colon. The latter is a long luminal organ with many folds, which impede the manipulation of the endoscope. The thin walls are easier to penetrate in comparison to the gastric wall. The insuflated gas during longer procedures may cause paradoxical movement of the endoscope. This situation occurs specifically in tumour, located above the sigmoid colon. It is difficult to find specific studies only on colon ESD. Therefore the presented data will cover also outcomes of colorectal ESD, bearing in mind that the rectal manipulations are easier due to the length of this segment. The rate of perforation of ESD is dramatically high when compared with that observed for endoscopic mucosal resection (EMR) [34–36] and has been reported to be 1.4–10.4%. According to several clinical studies the predicting factors for perforation are large lesions (>30 mm), fibrosis, colonic location and less experience with ESD [12, 22, 37, 38]. (**Table 2**).

The use of knife coagulation is considered the most common cause of perforation [39]. As described in the previous section, the obtuse knives such as DualKnife and the Flush Knife can easily cause perforation. In contrast the Hook Knife is able to hook up the mucosa, separate it from the submucosal layer and cut it safely. Other reasons for perforation include snare resection, coagulation by special haemostatic forceps with soft coagulation, endoscopic clipping onto coagulated submucosa [39]. The complications following ESD for colon tumour can be severe and even fatal in case of peritonitis. Alarming symptoms for perforation are abdominal tympanism, emphysema, and abdominal pain and muscle resistance. Most of the perforation cases are treated conservatively without emergency surgery. Although the closure of the mucus defect is practiced in several centres in Japan, this practice is currently considered impractical and technically challenging with the available devices, e.g. hemo-clips. Endoscopic clipping is possible for small perforation [40, 41]. The abdominal distention can be treated by decompression of the peritoneum via 20 Fr needle [10]. A new closure device which consists of clip with a loop may come in handy [42]. In some cases the perforation is not detected during endoscopy and only later on computed tomography. The possible explanation is that microperforations occur during ESD on deep injection by the needle. Those cases are not clinically significant and can be safely treated by conservative measures, such as stopping of oral intake. Another specific case of perforation is the delayed perforation. It accounts to 0.3% to 0.7% of the perforations [4, 5, 43] and is considered to be related to excessive coagulation in the muscularis propria. Usually delayed perforations are large in size and therefore require emergency surgery [4, 5, 43]. Bleeding after ESD is another common complication. The usual practice is to cut any vessel below 2 mm in diameter with a knife in coagulation mode. For vessels larger than 2 mm in diameter, a special haemostatic forceps should be used in soft coagulation mode. These forceps have the ability to gently catch the vessel and lift it upwards from muscularis propria. The surrounding mucosa around the vessel is also resected with the forceps. Removal of the coagulated vessel and the surrounding submucosa ensures safer and easier submucosal dissection. In cases when bleeding cannot be stopped by the knife the haemostatic forceps can be used as well with SOFT coagulation mode. The rate of postoperative haemorrhage in ESD is reported to be 0–12.0% (**Table 1**) [4, 5, 8–10, 22, 23, 25, 26, 44]. Most cases of postoperative haemorrhage are treated only by endoscopic clipping and withholding oral intake without emergency surgery or blood transfusion.

Author	Year	Country	Number of cases	Post-ESD perforation rate	Bleeding rate
Tamegai et al.	2007	Japan	71	–	1.4%
Hurlstone et al.	2007	UK	42	2.4%	9.5%
Fujishiro et al.	2007	Japan	200	6.0%	0.5%
Zhou et al.	2009	China	74	8.1%	1.4%
Isomoto et al.	2009	Japan	292	7.9%	0.7%
Saito et al.	2009	Japan	405	3.5%	1.0%
Iizuka et al.	2009	Japan	38	7.9%	–
Hotta et al.	2010	Japan	120	7.5%	–
Niimi et al.	2010	Japan	310	4.8%	1.6%
Yoshida et al.	2010	Japan	250	6.0%	2.4%
Toyonaga et al.	2010	Japan	512	1.8%	1.6%
Matsumoto et al.	2010	Japan	203	6.9%	–
Uraoka et al.	2011	Japan	202	2.5%	0.5%
Shono et al.	2011	Japan	137	3.6%	3.6%
Kim et al.	2011	Korea	108	20.4%	–
Lee et al.	2011	Korea	499	7.4%	–
Probst et al.	2012	Germany	76	1.3%	7.9%
Okamoto et al.	2013	Japan	30	0.0%	0.0%
Nawata et al.	2014	Japan	150	0.0%	0.0%

Table 2. Rate of complications after colorectal ESD from single center studies.

Another common effect after ESD is local inflammation to a certain degree. C-reactive protein level may rise to 5,82 ± 12.10 mg/L 2 days after the procedure in cases with perforation and

1.27 ± 2.00 mg/L in cases without perforation [45]. Fever and abdominal pain were also reported without perforation. A rare complication was acute colon obstruction after ESD of a colonic tumour located at the cecal base [46].

10. Clinical Studies on Colorectal ESD

Several large series on colorectal ESD have been published from Asian centres. However, most of the data are retrospective, and direct prospective comparative data on ESD versus EMR or surgery are not available. The Japan Society for Cancer of the Colon and Rectum conducted a multi-centre, observational study for all patients treated by conventional endoscopic resection and ESD for colorectal neoplasms exceeding 20 mm in size from October 2007 to December 2010 [9]. A total of 816 lesions were treated by ESD and the short-term outcomes were as follows. The mean lesion size was about 40 mm in diameter. *En bloc* resection was achieved in more than 90% of the cases, regardless of lesion size, with a perforation rate of 2.0% and delayed bleeding rate of 2.2%. None of the perforation cases needed emergency surgery as most

Author	Year Country	Number of cases	En bloc resection rate	Complete en bloc resection rate
Tamegai et al.	2007 Japan	71	98.6%	95.8%
Hurlstone et al.	2007 UK	42	78.6%	73.8%
Fujishiro et al.	2007 Japan	200	91.5%	70.5%
Zhou et al.	2009 China	74	93.2%	89.2%
Isomoto et al.	2009 Japan	292	90.1%	79.8%
Saito et al.	2009 Japan	405	86.9%	–
Iizuka et al.	2009 Japan	38	60.5%	57.9%
Hotta et al.	2010 Japan	120	93.3%	51.0%
Niimi et al.	2010 Japan	310	90.3%	74.5%
Yoshida et al.	2010 Japan	250	86.8%	81.2%
Toyonaga et al.	2010 Japan	512	98.2%	
Matsumoto et al.	2010 Japan	203	–	85.7%
Uraoka et al.	2011 Japan	202	90.6%	–
Shono et al.	2011 Japan	137	89.1%	85.4%
Kim et al.	2011 Korea	108	–	78.7%
Lee et al.	2011 Korea	499	95.0%	–
Probst et al.	2012 Germany	76	81.6%	69.7%
Okamoto et al.	2013 Japan	30	100.0%	–
Nawata et al.	2014 Japan	150	98.7%	97.3%

Table 3. Rate of en-bloc resections and complete en-bloc resections after colorectal ESD from single center studies.

iatrogenic perforations is very small, and can be successfully closed with endoscopic clip placement alone followed by intravenous antibacterial therapy (nothing *per os*).

A recent systematic review reported resection rates of 90.5% (61–98.2%) for endoscopic en bloc resection and of 76.9% (58–95.6%) for histologically confirmed complete resection, with associated local recurrence rates of 1.9% (0–11%) (**Table 3**) [30]. In addition, there are several studies with >500 ESD procedures, including large single centre series [47, 48], multi-centre surveys [49, 50], and a prospective multi-centre study [51]. These series confirm the high "en bloc" resection rates (up to 88.8% histologically confirmed complete resections) and the reported complication rates (perforation 4.8–5.4%, delayed perforation 0.4–0.7%, bleeding 1.5–1.7%). It was also demonstrated that ESD is feasible not only for the resection of adenoma or superficial cancers, but is also curative for submucosal invasive cancer. Thus, submucosal invasion limited to the upper 1,000 inlinegraphic m of the submucosal layer (sm1) is sufficiently treated with local resection if the tumour has a G1/G2 differentiation and no lymphatic or vascular invasion (L0, V0) [52–55]. When compared to EMR, data on ESD consistently show a higher en bloc resection rate/lower recurrence rate. Thus, in an analysis of 26 studies on EMR, en bloc resection for relatively smaller target lesions was possible in only 42.6% (19.2–91.8%) and recurrence rates were 17% (4.8–31.4%) for lesions resected in a piecemeal fashion [9]. In addition, several retrospective case series [35, 56–58], a matched case control analysis [59], and a meta-analysis [60] were published on the comparative analysis of EMR versus ESD. All these reports show a higher efficacy of ESD for the resection of larger sessile or flat lesions, resulting in a lower recurrence rate. When analysing risk factors for adenoma recurrence after EMR, associations were reported with size and morphology of the lesions (higher risk of incomplete resection for serrated adenoma/flat adenoma), piecemeal resection, and number of fragments [61–65]. Data on complications after EMR/ESD show similar bleeding rates (EMR 0–11.1%; ESD 0.5–9.5%), but the perforation rate is higher for ESD (1.3–20%) than for EMR (0–5.8%). However, the vast majority of perforations occurring during ESD are small and easily treated during the procedure, and thus the actual need for emergency surgery does not differ for EMR versus ESD [14, 18, 49, 66–68]. ESD is technically demanding and does require long procedure times. Thus, a recent study comparing 1,029 cases of conventional EMR with 816 ESD procedures showed a significantly higher procedure time for ESD (96 min) than for EMR (18 min). Procedure times increased with the size of the lesion, although for very large lesions a comparison to laparoscopic surgery would be more appropriate [66, 67]. Comparative data are available for ESD versus surgery, but again without a formal head-to-head study. Two smaller retrospective studies found no significant difference for efficacy (including procedure time) and safety between ESD versus transanal endoscopic microsurgery (TEM) for the treatment of early rectal cancer [69, 70]. A recently published systematic review and meta-analysis of 11 ESD and 10 TEM studies showed higher en bloc resection rates and a reduced need for additional surgery for TEM, while recurrence rates were significantly lower after ESD and no difference in the overall complication rate was observed [71]. Finally, a comparative retrospective study from the National Cancer Centre Tokyo found that ESD is equally effective as laparoscopic surgery for the treatment of early colorectal cancer, with significantly lower complication rates and shorter procedure times [72]. Indeed, the accompanying editorial called for an initiative to disseminate ESD for optimal treatment of early colorectal cancer [73]. While larger studies on colorectal ESD are almost exclusively from Asia, data on colorectal ESD from Western countries is mostly limited to the distal colon [9, 19, 74–77](**Table 1**). Taken together, there are considerable advantages of ESD over EMR for the resection of larger sessile or flat lesions, in particular high enbloc resection rates and low recurrence rates. The major problem of ESD is the technical challenge and the relatively long procedure time. Compared with surgery, ESD shows similar performance as TEM for rectal lesions, while a clear advantage – both for clinical outcome and procedure time – was observed in a single comparative study for ESD versus laparoscopic surgery for the treatment of T1 colorectal carcinoma. Nevertheless, there still is a need for prospective comparative trials to better define the role of ESD in comparison to EMR or surgery.

11. Conclusion

ESD is an attractive endoscopic treatment modality for larger sessile or flat adenomas/ superficial or slightly submucosal invasive colorectal cancers. ESD is a reliable method for achieving en bloc resection of relatively large colorectal superficial neoplasms, with superior curability. Still, ESD is associated with technical difficulties and complications, including perforation. Therefore patients should be selected for ESD only according to strict criteria, including tumour characteristics. The prerequisite for ESD is proper diagnosis, established by magnifying endoscopy, endoscopic ultrasound, etc. While colorectal ESD has recently become a standard procedure in major Asian endoscopy centres, propagation of ESD in Western countries will critically depend on opportunities for specialized training and probably also on technical developments to facilitate ESD and reduce procedure times.

Author details

Valentin Ignatov, Anton Tonev*, Nikola Kolev, Aleksandar Zlatarov, Shteryu Shterev, Tanya Kirilova and Krasimir Ivanov

*Address all correspondence to: teraton@abv.bg

Department of General and Operative Surgery, Medical University Varna, Bulgaria

References

[1] Shono T, Ishikawa K, Ochiai Y, Nakao M, Togawa O, Nishimura M, et al. Feasibility of endoscopic submucosal dissection: a new technique for en bloc resection of a large superficial tumor in the colon and rectum. Int J SurgOncol. 2011;2011:948293.

[2]   Toyonaga T, Tanaka S, Man-I M, East J, Ono W, Nishino E, et al. Clinical significance of the muscle-retracting sign during colorectal endoscopic submucosal dissection. EndoscInt Open. 2015 May 5;3(03):E246–251.

[3]   Fujishiro M, Kodashima S, Ono S, Goto O, Yamamichi N, Yahagi N, et al. Submucosal injection of normal saline can prevent unexpected deep thermal injury of Argon plasma coagulation in the in vivo porcine stomach. Gut Liver. 2008 Sep;2(2):95–98.

[4]   Fujishiro M, Yahagi N, Kakushima N, Kodashima S, Muraki Y, Ono S, et al. Outcomes of endoscopic submucosal dissection for colorectal epithelial neoplasms in 200 consecutive cases. ClinGastroenterolHepatol. 2007;5(6):678–683.

[5]   Isomoto H, Nishiyama H, Yamaguchi N, Fukuda E, Ishii H, Ikeda K, et al. Clinicopathological factors associated with clinical outcomes of endoscopic submucosal dissection for colorectal epithelial neoplasms. Endoscopy. 2009 Aug;41(8):679–683.

[6]   Matsumoto A, Tanaka S, Oba S, Kanao H, Oka S, Yoshihara M, et al. Outcome of endoscopic submucosal dissection for colorectal tumors accompanied by fibrosis. Scand J Gastroenterol. 2010;45(11):1329–1337.

[7]   Matsui N, Akahoshi K, Nakamura K, Ihara E, Kita H. Endoscopic submucosal dissection for removal of superficial gastrointestinal neoplasms: A technical review. World J GastrointestEndosc. 2012 Apr 16;4(4):123–136.

[8]   Tamegai Y, Saito Y, Masaki N, Hinohara C, Oshima T, Kogure E, et al. Endoscopic submucosal dissection: a safe technique for colorectal tumors. Endoscopy. 2007 May; 39(5):418–422.

[9]   Hurlstone DP, Atkinson R, Sanders DS, Thomson M, Cross SS, Brown S. Achieving R0 resection in the colorectum using endoscopic submucosal dissection. Br J Surg. 2007 Dec;94(12):1536–1542.

[10] Zhou P-H, Yao L-Q, Qin X-Y. Endoscopic submucosal dissection for colorectal epithelial neoplasm. Surg Endosc. 2009 Jul;23(7):1546–1551.

[11] Saito Y, Sakamoto T, Fukunaga S, Nakajima T, Kiriyama S, Kuriyama S, et al. Endoscopic submucosal dissection (ESD) for colorectal tumors. Dig Endosc Off J JpnGastroenterolEndosc Soc. 2009 Jul;21Suppl 1:S7–12.

[12] Iizuka H, Okamura S, Onozato Y, Ishihara H, Kakizaki S, Mori M. Endoscopic submucosal dissection for colorectal tumors. GastroentérologieClin Biol. 2009;33(10–11):1004–11.

[13] Hotta K, Oyama T, Shinohara T, Miyata Y, Takahashi A, Kitamura Y, et al. Learning curve for endoscopic submucosal dissection of large colorectal tumors. Dig Endosc. 2010;22(4):302–306.

[14] Niimi K, Fujishiro M, Kodashima S, Goto O, Ono S, Hirano K, et al. Long-term outcomes of endoscopic submucosal dissection for colorectal epithelial neoplasms. Endoscopy. 2010 Sep;42(09):723–729.

[15] Yoshida N, Naito Y, Kugai M, Inoue K, Wakabayashi N, Yagi N, et al. Efficient hemostatic method for endoscopic submucosal dissection of colorectal tumors. World J Gastroenterol WJG. 2010 Sep 7;16(33):4180–4186.

[16] Toyonaga T, Man-i M, Chinzei R, Takada N, Iwata Y, Morita Y, et al. Endoscopic treatment for early stage colorectal tumors: the comparison between EMR with small incision, simplified ESD, and ESD using the standard flush knife and the ball tipped flush knife. ActaChirIugosl. 2010;57(3):41–46.

[17] Uraoka T, Higashi R, Kato J, Kaji E, Suzuki H, Ishikawa S, et al. Colorectal endoscopic submucosal dissection for elderly patients at least 80 years of age. SurgEndosc. 2011 Sep;25(9):3000–3007.

[18] Kim ES, Cho KB, Park KS, Lee KI, Jang BK, Chung WJ, et al. Factors predictive of perforation during endoscopic submucosal dissection for the treatment of colorectal tumors. Endoscopy. 2011 Jul;43(7):573–578.

[19] Probst A, Golger D, Anthuber M, Märkl B, Messmann H. Endoscopic submucosal dissection in large sessile lesions of the rectosigmoid: learning curve in a European center. Endoscopy. 2012 Jul;44(7):660–667.

[20] Okamoto K, Kitamura S, Muguruma N, Takaoka T, Fujino Y, Kawahara Y, et al. Mucosectom2-short blade for safe and efficient endoscopic submucosal dissection of colorectal tumors. Endoscopy. 2013 Nov;45(11):928–930.

[21] Nawata Y, Homma K, Suzuki Y. Retrospective study of technical aspects and complications of endoscopic submucosal dissection for large superficial colorectal tumors. Dig Endosc Off J JpnGastroenterolEndosc Soc. 2014 Jul;26(4):552–555.

[22] Saito Y, Uraoka T, Matsuda T, Emura F, Ikehara H, Mashimo Y, et al. Endoscopic treatment of large superficial colorectal tumors: a case series of 200 endoscopic submucosal dissections (with video). GastrointestEndosc. 2007 Nov;66(5):966–973.

[23] Toyonaga T, Man-I M, Morita Y, Sanuki T, Yoshida M, Kutsumi H, et al. The new resources of treatment for early stage colorectal tumors: EMR with small incision and simplified endoscopic submucosal dissection. Dig EndoscOff J JpnGastroenterolEndosc Soc. 2009 Jul;21Suppl 1:S31–37.

[24] Fujishiro M, Kodashima S, Goto O, Ono S, Muraki Y, Kakushima N, et al. Technical feasibility of endoscopic submucosal dissection of gastrointestinal epithelial neoplasms with a splash-needle. SurgLaparoscEndoscPercutan Tech. 2008 Dec;18(6):592–597.

[25] Takeuchi Y, Uedo N, Ishihara R, Iishi H, Kizu T, Inoue T, et al. Efficacy of an endo-knife with a water-jet function (Flushknife) for endoscopic submucosal dissection of superficial colorectal neoplasms. Am J Gastroenterol. 2010 Feb;105(2):314–322.

[26] Yoshida N, Naito Y, Sakai K, Sumida Y, Kanemasa K, Inoue K, et al. Outcome of endoscopic submucosal dissection for colorectal tumors in elderly people. Int J Colorectal Dis. 2010 Apr;25(4):455–461.

[27] Saito Y, Kawano H, Takeuchi Y, Ohata K, Oka S, Hotta K, et al. Current status of colorectal endoscopic submucosal dissection in Japan and other Asian countries: progressing towards technical standardization. Dig Endosc Off J JpnGastroenterolEndosc Soc. 2012 May;24Suppl 1:67–72.

[28] Akahoshi K, Akahane H, Murata A, Akiba H, Oya M. Endoscopic submucosal dissection using a novel grasping type scissors forceps. Endoscopy. 2007 Dec;39(12):1103–1105.

[29] Jung YS, Park DI. Submucosal injection solutions for endoscopic mucosal resection and endoscopic submucosal dissection of gastrointestinal neoplasms. GastrointestInterv. 2013;2(2):73–77.

[30] Matsuda T, Fujii T, Saito Y, Nakajima T, Uraoka T, Kobayashi N, et al. Efficacy of the invasive/non-invasive pattern by magnifying chromoendoscopy to estimate the depth of invasion of early colorectal neoplasms. Am J Gastroenterol. 2008 Nov;103(11):2700–2706.

[31] Hayashi N, Tanaka S, Hewett DG, Kaltenbach TR, Sano Y, Ponchon T, et al. Endoscopic prediction of deep submucosal invasive carcinoma: validation of the narrow-band imaging international colorectal endoscopic (NICE) classification. GastrointestEndosc. 2013 Oct;78(4):625–632.

[32] Yoshida N, Yagi N, Naito Y, Yoshikawa T. Safe procedure in endoscopic submucosal dissection for colorectal tumors focused on preventing complications. World J Gastroenterol. 2010 Apr 14;16(14):1688–1695.

[33] Saito Y, Uraoka T, Matsuda T, Emura F, Ikehara H, Mashimo Y, et al. A pilot study to assess the safety and efficacy of carbon dioxide insufflation during colorectal endoscopic submucosal dissection with the patient under conscious sedation. GastrointestEndosc. 2007;65(3):537–542.

[34] Tanaka S, Haruma K, Oka S, Takahashi R, Kunihiro M, Kitadai Y, et al. Clinicopathologic features and endoscopic treatment of superficially spreading colorectal neoplasms larger than 20 mm. GastrointestEndosc. 2001 Jul;54(1):62–66.

[35] Saito Y, Fukuzawa M, Matsuda T, Fukunaga S, Sakamoto T, Uraoka T, et al. Clinical outcome of endoscopic submucosal dissection versus endoscopic mucosal resection of large colorectal tumors as determined by curative resection. SurgEndosc. 2010 Feb; 24(2):343–352.

[36] Iishi H, Tatsuta M, Iseki K, Narahara H, Uedo N, Sakai N, et al. Endoscopic piecemeal resection with submucosal saline injection of large sessile colorectal polyps. GastrointestEndosc. 2000 Jun;51(6):697–700.

[37] Jeong G, Lee JH, Yu MK, Moon W, Rhee P-L, Paik SW, et al. Non-surgical management of microperforation induced by EMR of the stomach. Dig Liver Dis Off J Ital SocGastroenterol Ital Assoc Study Liver. 2006 Aug;38(8):605–608.

[38] Seebach L, Bauerfeind P, Gubler C. "Sparing the surgeon": clinical experience with over-the-scope clips for gastrointestinal perforation. Endoscopy. 2010 Dec;42(12):1108–1111.

[39] Yoshida N, Wakabayashi N, Kanemasa K, Sumida Y, Hasegawa D, Inoue K, et al. Endoscopic submucosal dissection for colorectal tumors: technical difficulties and rate of perforation. Endoscopy. 2009 Sep;41(09):758–761.

[40] Fujishiro M, Yahagi N, Kakushima N, Kodashima S, Muraki Y, Ono S, et al. Successful nonsurgical management of perforation complicating endoscopic submucosal dissection of gastrointestinal epithelial neoplasms. Endoscopy. 2006 Oct;38(10):1001–1006.

[41] Uraoka T, Kawahara Y, Kato J, Saito Y, Yamamoto K. Endoscopic submucosal dissection in the colorectum: present status and future prospects. Dig Endosc. 2009;21:S13–16.

[42] Sakamoto N, Beppu K, Matsumoto K, Shibuya T, Osada T, Mori H, et al. "Loop Clip", a new closure device for large mucosal defects after EMR and ESD. Endoscopy. 2008 Sep;40Suppl 2:E97–98.

[43] Toyanaga T, Man-I M, Ivanov D, Sanuki T, Morita Y, Kutsumi H, et al. The results and limitations of endoscopic submucosal dissection for colorectal tumors. ActaChirIugosl. 2008;55(3):17–23.

[44] Tanaka S, Oka S, Kaneko I, Hirata M, Mouri R, Kanao H, et al. Endoscopic submucosal dissection for colorectal neoplasia: possibility of standardization. GastrointestEndosc. 2007;66(1):100–107.

[45] Yoshida N, Kanemasa K, Sakai K. Experience of endoscopic submucosal dissection (ESD) to colorectal tumor-especially about clinical course of cases with perforation. 2008 [cited 2016 Jan 8]; Available from: http://inis.iaea.org/Search/search.aspx?orig_q=RN:39103526

[46] Park SY, Jeon SW. Acute intestinal obstruction after endoscopic submucosal dissection: report of a case. Dis Colon Rectum. 2008 Jun 7;51(8):1295–1297.

[47] Yoshida N, Yagi N, Inada Y, Kugai M, Yanagisawa A, Naito Y. Prevention and management of complications of and training for colorectal endoscopic submucosal dissection. Gastroenterol Res Pract. 2013;2013:287173.

[48] Lee E-J, Lee JB, Lee SH, Kim DS, Lee DH, Lee DS, et al. Endoscopic submucosal dissection for colorectal tumors--1,000 colorectal ESD cases: one specialized institute's experiences. SurgEndosc. 2013 Jan;27(1):31–39.

[49] Tanaka S, Terasaki M, Kanao H, Oka S, Chayama K. Current status and future perspectives of endoscopic submucosal dissection for colorectal tumors. Dig Endosc. 2012;24(s1):73–79.

[50] Tanaka S, Tamegai Y, Tsuda S, Saito Y, Yahagi N, Yamano H. Multicenter questionnaire survey on the current situation of colorectal endoscopic submucosal dissection in Japan. Dig Endosc. 2010;22(s1):S2–8.

[51] Saito Y, Uraoka T, Yamaguchi Y, Hotta K, Sakamoto N, Ikematsu H, et al. A prospective, multicenter study of 1111 colorectal endoscopic submucosal dissections (with video). GastrointestEndosc. 2010 Dec;72(6):1217–1225.

[52] Oka S, Tanaka S, Kanao H, Ishikawa H, Watanabe T, Igarashi M, et al. Mid-term prognosis after endoscopic resection for submucosal colorectal carcinoma: summary of a multicenter questionnaire survey conducted by the colorectal endoscopic resection standardization implementation working group in Japanese Society for Cancer of the Colon and Rectum. Dig Endosc Off J JpnGastroenterolEndosc Soc. 2011 Apr;23(2):190–194.

[53] S Y, M W, H H, H B, K Y, J S, et al. The risk of lymph node metastasis in T1 colorectal carcinoma. Hepatogastroenterology. 2003 Dec;51(58):998–1000.

[54] Bosch SL, Teerenstra S, de Wilt JHW, Cunningham C, Nagtegaal ID. Predicting lymph node metastasis in pT1 colorectal cancer: a systematic review of risk factors providing rationale for therapy decisions. Endoscopy. 2013 Oct;45(10):827–834.

[55] Carrara A, Mangiola D, Pertile R, Ricci A, Motter M, Ghezzi G, et al. Analysis of risk factors for lymph nodal involvement in early stages of rectal cancer: When can local excision be considered an appropriate treatment? Systematic review and meta-analysis of the literature. Int J SurgOncol. 2012 Jun 19;2012:e438450.

[56] Lee E-J, Lee JB, Lee SH, Youk EG. Endoscopic treatment of large colorectal tumors: comparison of endoscopic mucosal resection, endoscopic mucosal resection–precutting, and endoscopic submucosal dissection. SurgEndosc. 2012 Jan 26;26(8):2220–2230.

[57] Terasaki M, Tanaka S, Oka S, Nakadoi K, Takata S, Kanao H, et al. Clinical outcomes of endoscopic submucosal dissection and endoscopic mucosal resection for laterally spreading tumors larger than 20 mm. J GastroenterolHepatol. 2012 Apr;27(4):734–740.

[58] Tajika M, Niwa Y, Bhatia V, Kondo S, Tanaka T, Mizuno N, et al. Comparison of endoscopic submucosal dissection and endoscopic mucosal resection for large colorectal tumors. Eur J GastroenterolHepatol. 2011 Nov;23(11):1042–1049.

[59] Kobayashi N, Yoshitake N, Hirahara Y, Konishi J, Saito Y, Matsuda T, et al. Matched case-control study comparing endoscopic submucosal dissection and endoscopic mucosal resection for colorectal tumors. J GastroenterolHepatol. 2012 Apr;27(4):728–733.

[60] Cao Y, Liao C, Tan A, Gao Y, Mo Z, Gao F. Meta-analysis of endoscopic submucosal dissection versus endoscopic mucosal resection for tumors of the gastrointestinal tract. Endoscopy. 2009 Sep;41(09):751–757.

[61] Pohl H, Srivastava A, Bensen SP, Anderson P, Rothstein RI, Gordon SR, et al. Incomplete polyp resection during colonoscopy—Results of the complete adenoma resection (CARE) Study. Gastroenterology. 2013;144(1):74–80.e1.

[62] Woodward TA, Heckman MG, Cleveland P, De Melo S, Raimondo M, Wallace M. Predictors of Complete Endoscopic Mucosal Resection of Flat and Depressed Gastrointestinal Neoplasia of the Colon. Am J Gastroenterol. 2012;107(5):650–4.

[63] Kim HH, Kim JH, Park SJ, Park MI, Moon W. Risk factors for incomplete resection and complications in endoscopic mucosal resection for lateral spreading tumors. Dig Endosc. 2012;24(4):259–266.

[64] Mannath J, Subramanian V, Singh R, Telakis E, Ragunath K. Polyp recurrence after endoscopic mucosal resection of sessile and flat colonic adenomas. Dig Dis Sci. 2011 Feb 16;56(8):2389–2395.

[65] Sakamoto T, Matsuda T, Otake Y, Nakajima T, Saito Y. Predictive factors of local recurrence after endoscopic piecemeal mucosal resection. J Gastroenterol. 2012 Jan 6;47(6):635–640.

[66] Ohata K, Nonaka K, Minato Y, Misumi Y, Tashima T, Shozushima M, et al. Endoscopic submucosal dissection for large colorectal tumor in a Japanese general hospital. J Oncol. 2013;2013:218670.

[67] Nakajima T, Saito Y, Tanaka S, Iishi H, Kudo S, Ikematsu H, et al. Current status of endoscopic resection strategy for large, early colorectal neoplasia in Japan. SurgEndosc. 2013 Sep;27(9):3262–3270.

[68] Lee E-J, Lee JB, Choi YS, Lee SH, Lee DH, Kim DS, et al. Clinical risk factors for perforation during endoscopic submucosal dissection (ESD) for large-sized, nonpedunculated colorectal tumors. SurgEndosc. 2012 Jun;26(6):1587–1594.

[69] Kawaguti FS, Nahas CSR, Marques CFS, Martins B da C, Retes FA, Medeiros RSS, et al. Endoscopic submucosal dissection versus transanal endoscopic microsurgery for the treatment of early rectal cancer. SurgEndosc. 2014 Apr;28(4):1173–1179.

[70] Park SU, Min YW, Shin JU, Choi JH, Kim Y-H, Kim JJ, et al. Endoscopic submucosal dissection or transanal endoscopic microsurgery for nonpolypoid rectal high grade dysplasia and submucosa-invading rectal cancer. Endoscopy. 2012 Nov;44(11):1031–1036.

[71] Arezzo A, Passera R, Saito Y, Sakamoto T, Kobayashi N, Sakamoto N, et al. Systematic review and meta-analysis of endoscopic submucosal dissection versus transanal endoscopic microsurgery for large noninvasive rectal lesions. SurgEndosc. 2014 Feb; 28(2):427–438.

[72] Kiriyama S, Saito Y, Yamamoto S, Soetikno R, Matsuda T, Nakajima T, et al. Comparison of endoscopic submucosal dissection with laparoscopic-assisted colorectal surgery for early-stage colorectal cancer: a retrospective analysis. Endoscopy. 2012 Nov;44(11): 1024–1030.

[73] Swanström LL. Treatment of early colorectal cancers: too many choices? Endoscopy. 2012 Nov;44(11):991–992.

[74] Farhat S, Chaussade S, Ponchon T, Coumaros D, Charachon A, Barrioz T, et al. Endoscopic submucosal dissection in a European setting. A multi-institutional report of a technique in development. Endoscopy. 2011 Aug;43(8):664–670.

[75] Repici A, Hassan C, Pagano N, Rando G, Romeo F, Spaggiari P, et al. High efficacy of endoscopic submucosal dissection for rectal laterally spreading tumors larger than 3 cm. GastrointestEndosc. 2013 Jan;77(1):96–101.

[76] Thorlacius H, Uedo N, Toth E. Implementation of endoscopic submucosal dissection for early colorectal neoplasms in Sweden. Gastroenterol Res Pract. 2013;2013:758202.

[77] Sauer M, Hildenbrand R, Bollmann R, Sido B, Dumoulin FL. Tu1426 Endoscopic Submucosal Dissection (ESD) of large sessile and flat neoplastic lesions in the colon: a single-center series with 83 procedures from Europe. GastrointestEndosc. 2014 May; 79(5):AB536.

10

Modulation of Apoptosis in Colon Cancer Cells by Bioactive Compounds

Marinela Bostan, Mirela Mihaila, Camelia Hotnog,
Coralia Bleotu, Gabriela Anton, Viviana Roman and
Lorelei Irina Brasoveanu

Abstract

A big challenge for a successful colon cancer treatment is the lack of eradication of the entire tumour cell population and consequent development of chemoresistance. Control of cell number from tissues and elimination of cells predisposed to malignant transformation, having an aberrant cell cycle or presenting DNA mutations, might be performed by a cellular 'suicide' mechanism — the programmed cell death, or apoptosis. Coordinated activation and execution of multiple subprograms are needed, added by a good knowledge of the basic components of the death machinery, besides their interaction to regulate apoptosis in a coordinated manner. Triggering apoptosis in target cells is a key mechanism by which chemotherapy promotes cell killing. Many anti-cancer drugs act during physiological pathways of apoptosis, leading to tumour cell destruction. New therapeutic approaches in cancer induce tumour cells to undergo apoptosis and break the cancer cell resistance to apoptosis commands. Administrations of natural compounds that prevent induction, inhibit or delay the progression of cancer, or induce inhibition or reversal of carcinogenesis at a premalignant stage represent chemoprevention strategies. Several natural compounds have been shown to be promising based on their anti-cancer effects and low toxicity; alternative approaches might be taken into account to obtain a stronger anti-tumour response when lower concentrations of anti-cancer drugs are used, and to diminish the undesirable side-effects.

Keywords: colon cancer, apoptosis, tumour evasion, bioactive compounds, combined therapy

1. Introduction

Cancer is a disease of cells that is thought to evolve along a multi-step process: the transformation of normal cells, tumour progression and advanced metastasis, that involve a complex series of events such as genetic alterations, aberrant progression of the cell cycle, resistance to growth inhibition, proliferation without dependence on growth factors, replication without limit, evasion of apoptosis, induction of angiogenesis and modification of cell adhesion [1]. For an accurate prediction, prevention, early detection and development of anti-cancer drugs, it is essential to identify the stages of development and use basic information [2]. The lack of eradication of the entire tumour cell population and the consequent development of chemoresistance represent main obstacles to a successful treatment in many malignancies, including colon cancer [3, 4]. The control of cell number from tissues and elimination of those predisposed to malignant transformation, having an aberrant cell cycle or presenting DNA mutations, might be performed by a cellular "suicide" mechanism, the programmed cell death or apoptosis [5, 6]. Elucidating the mechanisms of programmed cell death process seems to be of great importance for carcinogenesis, tumour evasion, and to have practical implications for anti-cancer therapy since many anti-cancer drugs act during physiological pathways of apoptosis, leading to tumour cell destruction [7, 8].

Several therapeutic agents used in colon cancer treatment, e.g. fluoropyrimidines, cisplatin, oxaliplatin, irinotecan have been shown to induce resistance in cancer cell killing, and their number are rapidly increasing, possibly through the modulation of survival cell components, such as proliferative or anti-apoptotic proteins [9, 10]. Triggering apoptosis in target cells represents a key mechanism by which chemotherapy promotes cell killing. Continuing efforts are made for discovering new molecular target-based molecules [11], and new therapeutic approaches in colon cancer involve restored cellular mechanisms responsible for the induction of apoptosis in tumour cells [12–15].

A main strategy in colon cancer treatment might be the combined multi-drug chemotherapy, the reason being the potential additive or synergistic tumour cytotoxicity produced [1]. The focus on finding new therapeutic strategies has recently shifted to natural products. Various plants and their bioactive compounds have been shown to have anti-carcinogenic and anti-proliferative effects towards the colon cancer cells. Studies have also reported positive correlation between the antioxidant activity of plants and their anti-proliferative effects, suggesting the potential action of antioxidants in inhibiting cancer cell growth. For example, the flavonoids display a wide range of biological activities, including anti-inflammatory and cytoprotective activities, and several are known to act as anti-cancer reagents [16].

The administration of synthetic or natural compounds that prevent induction of cancer, inhibit or delay its progression, or reverse carcinogenesis at a premalignant stage could represent useful strategies because of their potential clinical application in combined treatments with anti-cancer drugs [17]. By combining natural compounds with anti-cancer drugs, it might be obtained an increase of cancer treatment effects, specifically in highly invasive colon cancer cells, while in non-tumour cells the use of natural compounds could reduce the cytotoxic side effects [18].

2. Biology of colon cells: normal versus carcinogenic

Colorectal cancer (CRC) is the third most common malignancy worldwide, being frequently diagnosed in advanced stages. Recent data added to the molecular explanations of growth dysregulation, metastasis formation, extension of life span, and loss of maintenance of genomic and epigenetic integrity in cancer suggest models for their causal connection. The mechanisms of growth control, senescence, and anchorage dependence are linked at the molecular level [2].

The adult colon epithelium contains three cell types that arise from a multipotent stem cell: absorptive epithelial, enteroendocrine and Goblet cells. Colonic epithelial cells are configured in deep invaginations into the wall of the colon named crypts: from stem cells located at the base of the crypt, they arise and migrate to the luminal surface of the crypt where they are shed. Stem cells divide asymmetrically: the "old" DNA is retained in the stem cell population, and the new synthesised DNA is donated to daughter cells that migrate up the crypt and are ultimately shed. Stem cells are particularly vulnerable to developing mutations that might evolve into a malignant clone. Therefore, the cells located at the base of crypts, presumably stem cells, are highly prone to apoptosis, able to counteract dangerous mutations [19]. The result of the imbalance between cell proliferation and apoptosis determines colorectal tumour growth. Relatively undifferentiated tumours with higher proliferative potential are often more aggressive than well-differentiated ones [2]. The molecular mechanisms of cell division and apoptosis are similar in normal and tumour cells, but in tumour cells, these mechanisms are aberrantly regulated. Four cellular functions are inadequate regulated in tumour cells: (1) control of cell proliferation is inefficient; (2) genetic and chromosomal structure is destabilized; (3) cellular differentiation program is frequently altered; (4) the control of apoptosis is disturbed [20].

Multiple sequential genetic changes are needed to occur in order to ensure colorectal cancer evolution. During progression of normal epithelial to carcinoma cell in colorectal cancer, TP53, KRAS, BRAF and PIK3CA gene alterations play important roles. Gene alterations cause disruption of signalling pathways in which they are involved, accompanied by increased proliferative potential and decreased apoptosis of cells [21]. Along with genetic mutations, colon carcinogenesis is accompanied by epigenetic changes that lead to altered expression of key genes. Three major epigenetic regulatory mechanisms are described: (a) DNA methylation, (b) the covalent modifications of histones and (c) non-coding RNA interference [22].

3. Programmed cell death in normal versus carcinogenic colon cells

Apoptosis represents a cellular "suicide" mechanism which allows control of the number of cells from tissues and removal of cells that present DNA mutations or have an aberrant cell cycle, predisposed to malignant transformation [5]. Thus, elucidating the mechanisms of programmed cell death process seems to be of great importance for malignant transformation, tumour evasion, and therefore for anti-cancer therapy like restoration of cellular mechanisms responsible for the induction of apoptosis in tumour cells [23, 24]. Abnormalities in apoptotic function contribute to both pathogenesis of colorectal cancer, and its resistance to chemotherapeutics and radiotherapy [19].

3.1. Apoptosis pathways

Apoptosis is an active, specialized form of cell death with distinct biochemical and genetic pathways that play a critical role in normal tissue homeostasis and development. Under stress, such as precancerous lesions, the mechanisms involved in repairing DNA damage are activated and potentially harmful cells are removed, and carcinogenesis is blocked [25]. Lack of regulation of the apoptosis pathways may promote tumorigenesis and induce resistance to treatment in cancer cells [19].

The apoptotic process displays morphological features of the cells: cellular shrinkage with nuclear chromatin condensation and nuclear fragmentation, membrane blebbing, and cell-self-fragmentation into apoptotic bodies. Apoptosis is initiated by two basic signalling pathways: **the extrinsic pathway**, initiated by external stimuli and via activation of death receptors on the cell surface, such as tumour necrosis factor-α (TNF-α), Fas (CD95/APO1) and TNF-related apoptosis-inducing ligand (TRAIL) receptors, and **the intrinsic** (or mitochondrial) **pathway,** activated by intracellular stimuli and characterized by mitochondrial outer membrane permeabilization and release of mitochondrial cytochrome c (cyt-c) [26]. There is an overlap between the two apoptotic pathways: the extrinsic pathway usually also activates the intrinsic pathway, and both pathways result in the recruitment and activation of cysteine-aspartic acid proteases (caspases) [27, 28]. Upon receiving specific signals instructing the cells to undergo apoptosis, the caspase family of proteins is typically activated and cleaves key cellular components required for normal cellular function, including structural proteins in the cytoskeleton and nuclear proteins such as DNA repair enzymes [29]. Caspases can directly signal apoptosis or use mitochondria as an intermediate and additional point of regulation in apoptosis signalling [30].

(a) the mitochondrial pathway (the intrinsic pathway) is activated by a wide variety of cytotoxic drugs, DNA damage, growth factor deprivation, oxidative stress, Ca^{2+} overload and oncogene activation [29, 30]. It is regulated by formation of the mitochondrial permeability transition pore (MPTP), composed by Bcl-2 family members and voltage-dependent anion channels on the outer mitochondrial membrane [31], leading to mitochondrial outer membrane permeabilization (MOMP). The drop of mitochondrial membrane potential initiates the osmotic swelling of the matrix by water influx and release of cytochrome c from mitochondrial intermembrane space into the cytoplasm. Cytochrome c then associates with apoptotic protease-activating factor 1 (APAF-1) and caspase-9 forming apoptosome complex. The activation of caspase-9 and/or caspase-8 leads to caspase-3 cleavage, endonuclease activation, and ultimately nuclear DNA fragmentation, which is the hallmark of apoptosis [31, 32]. B cell leukaemia/lymphoma 2 (Bcl-2) family proteins are central regulators of the intrinsic pathway, which either suppress or promote changes in mitochondrial membrane permeability required for the release of cyt-c and other apoptogenic proteins [33].

(b) the extrinsic pathway starts with the stimulation of specific death receptors upon binding of their ligands, like tumour necrosis factor (TNF), tumour necrosis factor-related apoptosis-inducing ligand (TRAIL) and CD95 (Fas or APO1) [34]. Death receptors are transmembrane proteins with a death domain in their cytosolic region; the ligands binding causes oligomerization of these receptors, exposing their death domains (DD) in their cytosolic tail, which rapidly bind to Fas-Associated Death Domain (FADD). Several of the DD-containing TNF-family receptors use caspase activation as a signalling mechanism, including TNFR1/CD120a, Fas/APO1/CD95, DR3/Apo2/Weasle, DR4/TrailR1, DR5/TrailR2, and DR6 [35, 36]. Binding of these receptors at the cell surface results in the recruitment of several intracellular proteins, including some procaspases, to the cytosolic domains of these receptors, forming a "death-inducing signalling complex" (DISC) that triggers caspase-8 activation [37, 38]. In the case of TNFR1, after the ligand binds to TNFR1, the cytosolic region of the receptor does not bind FADD, but TRADD adaptor, as well as several other signalling proteins, some of them being involved in the activation of NF-κB transcription factor. The initial complex is then released from the receptor, TRADD binds to FADD in the cytosol, and caspase-8 is recruited. The downstream signalling depends on additional interactions with proteins like FLICE-like inhibitory proteins (c-FLIP), forming a complex that contains heterodimers of caspase-8 and c-FLIP that will inhibit apoptosis. However, if NF-κB activity is blocked or disrupted, or c-FLIP expression is inhibited, caspase-8 is activated and cell undergoes apoptosis [30, 39]. Between the death receptor pathway and the mitochondrial pathway of apoptosis, there is an overlap. Caspase-8 has another substrate in the cell, BID, a BH3-only protein: when caspase-8 cleaves BID, the protein is translocated to the mitochondria to promote MOMP and to initiate mitochondria-dependent apoptosis [40].

3.2. Evasion mechanisms of apoptosis in colon cancer

Apoptosis is subverted during tumorigenesis through the systematic loss of regulatory control mechanisms, ultimately resulting in the generation of a malignant phenotype and resistance to chemotherapy and radiation therapy. Several potential mechanisms and factors involved were taken into account to explain the defects in apoptotic signalling and the increased activation of anti-apoptotic pathways that were observed in colon cancer cells:

(a) Disrupted balance between pro- and anti-apoptotic proteins

Many proteins exert pro- or anti-apoptotic activity in cells, and the ratio between them plays an important role in the regulation of cell death. Over- or under-expressed genes were also found to contribute to carcinogenesis by reducing apoptosis in cancer cells. Key regulatory proteins of apoptotic machinery, such as Bcl-2 (including Bcl-xl and Bax) and IAP family, undergo changes in expression during the transition from adenoma to carcinoma, and therefore, they were used as prognostic biomarkers [7]. Pro- and anti-apoptotic mediators can regulate mitochondrial outer membrane permeability and release of cytochrome *c* from the mitochondria into the cytoplasm [41] (**Figure 1**).

When there is a disruption in the balance of anti-apoptotic and pro-apoptotic members of the **Bcl-2 family**, the result is a dysregulation of apoptosis in the affected cells. This can be due to the overexpression of one or more anti-apoptotic proteins, or the underexpression of one or more pro-apoptotic proteins, or both [42, 43]. In colorectal cancer, the dysregulated expression of Bcl-2 family members may be associated with disease outcomes. Bcl-2 expression is restricted to the basal epithelial cells in normal and hyperplastic mucosa, but in dysplastic polyps and carcinomas, it is extended to the parabasal and superficial regions. Bcl-2 expression is increased in hyperplastic polyps and markedly increased in almost all adenomas, while carcinomas show weaker Bcl-2 expression, indicating the decrease of apoptosis during progression from adenoma to carcinoma [44, 45].

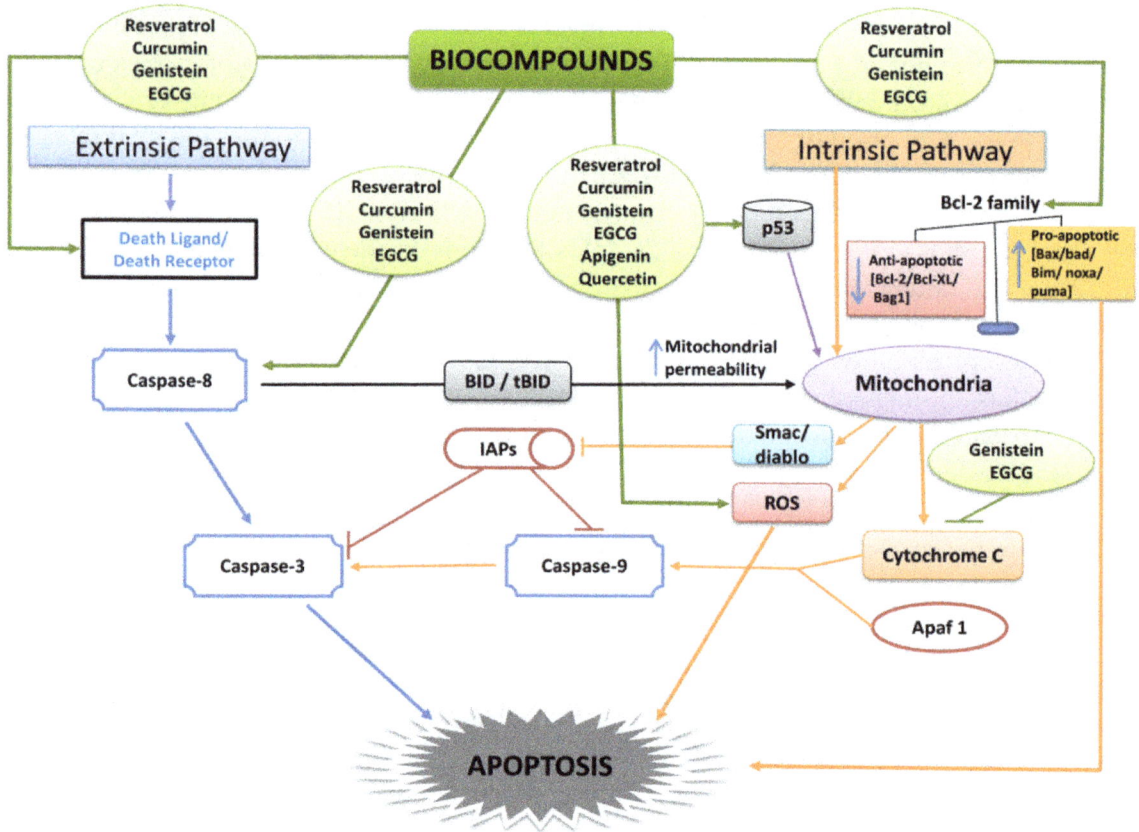

Figure 1. Role of biocompounds in modulation of intrinsic and extrinsic pathways of apoptosis.

Overexpression of the anti-apoptotic Bcl-2 family member Bcl-XL predicts poor prognosis in patients with colonic adenocarcinomas, conferring a multidrug resistance phenotype [46, 47]. Bcl-w, another anti-apoptotic Bcl-2 family protein, plays a general role in the progression from adenoma to adenocarcinoma in the colorectal epithelium; it is frequently expressed in colorectal adenocarcinomas at significant higher levels in TNM stage III tumours, positive correlated with node involvement [42]. In primary colorectal adenocarcinomas, elevated levels of expression for Bcl-xL and Bcl-w were reported to be associated with reduced expression of Bax [42]. Regarding the pro-apoptotic members of Bcl-2 family like Bcl-10, Bax, Bak, Bid, Bad, Bim, Bik, and Blk, increasing evidences suggest the involvement of Bak and Bax in the release of cytochrome *c*, based on phosphorylation of both Bak and Bax that facilitate their homo-oligomerization and subsequently the localization in mitochondria [29, 48]. Mutations in both

Bax and Bak genes confer cells the resistance to apoptosis [49, 50]. In colon cancer, Bax gene is frequently mutated in hereditary non-polyposis colorectal cancers [51] and microsatellite mutator phenotype [52, 53]. Decreased Bax expression was correlated with poor prognosis and progression towards metastasis [54].

One of the best known tumour suppressor proteins is **p53**, encoded by the tumour suppressor gene TP53 located on the short arm of chromosome 17 (17p13.1). The oncogenic property is due to a p53 mutations [55, 56], and half of all colorectal cancer cases show mutations in TP53 gene that were correlated with adenoma-to-carcinoma transitions and aggressive subsets of colorectal cancer [57, 58]. TP53 is a tumour suppressor gene in the mitochondrial apoptotic pathway, and one of the key regulators of cell-cycle control and apoptosis. Tumour cells presenting p53 mutations are defective in the induction of apoptosis. Its expression is down-regulated by survivin and Bcl-2 [59]. The molecular mechanisms that are employed by p53 to induce cell death in the context of suppressing cancer progression include the transcriptional regulation of pro-apoptotic PUMA expression, the generation of oxidative free radicals within mitochondrial components, the reduction of COX-2/PGE2 synthesis, and the induction of death receptor 5 [60, 61] (**Figure 1**).

Inhibitors of apoptosis (IAPs family) suppress apoptosis through inhibition of effector caspases [62]. The expression of inhibitor of apoptosis proteins (IAPs) is dysregulated in colorectal cancer. The anti-apoptotic regulators belonging to the IAP family, including XIAP, cIAP, and survivin, bind to caspase-3 and caspase-9 and thereby inhibit c aspase activity (**Figure 1**). Moreover, XIAP-associated factor 1 (XAF1) negatively regulates the anti-apoptotic function of XIAP. Molecules like c-FLIP, XIAP, cIAP2, and survivin have increased expression levels in colon cancer patients, and this has been correlated with disease progression and poor survival [47, 63, 64].

(b) Reduced caspase activity

During apoptosis process, the caspases implicated are either **initiator caspases** (e.g. caspase-2, caspase-8, caspase-9 and caspase-10) which are primarily responsible for the initiation of the apoptotic pathway, or **effector caspases** (caspase-3, caspase-6 and caspase-7), which are responsible in the actual cleavage of cellular components during apoptosis [65]. In the initiation and execution of apoptosis, caspases remain important players; therefore, low levels of caspases or impairment in caspase function may lead to a decrease in apoptosis and carcino-genesis [66, 67]. More than one caspase can be downregulated, contributing to colon cancer cell growth and development. Studies on differential expression by cDNA array showed a downregulation of both capase-8 and caspase-10, phenomenon that influences the pathogen-esis of carcinomas [68].

(c) Impaired death receptor signalling

Several receptors and ligands that modulate the programmed cell death were described: TNF receptor superfamily, Fas/Fas-L, CD27, death receptors and ligands, receptors phosphatases. Signalling via death receptors could be impaired in human cancers via downregulation of receptor surface expression as part of an adaptive stress response. Death receptors and their ligands are key players in the extrinsic pathway of apoptosis. The extrinsic signalling pathway leading to apoptosis involves transmembrane death receptors that are members of the tumour necrosis factor (TNF) receptor gene superfamily [69]. Several abnormalities in the death signalling pathways that can lead to evasion of the extrinsic pathway of apoptosis have been identified: the downregulation of receptor expression, the impairment of its function, as well as a reduced level in the death signals, all of which contribute to impaired signalling and a reduction of apoptosis. Reduced membrane expression of death receptors and abnormal expression of decoy receptors have also been reported to play a role in the evasion of the death signalling pathways in various cancers [12, 70] (**Figure 1**).

(d) Altered redox status in apoptosis induction

The oxidative stress process is characterized by an increased generation of reactive oxygen species (ROS) accompanied by a dysfunction of the antioxidant systems which exist in every cell, dependent on the metabolic state of the cell [71, 72]. The increased metabolic activity, mitochondrial dysfunction, peroxisome activity, oncogene activity, increased activity of oxidases, cyclooxygenases, lipoxigenases could be responsible for the generation and release of reactive oxygen species in tumour cells [73–75]. Low levels of ROS may influence processes like angiogenesis, cell proliferation and survival, while intermediate levels of ROS cause transient or permanent cell-cycle arrest and induce cell differentiation. When ROS production does not irreversibly alter cell viability, they can act as primary messengers, modulating several intracellular signalling cascades that lead to cancer progression [76]. High levels of ROS induce cell apoptosis or necrosis by causing an alteration of membrane permeability, a genetic instability, oxidative modifications that lead to less active enzymes or proteins more susceptible to proteolytic degradation [77]. Furthermore, ROS plays a crucial role in regulating expression of genes associated with cancer cell proliferation, angiogenesis, invasion and metastasis by activating transcription factors such as NF-κB, activator protein-1 (AP-1) and hypoxia inducible factor-1 (HIF-1α) [78].

Excessive production of ROS in tumour cells induces apoptosis or necrosis, and acts as an important inhibitor of cancer cell proliferation. Fas ligand mediates the induction of ROS, essential for the initiation of apoptotic signalling cascade and activation of the intrinsic apoptotic machinery by disruption of mitochondrial membrane integrity [79] (**Figure 1**). The transformed cells use ROS signals to drive proliferation to tumour progression. Tumour cells present an increased basal oxidative stress, making them vulnerable to chemotherapeutic agents that further augment ROS generation or weaken antioxidant defences of the cell [80]. Human colorectal tumours have increased levels of different markers of oxidative stress, such as ROS, nitric oxide (NO), lipid peroxides, glutathione peroxidase (GPx), catalase (CAT), and decreased cytosine DNA methylation [81–83].

ROS-sensitive signalling pathways are persistently elevated in many types of cancers, including colon cancer [84]. Reactive oxygen species can act as second messengers in cellular signalling. For example, hydrogen peroxide (H_2O_2) regulates protein activity through reversible oxidation of its targets, including protein tyrosine phosphatases, protein tyrosine kinases, receptor tyrosine kinases and transcription factors [85, 86]. The mitogen-activated protein (MAP) kinase/Erk cascade, phosphoinositide-3-kinase (PI3K)/Akt-regulated signalling cascades, as well as the IκB kinase (IKK)/nuclear factor κ-B (NF-κB)-activating pathways are regulated by ROS. The extracellular signal-regulated kinase pathway (ERK) mediates signal transduction involved in cell proliferation, differentiation, and migration [87]. Activation of ERK in tumour cells by biocompounds (e.g. resveratrol, quercetin) results in anti-proliferative effects, such as apoptosis, senescence, or autophagy [88–91]. Then, ERK can activate apoptotic enzymes or phosphorylate transcription factors that regulate the expression of pro-apoptotic genes [92]. Cell death in tumour cells treated with resveratrol and quercetin was accompanied by increased ROS levels and p53 expression, decreased Bcl-2 expression, depolarization of the mitochondrial membrane, cleaved caspase-3, and DNA fragmentation [93]. Elevated levels of ROS triggered by treatment with biocompounds might inhibit dual-specificity phosphatases (DUSPs) that dephosphorylate and inactivate MAPKs, leading to ERK activation and promoting cancer cell death. Therefore, biocompounds might induce apoptosis in colon cancer cells via activation of the MEK/ERK pathway [94].

Mitochondrial release of H_2O_2 and NO upon apoptotic signals leads to the activation of c-Jun N-terminal kinases (JNKs). In response to ROS, JNKs catalyze the phosphorylation and downregulation of anti-apoptotic proteins such as Bcl-2 and Bcl-XL. JNK influences the composition of the Bax/Bcl-2 complex by increasing the expression of Bax, leading to the formation of Bax homodimers and dissipation of mitochondrial membrane integrity [95, 96]. In response to the increased generation of ROS, the MAPK family member p38MAP is also implicated in apoptotic signalling [97].

In addition, ROS play an important role in the regulation of IKK/NF-κB pathway. NF-κB is a redox-regulated sensor for oxidative stress that is activated by low doses of hydrogen peroxide. The activation of NF-κB is mediated through the NF-κB-inducing kinase (NIK) and IκB kinase (IKK) complexes. Degradation of IκB translocates NF-κB to the nucleus, where it acts as a transcription factor to induce the expression of anti-apoptotic and anti-inflammatory genes [98]. Peroxisome proliferator-activated receptor-gamma (PPARγ) has been shown to exert an inhibitory effect on cell growth in most cell types. The expression of PPARγ was significantly increased in tumour tissues from human colon cancer, and the occurrence of apoptosis induced by PPARγ ligands was sequentially accompanied by reduced levels of NF-κB and Bcl-2. PPARγ-Bcl-2 feedback loop might control the life–death continuum in colonic cells, while a deficiency in generation of PPARγ ligands could precede the development of human colon cancer [99].

4. Bioactive compounds and colon cancer

Recent studies focused on the discovery of new chemotherapeutic agents among natural products since many plants and their bioactive compounds displayed anti-carcinogenic and anti-proliferative effects towards colon cancer cells [13]. Positive correlations between antioxidant activities of plants and their anti-proliferative effects, suggesting the potential action of antioxidants in inhibiting cancer cell growth, were also reported [13]. Among them, over 5000 flavonoids were found in vegetables and fruits, wines, seeds, nuts, grains and teas, herbs, and represent a class of plant secondary metabolites, known for their antioxidant properties [100]. The position of hydroxyl groups and other features in the chemical structure of flavonoids are important for their antioxidant and free radical scavenging activities [70]. The dietary compounds could interfere with specific stages of the carcinogenic process, inhibiting cell proliferation and inducing apoptosis in different types of cancer cells [101]. In addition, they might affect the expression of several detoxifying enzymes and their ability to modulate protein-signalling cascades [102].

4.1. Dietary sources and functional features

Since the 1950s, despite extensive clinical trials, mortality from colon cancer is a major public health problem in developed countries as a result of high consumption of animal fat or red meat and low intake of fibres or vegetables [103]. Protective factors include physical activity and increased intakes of dietary fibre, fish, nuts, dairy products, fruits and vegetables, while other factors, including weight and obesity, waist circumference, smoking, alcohol consumption, and red and processed meat intakes increase the risk of colorectal cancer [104, 105]. Using simple lifestyle modifications, changing the diet might substantially reduce the risk of colorectal cancer and could complement screening, so that CRC could be preventable in 90% of cases [106]. Over the last decade, different drugs and nutritional elements have been studied in preclinical as well as clinical trials and proved to have potential benefit in the field of CRC prevention [107]. Chemoprevention, the use of drugs or other agents to inhibit the development or progression of malignant changes in cells represents an alternative approach to reduce the mortality from colorectal cancer as well as other cancers [108].

Biocompounds	Source	Mechanisms of action	Refs.
Resveratrol	Grapes and red wine, mulberries, peanuts, seeds	Caspase activation NF-κB inhibition FasL induction Activation of MEK/ERK pathway Bcl-2 downregulation Increase of ROS and p53 levels	[92–94, 111, 137, 166, 167]
Genistein	Soybeans, fava beans, lupin, coffee	NF-κB inhibition Caspase activation Inhibition of PTK Inhibition of AKT pathway mdm2 downregulation	[113, 114]
Quercetin	Vegetables (capers, radish	Bcl-2, EGFR downregulation	[91–94,

Biocompounds	Source	Mechanisms of action	Refs.
	leaves, dill, cilantro, fennel, red onion, radicchio, kale), fruits (cranberry, black plums, blueberry, apples), seeds, nuts, tea, red wine	Cyclin D1, survivin inhibition Inhibition of Wnt/beta-catenin signalling pathway Increase of ROS and p53 levels Activation of MEK/ERK pathway	164]
Curcumin	Turmeric, curry, mustard	NF-κB inhibition ROS induction Modulation of MAPK pathway Downregulation of survivin and IGF-1 expression	[141–143, 146, 147]
Apigenin	Parsley, celery, dandelion, coffee, chamomile tea	Modulation of survival and death effectors (PI3K, AKT, ERK, STAT3, JNK, Mcl-1)	[119, 168]
Epigallocatechin gallate (EGCG)	Green tea, white tea, black tea	Modulation of ROS production NF-κB inhibition Inhibition of growth factor-dependent signalling (EGF, VEGF, IGF-I) Inhibition of MAPK and p21 pathways Downregulation of survivin	[148, 149, 151–155, 157, 176]
Silibinin	Milk thistle seeds	Bcl-2 downregulation Bax upregulation Decrease of cyclin D1 and c-myc expression Upregulation of death receptors DR4, DR5	[17, 127, 136, 138, 139]
Naringenin	Grapefruits, oranges and tomatoes (skin)	Losses in mitochondrial membrane potential Caspase-3 activation Intracellular ROS production Sustained ERK activation	[129, 163]
Pomegranate juice	Pomegranate	Downregulation of Bcl2-XL Caspase-3 and caspase-9 activation NF-κB inhibition Suppression of AKT pathway	[131, 132, 158, 160]

Biocompounds	Source	Mechanisms of action	Refs.
Sulforaphane	Broccoli, Brussels sprouts, cabbage, cauliflower, kale, collards, kohlrabi, mustard, turnip, radish, arugula, watercress	Upregulation of Bax, p21 G_2/M cell-cycle arrest	[121, 122, 177, 178]
Ellagic acid	Strawberries, walnuts, pecans	Disruption in mitochondrial membrane potential Activation of caspase-3, caspase-8 and caspase-9 Inactivation of PI3K/Akt pathway Bax upregulation; Bcl-2 downregulation Increase of ROS production	[169, 170]
Lycopene	Tomatoes, red carrots, watermelons, papayas	Bax and FasL upregulation; Bcl-2 and Bcl-XL downregulation Downregulation of Akt, NF-κB	[171, 172]

Table 1. Biocompounds—dietary sources and mechanisms of action involved in modulation of apoptosis.

Different natural compounds display a wide range of biological activities, including anti-inflammatory and cytoprotective activities, and several are known to act as anti-cancer reagents. Curcumin from turmeric, genistein from soybean, tea polyphenols like epigalloca-techin gallate from green tea, resveratrol from grapes, sulforaphane from broccoli, isothiocya-nates from cruciferous vegetables, silymarin from milk thistle, diallyl sulphide from garlic, lycopene from tomato, rosmarinic acid from rosemary, apigenin from parsley, gingerol from ginger and quercetin (**Table 1**) have high antioxidant activities, and demonstrated anti-proliferative effects against various cancer cell lines [13].

Resveratrol (RSV, trans-3,4′,5-trihydroxystilbene), a naturally occurring polyphenol phytoa-lexin, is abundant in a wide variety of plants and their products, including grapes and red wine, mulberries, peanuts, seeds, and has anti-inflammatory, antioxidant, anti-neoplastic, anti-carcinogenic, anti-tumorigenic, cardioprotective, neuroprotective, anti-aging and antiviral effects [102, 109]. Resveratrol exhibited anti-colon cancer properties by inhibiting cell prolif-eration, inducing apoptosis, decreasing angiogenesis, and causing cell-cycle arrest [110, 111].

Genistein (GST, 4′,5,7-trihydroxyisoflavone) is a natural compound found in lupin, fava beans, soybeans, coffee and occurs in Asian diet, rich in soy products [112]. It is a strong topoisomerase inhibitor, similarly to etoposide and doxorubicin. It has a wide spectrum of activity, expressed in protecting cells from malignant transformation, reducing proliferation of tumour cells and stimulating apoptosis [113, 114].

Quercetin (QCT, 3,3',4',5,7-pentahydroxyflavone) is an important dietary flavonoid, which presents in different vegetables (e.g. capers, radish leaves, dill, cilantro, fennel, red onion, radicchio, kale), fruits (cranberry, black plums, blueberry, apples), seeds, nuts, tea and red wine. It is involved in suppression of tumour-related processes, including oxidative stress, proliferation and metastasis. QCT has also received greater attention as pro-apoptotic flavonoid with a specific and almost exclusive activity on tumour cell lines rather than normal, non-transformed cells [115]. The anti-tumour effect found in SW480 colon cancer cell line was related to the inhibition of Cyclin D (1) and survivin expression, as well as Wnt/beta-catenin signalling pathway [116].

Curcumin (CRM, 1,7-bis-(4-hydroxy-3-methoxyphenyl)-1,6-heptadiene-3,5-dione) is a diarylheptanoid and the principal curcuminoid of turmeric, extracted from *Curcuma longa*; it possesses anti-inflammatory and antioxidant properties, and has a strong inhibitory effect on cell proliferation in the HT-29 and HCT-15 human colon cancer cell lines [117, 118].

Apigenin (APG, 4',5,7-trihydroxyflavone) is one of the most common flavonoids widely distributed in fruits and vegetables, such as parsley, celery, dandelion coffee and chamomile tea. However, apigenin only showed a modest anti-tumour activity towards cancer cells. New strategies are needed to enhance apigenin's anti-tumour efficacy [119].

Epigallocatechin 3-O-gallate (EGCG) [(2R,3R)-5,7-dihydroxy-2-(3,4,5-trihydroxyphenyl)-3,4-dihydro-2H-1-benzopyran-3-yl 3,4,5-trihydroxybenzoate] is the most abundant catechin in tea, a polyphenol found in high quantities in the dried leaves of white tea, green tea and, in smaller content in black tea [120]. EGCG was found to exert profound anti-inflammatory, antioxidant, anti-infective, anti-cancer, anti-angiogenic, and chemopreventive effects [120].

Sulforaphane (1-Isothiocyanato-4-methylsulfinylbutane) is found in cruciferous vegetables such as broccoli, Brussels sprouts, cabbage, cauliflower, bok choy, kale, collards, Chinese broccoli, broccoli raab, kohlrabi, mustard, turnip, radish, arugula and watercress. Young sprouts of broccoli and cauliflower are particularly rich in glucoraphanin. It is produced when the enzyme myrosinase transforms glucoraphanin, a glucosinolate, into sulforaphane upon damage to the plant which allows the two compounds to mix and react [121]. Sulforaphane (SFN) is a naturally occurring chemopreventive agent, inducing the cell-cycle arrest and apoptosis in colon cancer. However, little is known about the differential effects of SFN on colon cancer and normal cells [122].

Lycopene is a bright carotenoid pigment and phytochemical found in tomatoes, red carrots, watermelons and papayas. Although lycopene is chemically a carotene, it has no vitamin A activity. Also foods that are not red may contain lycopene, such as asparagus or parsley. Lycopene exhibited potential anti-carcinogenic activity, and the consumption of tomatoes was associated with reduced risk of several types of human cancer, including colon cancer [123, 124].

Glucobrassicin is a type of glucosinolate found in cabbages, broccoli, mustards, horseradish and woad. The main hydrolysis product after glucobrassicin is degraded by myrosinase is indole-3-carbinol, which was found to have apoptosis-inducing effects in a concentration- and time-dependent manner in human colon cancer cells [125, 126].

Silibinin is the major active constituent of **silymarin**, a standardized extract of the milk thistle seeds, that contains a mixture of flavonolignans and was shown to induce apoptosis in colon cancer cells [127, 128].

Naringenin (5,7-dihydroxy-2-(4-hydroxyphenyl)chroman-4-one) is a flavanone, considered to have a bioactive effect on human health as antioxidant, free radical scavenger, anti-inflammatory, carbohydrate metabolism promoter and immune system modulator. It can be found in grapefruits, oranges and tomatoes (skin) [129].

Pomegranate juice obtained from Punica granatum is rich in polyphenol compounds such as gallo, ellagitannin and flavonoid classes. It possesses therapeutic activity such as anti-atherogenic, anti-parasitic, anti-microbial, antioxidant, anti-carcinogenic and anti-inflammatory effects [130]; in preclinical animal studies, oral consumption of pomegranate extract inhibited the growth of lung, skin, colon and prostate tumours [131]. It was shown that pomegranate juice derivatives promote apoptosis of colon cancer cells by inducing the intrinsic pathway, but no effect was shown on the extrinsic pathway [132].

5. Bioactive compounds and their role in modulation of apoptosis in colon cancer

Results of clinical trials revealed that colon cancer can be successfully treated by chemotherapy, if the tumour selective detection can be substantial increased. In this regard, there is an increasing demand for biomarkers for risk assessment, early detection, prognosis and surrogate end points. This will be possible by the introduction of new drugs with more precise mechanisms of action, such as those acting specifically upon well-known aberrant pathways (e.g. apoptosis, cell signalling) [133]. New drugs can initiate or modulate the apoptosis cascade acting on caspases, Fas, Bax, Bid, APC or molecules which promote colon cancer cell survival (p53 mutants, Bcl-2 or COX-2) [134].

The implementation of new treatment options (and the management of metastatic colon cancer) must take into account the role of apoptosis in colon tumorigenesis with a highlight on the mechanisms leading to chemotherapeutic resistance as well as immune system evasion [69]. From this point of view, apoptosis can be considered as a potential target for cancer treatment at various stages of tumour progression, while chemoprevention as well as the apoptotic mechanisms could be utilized in the prevention and management of tumorigenesis [35, 135].

5.1. Mechanisms and targets involved

Grape seed extract that consists in a mixture of polyphenols was able to decrease cyclin D1, and c-myc expression, preventing cycle cell disruption, reduce expression of iNOS and COX-2 decreasing oxidative cellular stress [136]. On the other hand, *in vitro* studies performed on CRC cell lines showed that grape seed extract induces apoptosis via activation of caspase-3, caspase-8, and caspase-9, and also generation of ROS. It is worth mentioning that proapoptotic activity of grape seed extract has no effect in normal colonocytes [107].

Resveratrol has anti-CRC effects by inhibiting tumour initiation and progression by affecting caspase activation, NF-κB inhibition and FasL induction. Resveratrol could suppress inflammatory responses through decreasing nitric oxide levels and inhibiting the phosphorylation of the IκB enzyme complex, thus suppressing the activation of NF-κB dependent mechanisms [111, 137]. It was also described to interfere with mitochondrial functions by inhibiting mitochondrial ATP synthesis through its binding to F_1-ATPase. In addition, resveratrol can antagonize anti-apoptotic proteins that prevent the induction of apoptosis in cancer cells. Resveratrol induces p53-independent upregulation of p21, p21-triggered cell-cycle arrest and subsequently cell-cycle-dependent depletion of the anti-apoptotic protein survivin, thereby sensitizing cancer cells to TRAIL-induced apoptosis. Moreover, it suppresses expression levels of additional anti-apoptotic proteins (e.g. Bcl-x_L and MCL-1). The anti-tumour activities of resveratrol are also due to its ability to interfere with the phosphatidylinositol-3 kinase (PI-3K)/AKT and the MAPK pathways [13] (**Table 1**).

Silibinin: Studies *in vitro* and *in vivo* have shown a chemopreventive role in CRC by interfering in proliferation, signalling pathway and inflammation processes [17]. It was also found to cause decrease of cyclin D1 and c-myc expression [127]. Moreover, silibinin modulates the expression of anti-apoptotic proteins (Bcl-2, Mcl-1, X-linked inhibitor of apoptosis protein, and survivin) [136]. Silibinin can induce apoptosis by downregulation of the anti-apoptotic protein Bcl-2 and upregulation of the pro-apoptotic protein Bax, inverting the Bcl-2/Bax ratio. Sibilin also promotes apoptosis by upregulating transcription of the death receptors DR4 and DR5 [138], inhibits TNF-α activation of NF-κB, decreases expression of COX-2 and iNOS [139]. Silibinin decreased the expression of IL-1, TNF-alpha and their downstream target MMP7, all of them being upregulated during colon carcinogenesis [127, 138]. In a study evaluating silibinin pharmacodynamics, Hoh et al. [140] showed that silibinin is not toxic to normal colonic epithelium (**Table 1**).

Curcumin is effective in apoptosis triggering, inhibiting DNA mutations, cancer cell proliferation, metastasis and inflammation. Curcumin induces the production of ROS in concentration that leads to p21 protein upregulation, and consequently inhibiting cancer cell growth [141]. Moreover, curcumin interferes with the protein kinase (MAPK) pathway, which in turn decreases production of TNF-α and COX-2 as well as downregulates the expression of NF-κB and IL-6 [142, 143]. The downregulation of NF-κB levels has also effect on expression level of c-myc, cyclin D1 and Bcl-2 genes, and finally modulates the cell cycle [144]. It promotes cancer cell apoptosis by inducing expression of proapoptotic proteins (Bax, Bim, Bak, Noxa) and inhibiting expression of anti-apoptotic proteins (Bcl-2, Bcl-xl) [143]. Curcumin prevents the formation of metastases by decreasing vascular endothelial growth factor (VEGF) and matrix metalloproteinase 9 expression [144]. In recent in vitro study in CRC cells, Patel et al. [145] have shown that curcumin inhibits the receptor expression of HER2 and insulin-like growth factor 1 (IGF-1) which is well known to create resistance to 5-fluorouracil and oxaliplatin. Curcumin downregulates the expression of survivin and IGF-1 by activating the expression of p53 and reducing TNF-α levels, leading to activation of apoptotic signal [146, 147] (**Table 1**).

Epigallocatechin 3-Gallate Epigallocatechin 3-gallate (EGCG) has a strong antioxidant activity preventing ROS formation, blocking cancer cell proliferation and metastasis formation by down-regulating the expression of growth factors (epidermal growth factor, IGF-1, VEGF) [148]. EGCG blocks the cell cycle through the modulation of both MAPK and p21 pathways [149]. Furthermore, by upregulation of p53, EGCG induces apoptosis in CRC cells [150]. EGCG promotes cell growth arrest and induces apoptosis by affecting regulatory proteins of the cell cycle and inhibition of NFκB [151–153]. Some reports point out that the ROS-related effects may contribute to the anti-proliferative and pro-apoptotic activity of EGCG [154]. The effects are associated with modulation of reactive oxygen species (ROS) production. Although EGCG has a dual function of antioxidant and pro-oxidant, EGCG-mediated modulation of ROS production is reported to be responsible for its anti-cancer effects. The EGCG-mediated inhibition of NF-κB signalling is also associated with inhibition of migration, angiogenesis and cell viability [155]. Furthermore, it inhibits growth factor-dependent signalling (e.g. EGF, VEGF and IGF-I), the MAPK pathway, proteasome-dependent degradation and expression of COX-2. EGCG seems to directly interact with and modulate the character of membrane lipid rafts, which explains the ability to alter signalling processes of growth factor receptors. Furthermore, EGCG inhibits telomerase, topoisomerase II and DNA methyltransferase 1, thereby affecting the functions of chromatin [153, 156]. EGCG has a protective effect against NO-induced apoptosis in HDPC by scavenging ROS and modulating the Bcl-2 family [157] (**Table 1**).

Pomegranate may inhibit cancer cell proliferation and apoptosis through the modulation of cellular transcription factors and signalling proteins. In previous studies, pomegranate juice and its derivate inhibited proliferation and induced apoptosis in colon cancer cells, significantly suppressed TNF-α-induced COX-2 protein expression. It also reduced phosphorylation of the p65 subunit and binding to NF-κB, and abolished TNF-α induced AKT activation, playing an important role in the modulation of cell signalling in colon cancer cells [158]. The pomegranate juice exhibited a dose- and time-dependent decrease in cell proliferation, inducing cell-cycle arrest in the G_0/G_1 and G_2/M stages of the cell cycle, followed by apoptosis [159]. In the same regard, Larrosa et al. [160] have shown that induction of apoptosis was due to the downregulation of Bcl2-XL protein as well as activation of caspase-3 and caspase-9, but not caspase-8 (**Table 1**).

Citrus flavonoids: Volatile oil of *Citrus aurantifolia*, showed 78% growth inhibition of human colon cancer cells, induced the characteristic pattern of DNA fragmentation, via caspase-3 dependent pathway along with modulation of apoptosis-related protein expression [161].

Orange (*Satsuma mandarin*) juice contains a lot of flavonoids, which are potential chemoprotective compounds, with the capacity to suppress the expression of several cytokines (TNF-α, IL-1β, IL-6) as well as inflammatory enzymes (COX-2 and iNOS). In human colon cancer cell lines, the mechanism that induced the inhibition of their growth acted by blocking the cell cycle in G_0/G_1 phase and reducing levels of cyclins (A, D1 and E) [162].

Naringenin: Treatment with naringenin derivates resulted in significant apoptosis-inducing effects concomitant with losses in mitochondrial membrane potential, caspase activation, intracellular ROS production and sustained ERK activation [129]. In human colon adenocarcinomas, it induced activation of p38/MAPK, leading to the pro-apoptotic caspase-3 activation and poly (ADP-ribose) polymerase cleavage [163] (**Table 1**).

Quercetin plays a role in inhibiting tumorigenesis in colon cells through antioxidant, anti-inflammatory, anti-proliferative and pro-apoptotic mechanisms. Quercetin downregulated Bcl-2 through the inhibition of NF-κB and inhibited phosphorylation of EGFR suppressing downstream signalling in colon carcinoma cells. It augments TRAIL-induced apoptotic death and inhibits cyclin D1, survivin expression and Wnt/beta-catenin signalling pathway [91, 164] (**Table 1**).

Apigenin: Studies have shown that apigenin induces cell-cycle arrest and causes apoptosis in different cancer cells including colon cancer through modulation of various survival and death effectors, such as PI3K, AKT, ERK, STAT3, JNK and Mcl-1 [119] (**Table 1**).

Genistein inhibits the activation of NF-κB and Akt signalling pathways, both of which are known to maintain a homeostatic balance between cell survival and apoptosis; antagonizes estrogen- and androgen-mediated signalling pathways in the processes of carcinogenesis [114]. It has antioxidant properties, being a potent inhibitor of angiogenesis and metastasis. Genistein is a known inhibitor of protein-tyrosine kinase (PTK), which may attenuate the growth of cancer cells by inhibiting PTK-mediated signalling mechanisms. Genistein also inhibits topoisomerase I and II, 5α-reductase and protein histidine kinase, all of which may contribute to the anti-proliferative or pro-apoptotic effects [113]. It also down-regulates mdm2 at both transcriptional and post-translational levels [165] (**Table 1**).

5.2. Epigenetic mechanisms related to apoptosis, influenced by natural compounds

Several papers pointed the role of various natural compounds that target the **epigenetic mechanisms** in order to modulate the biologic activities, including apoptosis [173]. Epigenetic control mechanisms are reversible and natural compounds that target them may contribute to the development of new and attractive therapeutic strategies. A review of some natural compounds that target apoptosis through epigenetic mechanisms is presented below.

EGCG has a role in inhibiting histone deacetylases (HDACs) [174]. Site-specific acetylation of histones is essential to switch between permissive and repressive chromatin structures. Chromatin remodelling allows the regulation of gene expression, and it takes place under the action of enzymes responsible for acetylation (histone acetyl transferase, HAT) and deacety-lation (histone deacetyl transferase, HDAC) [175]. An increased HDAC activity is characteristic to many cancers and is associated with alterations of several cellular mechanisms, including apoptosis. Therefore, by targeting HDACs, it is possible to modulate several cell processes like cell cycle, cell differentiation and apoptosis. Combined treatments of EGCG and sodium butyrate (NaB), in physiologically achievable concentrations, were shown to promote apop-tosis and induce cell-cycle arrest in RKO, HCT-116 and HT-29 colon cell lines [176]. Both EGCG and NaB are epigenetic regulators, and treatment with these two compounds reduced both the expression of survivin (which has anti-apoptotic activity), as well as the expression of enzymes involved in epigenetic regulation (HDAC and DNA methyltransferase- DNMT) [176].

HDAC activity is also inhibited by **sulforaphane** (SFN) and induces an increased histone acetylation, mainly at p21 and Bax 2 promoters, events that lead to G_2/M cell-cycle arrest and apoptosis [177]. Oral administration of SFN in mice increased p21 expression via HDAC inhibition, while in APC-knock-out mice the same treatment leaded to specific increase of acetylation in H3 and H4 with decrease of intestinal polyps [178]. Moreover, SFN was found to inhibit DNMTs (enzymes responsible for DNA methylation) in CaCo-2 colon cancer cell line [179]. Another epigenetic mechanism used by SFN to exert its activity is through miRNAs: in NCM460 and NCM356 normal colon epithelial cells SFN upregulated 15 miRNAs, among which several were involved in apoptosis (miR-9, miR-135b) [180].

Resveratrol activates type III HDAC inhibitors, sirtuin 1 (SIRT1) and p300 [181] which in turn negatively modulates the expression of survivin. On the other hand, in colon cancer cells, resveratrol inhibits the cell growth and induces apoptosis through miRNAs [182, 183]. Combined treatment of quercetin and resveratrol induced apoptosis in colorectal cancer cells through downregulation of miR-27a [184].

6. Combined therapy of colon cancer: current strategies and future directions

Conventional therapeutic approaches, including chemotherapy, radiotherapy and surgery, are limited for the treatment of advanced colon cancer, in prevention of the disease recurrence, and are associated with a high risk of complications, highlighting the need to develop new therapeutic strategies. The majority of CRC patients receive chemotherapy using multiple agents that are currently approved for the treatment in the appropriate setting, but many patients have tumours intrinsically resistant to them. However, it is a complex process to select the optimal chemotherapy for each patient, and the difference between theory and practice is still a problem. That's why new concepts and modern technologies are promoted by precision medicine in order to achieve a personalized treatment for cancer patients.

6.1. RTCA: useful tool for screening biocompounds and drugs

Contrast data are available on the anti-cancer effects of biocompounds in colon cancer, whether they could influence the effects of oncolytic drugs against the cell growth and apoptosis of human colon cancer cells, or which might be the proper concentrations of the compounds with cytotoxic or cytostatic potential. Real-time impedance data obtained by the xCELLigence System (ACEA Biosciences) might be used to generate compound-specific profiles which are dependent on the biological mechanisms of action of each compound used. The actual kinetic response of the cells within an assay prior or subsequent to certain manipulations provides important information regarding the biological status of the cell, such as cell growth, cell arrest, morphological changes and apoptosis [185]. Changes in a cell status, such as cell morphology, cell adhesion or cell viability lead to a change in cell index (CI), which is a quantitative measure of cell number present in a well. For example, the cytotoxicity versus proliferative capacity of genistein, resveratrol or 5-fluorouracil was assessed in LoVo colon cancer cell line in order to modulate the chemosensitivity of colon cancer cells to drug treatment, and overcome the chemo-resistance. The entire length of the assay was presented, allowing informed decisions regarding the timing of certain manipulations or treatments, choice of the proper concentrations for further end-point assays, such as flow-cytometry techniques or molecular biology approaches [186, 187].

6.2. Modulation of apoptosis by combined therapy

Many anti-cancer drugs act during physiological pathways of apoptosis, leading to tumour cell destruction. By combining natural compounds with anti-cancer drugs, an increase of the effects might be obtained, specifically in highly invasive cancer cells, while in non-tumoral cells the natural compounds could reduce the cytotoxic side effects [115] (**Figure 2**).

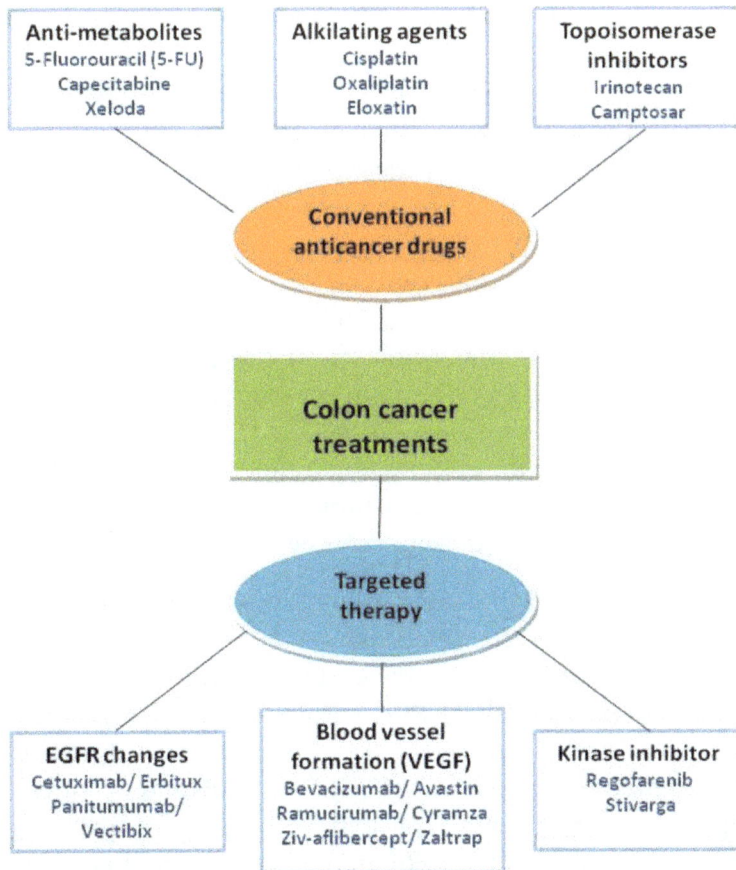

Figure 2. Available colon cancer therapeutic agents with disparate mechanisms of action.

A wide variety of currently available cancer therapeutical agents (**Figure 2**), with disparate mechanisms of actions, lead to the same mode of cell death [188]:

a.   5-Fluorouracil (5-FU) that blocks the thymidylate synthase (TS), which is essential for DNA synthesis;

b.   Capecitabine that blocks thymidylate synthase (orally administered prodrug converted to 5-FU)

c.   Oxaliplatin that inhibits DNA replication and transcription by forming inter- and intra-strand DNA adducts/cross-links;

d.   Irinotecan that inhibits topoisomerase I, an enzyme that facilitates the uncoiling and recoiling of DNA during replication;

e.   Bevacizumab, a monoclonal antibody, which binds to vascular endothelial growth factor (VEGF) ligand;

f.   Cetuximab, a monoclonal antibody to epidermal growth factor receptor (EGFR) (chimeric), that blocks the ligand-binding site;

g.   Panitumumab, a monoclonal antibody to EGFR (fully humanized), that blocks the ligand-binding site [188].

Several anti-cancer drugs act during physiological pathways of apoptosis, leading to tumour cell destruction [23, 189]. The pattern and extent of the cell damage induced by chemotherapeutics, like fluoropyrimidines, in human cancer cells have been suggested to depend also on the pathways downstream from drug-target interactions that once triggered will initiate programmed cell death (apoptosis) [190, 191]. 5-Fluorouracil (5-FU) is one of the widely used chemotherapeutic drugs targeting various cancers, but its chemoresistance remains as a major obstacle in clinical settings. Several groups reported the induction of apoptosis by 5-fluorouracil (5-FU) in HT29 [192] or LoVo human colon cancer cell lines [186, 187]. The long exposure of colon cells to 5-FU treatments influences both pro- and anti-apoptotic molecules like P53 and Bax, or Bcl-2 and Bcl-XL [193]. Several studies showed that 5-FU inhibits DNA proliferation in colon cancer cells by inhibiting the enzyme thymidylate synthase, leading to apoptosis, a mechanism of active cell death characterized by rapid loss of plasma membrane integrity, DNA fragmentation and altered expression of numerous genes [46, 52, 104] **(Figure 2)**.

The biocompounds extracted from botanicals may be used as chemopreventive and therapeutic agents for various human cancers, inclusive colon cancer [94]. The active biocompounds might induce cancer-selective cell death by increasing production of reactive oxygen species. The cancer cells have increased levels of ROS accompanied by a highly active antioxidant defense system; therefore, the tumour cells are unable to recover from additional oxidative stress and die. It is accepted that mitochondria-derived ROS play a critical role in their pro-death and chemopreventive responses. The natural biocompounds inhibit mitochondrial electron transport chains causing ROS production, thus triggering apoptotic cell death [80]. By combining flavonoids with anti-cancer drugs, it might be obtained an increase of the desired effects, specifically in highly invasive cancer cells, while in non-tumour cells the cytotoxic side effects could be reduced [186]. In vitro, studies showed that LoVo colon cancer cells were markedly sensitized to apoptosis by both 5-FU and genistein compared to the 5-FU treatment alone. When time of incubation was increased, treatments with GST and/or 5-FU had much stronger effects on the induction of apoptosis in LoVo cells, evaluated by using annexin-V/FITC and PI double staining, followed by flow-cytometry analysis [186]. Similar studies demonstrated the additive effect of GST to anti-cancer drug treatment, and in reversing the multi-drug resistance [13, 14].

Experimental assays showed that resveratrol (RSV) induced higher levels of early and late apoptosis compared to untreated or 5-FU-treated LoVo cells. When treatments were prolonged to 72 h, stronger effects were observed both for RSV alone and combined treatments with 5-FU [187]. Flow-cytometry analyses showed that treatments with 25 µM 5-FU or 50 µM RSV slightly increased the expression of the pro-apoptotic molecules p53 and Bax. The combined treatments of 50 µM RSV and 25 µM 5-FU induced a higher increase of p53 expression compared to the non-treated cells. Also the increase of Bax expression was much higher for the combined treatments compared to non-treated cells or treated cells with 5-FU alone. Both RSV and 5-FU treatments seemed to decrease Bcl-2 expression, but the effect was stronger for the combined treatments. Combined treatments induced a higher increase of pro-apoptotic antigen expression, both for P53 and Bax, compared to 5-FU treatment [187].

Therefore, addition of flavonoids and other natural compounds might be an alternative approach in order to obtain the same or a stronger anti-tumour response, enhance the chemosensitivity of tumours to anti-cancer drugs, or diminish the undesirable side effects by using lower concentrations [194, 195].

7. Conclusions

A big challenge for a successful treatment of colon cancer is the lack of eradication of the entire tumour cell population and the consequent development of chemoresistance. Since many anti-cancer drugs act during physiological pathways of apoptosis, leading to tumour cell destruction, elucidation of the mechanisms that govern the programmed cell death process seems to be of great importance for carcinogenesis, tumour evasion, and to have practical implications for anti-cancer therapy. Many therapeutic drugs used in cancer treatment proved to induce resistance in cancer cell killing, and their number are rapidly increasing, possibly through the modulation of survival cell components such as proliferative or anti-apoptotic proteins. Contrast data are available on the anti-cancer effects of natural compounds in colon cancer, whether they could influence the effects of oncolytic drugs against the growth and apoptosis of human colon cancer cells, or which might be the proper concentrations of compounds with cytotoxic or cytostatic potential. From a large number of natural compounds investigated, several have been shown to be promising, based on their anti-cancer effects related to apoptosis. A newly arising field involves therapeutic approaches in cancer in order to induce tumour cells to undergo apoptosis and break the cancer cell resistance to apoptosis commands. Therefore, manipulation of the mechanisms of programmed cell death process could be of outstanding importance for malignant transformation, and alternative approaches might be used to obtain a stronger anti-tumour response, and/or diminish the undesirable side effects by using lower concentrations of anti-cancer drugs. Thus, new concepts and modern technologies are promoted by precision medicine in order to achieve a personalized treatment for cancer patients.

Author details

Marinela Bostan[1], Mirela Mihaila[1], Camelia Hotnog[1], Coralia Bleotu[2], Gabriela Anton[3], Viviana Roman[1] and Lorelei Irina Brasoveanu[1*]

*Address all correspondence to: luli_brasoveanu@yahoo.com

1 Center of Immunology Dept., "Stefan S. Nicolau" Institute of Virology, Bucharest, Romania

2 Cellular and Molecular Pathology Dept., "Stefan S. Nicolau" Institute of Virology, Bucharest, Romania

3 Molecular Virology Dept., "Stefan S. Nicolau" Institute of Virology, Bucharest, Romania

References

[1] Jemal, A., R. Siegel, E. Ward, Y. Hao, J. Xu, T. Murray (2008) Cancer statistics. *CA Cancer J Clin*. 58:71–96.

[2] Weber, G.F. Molecular mechanisms of cancer. Dordrecht, The Netherlands: Springer; 2007. 645 p. (p. 39, 45–54, 93–99).

[3] Desoize, B., J. Jardillier (2000) Multicellular resistance: a paradigm for clinical resistance? *Crit Rev Oncol Hematol*. 36(2–3):193–207.

[4] Gottesman, M.M. (2002) Mechanisms of cancer drug resistance. *Annu Rev Med*. 53:615–627.

[5] Zimmermann, K.C., C. Bonzon, D.R. Green (2001) The machinery of programmed cell death. *Pharmacol Ther*. 92:57–70.

[6] Townson, J.L., G.N. Naumov, A.F. Chambers (2003) The role of apoptosis in tumor progression and metastasis. *Curr Mol Med*. 3:631–42.

[7] Miura, K., W. Fujibuchi, K. Ishida, T. Naitoh, H. Ogawa, T. Ando, N. Yazaki, K. Watanabe, S. Haneda, C. Shibata, I. Sasaki (2011) Inhibitor of apoptosis protein family as diagnostic markers and therapeutic targets of colorectal cancer. *Surg Today*. 41:175–182.

[8] Meadows, G.G. (2012) Diet, nutrients, phytochemicals, and cancer metastasis suppressor genes. *Cancer Metastasis Rev*. 31(3–4):441–454.

[9] Mattern, J. (2003) Drug resistance in cancer: a multifactorial problem. *Anticancer Res*. 23(2C):1769–1772.

[10] De Angelis, P.M., D.H. Svendsrud, K.L. Kravik, T. Stokke (2006) Cellular response to 5-fluorouracil (5-FU) in 5-FU-resistant colon cancer cell lines during treatment and recovery. *Mol Cancer.* 5:20–45.

[11] Gerhauser, C. (2013) Cancer chemoprevention and nutri-epigenetics: state of the art and future challenges. *Top Curr Chem.* 329:73–132.

[12] Fulda, S. (2010) Evasion of apoptosis as a cellular stress response in cancer. *Int J Cell Biol.* 2010; 2010:370835–370841.

[13] Fulda, S. (2010) Modulation of apoptosis by natural products for cancer therapy. *Planta Med.* 76:1075–1079.

[14] Shu, L., K.L. Cheung, T.O. Khor, C. Chen, A.N. Kong (2010) Phytochemicals: cancer chemoprevention and suppression of tumor onset and metastasis. *Cancer Metastasis Rev.* 29:483–502.

[15] Thornthwaite, J.T., H.R. Shah, P. Shah, W.C. Peeples, H. Respess (2013) The formulation for cancer prevention & therapy. *Adv Biol Chem.* 3:356–387.

[16] Russo, M., C. Spagnuolo, I. Tedesco, G.L. Russo (2010) Phytochemicals in cancer prevention and therapy: truth or dare? *Toxins.* 2:517–551.

[17] Rajamanickam, S., R. Agarwal (2008) Natural products and colon cancer: current status and future prospects. *Drug Dev Res.* 69(7):460–471.

[18] Fox, J.T., S. Sakamuru, R. Huang, N. Teneva, S.O. Simmons, M. Xia, R.R. Tice, C.P. Austin, K. Myung (2012) High-throughput genotoxicity assay identifies antioxidants as inducers of DNA damage response and cell death. *Proc Natl Acad Sci. USA* 109(14): 5423–5428.

[19] Watson, A.J.M. (2004) Apoptosis and colorectal cancer. *Gut.* 53:1701–1709.

[20] Pritchard, C.C., W.M. Grady (2011) Colorectal cancer molecular biology moves into clinical practice. *Gut.* 60(1):116–29.

[21] Tejpar, S., M. Bertagnolli, F. Bosman, H.J. Lenz, L. Garraway, F. Waldman, R. Warren, A. Bild, D. Collins-Brennan, H. Hahn, D.P. Harkin, R. Kennedy, M. Ilyas, H. Morreau, V. Proutski, C. Swanton, I. Tomlinson, M. Delorenzi, R. Fiocca, E. Van Cutsem, A. Roth (2010) Prognostic and predictive biomarkers in resected colon cancer: current status and future perspectives for integrating genomics into biomarker discovery. *Oncologist.* 15(4):390–404.

[22] Samowitz, W.S. (2008) Genetic and epigenetic changes in colon cancer. *Exp Mol Pathol.* 85(1):64–67.

[23] Kim, R., K. Tanabe, Y. Uchida, M. Emi, H. Inoue, T. Toge (2002) Current status of the molecular mechanisms of anticancer drug-induced apoptosis. The contribution of molecular-level analysis to cancer chemotherapy. *Cancer Chemother Pharmacol.* 50:343–352.

[24] Kaufmann, S.H., D.L. Vaux (2003) Alterations in the apoptotic machinery and their potential role in anticancer drug resistance. *Oncogene.* 22(47):7414–7430.

[25] Negrini, S., V.G. Gorgoulis, T.D. Halazonetis (2010) Genomic instability an evolving hallmark of cancer. *Nat Rev Mol Cell Biol.* 11(3):220–228.

[26] Su, Z., Z. Yang, Y. Xu, Y. Chen, X. Yu (2015) Apoptosis, autophagy, necroptosis, and cancer metastasis. *Mol Cancer.* 14:48.

[27] Elmore, S. (2007) Apoptosis: a review of programmed cell death. *Toxicol Pathol.* 35(4): 495–516.

[28] Taylor, R.C., S.P. Cullen, S.J. Martin (2008) Apoptosis: controlled demolition at the cellular level. *Nat Rev Mol Cell Biol.* 9(3):231–241.

[29] Hassan, M., O. Feyen, E. Grinstein (2009) Fas-induced apoptosis of renal cell carcinoma is mediated by apoptosis signal-regulating kinase 1 via mitochondrial damage-dependent caspase-8 activation. *Cell Oncol.* 31(6):437–456.

[30] Mendelsohn J., P.M. Howley, M.A. Israel, J.W. Gray, C.B. Thompson, editors. The Molecular Basis of Cancer. 4th ed. Philadelphia (PA): Elsevier; 2015. 863 p.

[31] Yang, S.Y., K.M. Sales, B. Fuller, A.M. Seifalian, M.C. Winslet (2009) Apoptosis and colorectal cancer: implications for therapy. *Trends Mol Med.* 15:225–233.

[32] Giansanti, V., A. Torriglia, A.I. Scovassi (2011) Conversation between apoptosis and autophagy: is it your turn or mine? *Apoptosis.* 16(4):321–333.

[33] Danial, N.N., S.J. Korsmeyer (2004) Cell death: critical control points. *Cell.* 116:205–219.

[34] Locksley, R.M., N. Killeen, M.J. Lenardo (2001) The TNF and TNF receptor superfamilies: integrating mammalian biology. *Cell.* 104(4):487–501.

[35] Ashkenazi, A., V.M. Dixit (1998) Death receptors: signaling and modulation. *Science.* 281(5381):1305–1308.

[36] Walczak, H., P.H. Krammer (2000) The CD95 (APO-1/Fas) and the TRAIL (APO-2L) apoptosis systems. *Exp Cell Res.* 256(1):58–66.

[37] Kuwana, T., L. Bouchier-Hayes, J.E. Chipuk (2005) BH3 domains of BH3-only proteins differentially regulate Bax-mediated mitochondrial membrane permeabilization both directly and indirectly. *Mol Cell.* 2005;17(4):525–535.

[38] Hassan, M., H. Watari, A. AbuAlmaaty, Y. Ohba, N. Sakuragi (2014) Apoptosis and Molecular Targeting Therapy in Cancer. *BioMed Res Int* (2014) Article ID 150845, 23 p., http://dx.doi.org/10.1155/2014/150845: 150845.

[39] Lavrik, I., A. Golks, P.H. Krammer (2005) Death receptor signaling. *J Cell Sci.* 118(2): 265–267.

[40] Su, M., Y. Mei, S. Sinha (2013) Role of the Crosstalk Between Autophagy and Apoptosis in Cancer. *J Oncology* (2013) Article ID 102735, 14 p., http://dx.doi.org/10.1155/2013/102735.

[41] Igney, F.H., P.H. Krammer (2002) Death and anti-death: tumour resistance to apoptosis. *Nat Rev Cancer.* 2(4):277–288.

[42] Wilson, J.W., M.C. Nostro, M. Balzi, P. Faraoni, F. Cianchi, A. Becciolini, C.S. Potten (2000) Bcl-w expression in colorectal adenocarcinoma. *Br J Cancer.* 82(1):178–85.

[43] Certo, M., V. Del Gaizo Moore, M. Nishino (2006) Mitochondria primed by death signals determine cellular addiction to antiapoptotic BCL-2 family members. *Cancer Cell.* 9:351–365.

[44] Kikuchi, Y., W.N. Dinjens, F.T. Bosman (1997) Proliferation and apoptosis in proliferative lesions of the colon and rectum. *Virchows Arch.* 431(2):111–7.

[45] Ilyas, M., X.P. Hao, K. Wilkinson, I.P. Tomlinson, A.M. Abbasi, A. Forbes, W.F. Bodmer, I.C. Talbot (1998) Loss of Bcl-2 expression correlates with tumour recurrence in colorectal cancer. *Gut.* 43:383–387.

[46] Zhang, Y.L., L.Q. Pang, Y. Wu, X.Y. Wang, C.Q. Wang, Y. Fan (2008) Significance of Bcl-xL in human colon carcinoma. *World J Gastroenterol.* 14(19):3069–3073.

[47] Huang, C.Y., L. Chia-Hui Yu (2015) Pathophysiological mechanisms of death resistance in colorectal carcinoma. *World J Gastroenterol.* 21(41):11777–11792.

[48] Wei, M.C., W.X. Zong, E.H. Cheng, T. Lindsten, V. Panoutsakopoulou, A.J. Ross, K.A. Roth, G.R. MacGregor, C.B. Thompson, S.J. Korsmeyer (2001) Proapoptotic BAX and BAK: a requisite gateway to mitochondrial dysfunction and death. *Science.* 292(5517):727–730.

[49] Kondo, S., Y. Shinomura, Y. Miyazak, T. Kiyohara, S. Tsutsui, S. Kitamura, Y. Nagasawa, M. Nakahara, S. Kanayama, Y. Matsuzawa (2000) Mutations of the bak gene in human gastric and colorectal cancers. *Cancer Res.* 60:4328–4330.

[50] Ionov, Y., H. Yamamoto, S. Krajewski, J.C. Reed, M. Perucho (2000) Mutational inactivation of the proapoptotic gene BAX confers selective advantage during tumor clonal evolution. *Proc Natl Acad Sci USA.* 97:10872–10877.

[51] Yagi, O.K., Y. Akiyama, T. Nomizu, T. Iwama, M. Endo, Y. Yuasa (1998) Proapoptotic gene BAX is frequently mutated in hereditary nonpolyposis colorectal cancers but not in adenomas. *Gastroenterology.* 114:268–274.

[52] De Angelis, P.M., T. Stokke, L. Thorstensen, R.A. Lothe, O.P. Clausenn (1998) Apoptosis and expression of Bax, Bcl-x, and Bcl-2 apoptotic regulatory proteins in colorectal carcinomas, and association with p53 genotype/phenotype. *Mol Pathol.* 51:254–261.

[53] Rampino, N., H. Yamamoto, Y. Ionov, Y. Li, H. Sawai, J.C. Reed, M. Perucho (1997) Somatic frameshift mutations in the BAX gene in colon cancers of the microsatellite mutator phenotype. *Science*. 275:967–969.

[54] Jansson, A., X.F. Sun (2002) Bax expression decreases significantly from primary tumor to metastasis in colorectal cancer. *J Clin Oncol*. 20:811–816.

[55] Bai, L., W.G. Zhu (2006) p53: structure, function and therapeutic applications. *J Cancer Mol*. 2(4):141–153.

[56] Vikhanskaya, F., M.K. Lee, M. Mazzoletti, M. Broggini, K. Sabapathy (2007) Cancer-derived p53 mutants suppress p53-target gene expression—potential mechanism for gain of function of mutant p53. *Nucl Acids Res*. 35(6):2093–2104.

[57] Russo, A., V. Bazan, B. Iacopetta, D. Kerr, T. Soussi, N. Gebbia (2005) The TP53 colorectal cancer international collaborative study on the prognostic and predictive significance of p53 mutation: influence of tumor site, type of mutation, and adjuvant treatment. *J Clin Oncol*. 23:7518–7528.

[58] Katkoori, V.R., C. Shanmugam, X. Jia, S.P. Vitta, M. Sthanam, T. Callens, L. Messiaen, D. Chen, B. Zhang, H.L. Bumpers, T. Samuel, U. Manne (2012) Prognostic significance and gene expression profiles of p53 mutations in microsatellite-stable stage III colorectal adenocarcinomas. *Plos One*. 7:e30020.

[59] Huerta, S., E.J. Goulet, E.H. Livingston (2006) Colon cancer and apoptosis. *Am J Surg*. 191:517–526.

[60] Nyiraneza, C., A. Jouret-Mourin, A. Kartheuser, P. Camby, O. Plomteux, R. Detry, K. Dahan, C. Sempoux (2011) Distinctive patterns of p53 protein expression and microsatellite instability in human colorectal cancer. *Hum Pathol*. 42(12):1897–910.

[61] Edagawa, M., J. Kawauchi, M. Hirata, H. Goshima, M. Inoue, T. Okamoto, A. Murakami, Y. Maehara, S. Kitajima (2014) Role of activating transcription factor 3 (ATF3) in endoplasmic reticulum (ER) stress-induced sensitization of p53-deficient human colon cancer cells to tumor necrosis factor (TNF)-related apoptosis inducing ligand (TRAIL)-mediated apoptosis through upregulation of death receptor 5 (DR5) by zerumbone and celecoxib. *J Biol Chem*. 289:21544–21561.

[62] Wu, W.K., X.J. Wang, A.S. Cheng, M.X. Luo, S.S. Ng, K.F. To, F.K. Chan, C.H. Cho, J.J. Sung, J. Yu (2013) Dysregulation and crosstalk of cellular signaling pathways in colon carcinogenesis. *Crit Rev Oncol Hematol*. 86(3):251–277.

[63] Mita, A.C., M.M. Mita, S.T. Nawrocki, F.J. Giles (2008) Survivin: key regulator of mitosis and apoptosis and novel target for cancer therapeutics. *Clin Cancer Res*. 14(16):5000–5005.

[64] Olsson, M., B. Zhivotovsky (2011) Caspases and cancer. *Cell Death Differ*. 18:1441–1449.

[65] Fink, S.L., B.T. Cookson (2005) Apoptosis, pyroptosis, and necrosis: mechanistic description of dead and dying eukaryotic cells. *Infect Immun.* 73(4):1907–1916.

[66] Devarajan, E., A.A. Sahin, J.S. Chen, R.R. Krishnamurthy, N. Aggarwal, A.M. Brun, A. Sapino, F. Zhang, D. Sharma, X.H. Yang, A.D. Tora, K. Mehta (2002) Downregulation of caspase 3 in breast cancer: a possible mechanism for chemoresistance. *Oncogene.* 21(57):8843–8851.

[67] Shen, X.G., C. Wang, Y. Li, L. Wang, B. Zhou, B. Xu, X. Jiang, Z.G. Zhou, X.F. Sun (2010) Downregulation of caspase-9 is a frequent event in patients with stage II colorectal cancer and correlates with poor clinical outcome. *Colorectal Dis.* 12(12):1213–1218.

[68] Fong, P.C., W.C. Xue, H.Y.S. Ngan, P.M. Chiu, K.Y.K. Chan, G.S.W. Tsao, A.N.Y. Cheung (2006) Caspase activity is downregulated in choriocarcinoma: a cDNA array differential expression study. *J Clin Pathol.* 59(2):179–183.

[69] Fulda, S., K.M. Debatin (2006) Extrinsic versus intrinsic apoptosis pathways in anti-cancer chemotherapy. *Oncogene.* 25:4798–4811.

[70] Fulda, S., L. Galluzzi, G. Kroemer (2010) Targeting mitochondria for cancer therapy. *Nat Rev Drug Dis.* 9(6):447–464.

[71] Acharya, A., I. Das, D. Chandhok, T. Saha (2010) Redox regulation in cancer: a double-edged sword with therapeutic potential. *Oxid Med Cell Longev.* 3:23–34.

[72] Circu, M.L., T.Y. Aw (2010) Reactive oxygen species, cellular redox systems, and apoptosis. *Free Radic Biol Med.* 48:749–762.

[73] Storz, P. (2005) Reactive oxygen species in tumor progression. *Front Biosci.* 10:1881–96.

[74] Afanas'ev, I. (2011) Reactive oxygen species signaling in cancer: comparison with aging. *Aging Dis.* 2(3):219–30.

[75] Dickinson, B.C., C.J. Chang (2011) Chemistry and biology of reactive oxygen species in signaling or stress responses. *Nat Chem Biol.* 7(8):504–11.

[76] Liou, G.Y., P. Storz (2010) Reactive oxygen species in cancer. *Free Radic Res.* 44(5):1–31.

[77] Waris, G, H. Ahsan (2006) Reactive oxygen species: role in the development of cancer and various chronic conditions. *J Carcinog.* 5:14.

[78] Gupta, R.A., R.N. DuBois, M.C. Wallace (2002) New avenues for the prevention of colorectal cancer: targeting cyclo-oxygenase-2 activity. *Best Pract Res Clin Gastroenterol.* 16:945–56.

[79] Martindale, J.L., N.J. Holbrook (2002) Cellular response to oxidative stress: signaling for suicide and survival. *J Cell Physiol.* 192(1):1–15.

[80] Trachootham, D., J. Alexandre, P. Huang (2009) Targeting cancer cells by ROSmediated mechanisms: a radical therapeutic approach? *Natl Rev Drug Dis.* 8:579–591.

[81] Oberreuther-Moschner, D.L., G. Rechkemmer, B.L. PoolZobel (2005) Basal colon crypt cells are more sensitive than surface cells toward hydrogen peroxide, a factor of oxidative stress. *Toxicol Lett.* 159(3):212–218.

[82] Rainis, T., I. Maor, A. Lanir, S. Shnizer, A. Lavy (2007) Enhanced oxidative stress and leucocyte activation in neoplastic tissues of the colon. *Dig Dis Sci.* 52(2):526–530.

[83] Slattery, M.L., A. Lundgreen, B. Welbourn, R.K. Wolff, C. Corcoran (2012) Oxidative balance and colon and rectal cancer: interaction of lifestyle factors and genes. *Mutat Res.* 734(1–2):30–40.

[84] Colin, D.J., E. Limagne, K. Ragot, G. Lizard, F. Ghiringhelli, É. Solary, B. Chauffert, N. Latruffe, D. Delmas (2014) The role of reactive oxygen species and subsequent DNA-damage response in the emergence of resistance towards resveratrol in colon cancer models. *Cell Death Dis.* 5:1533–1546.

[85] Chiarugi, P, T. Fiaschi (2007) Redox signalling in anchorage-dependent cell growth. *Cell Signal.* 19(4):672–82.

[86] Guo, Z., S. Kozlov, M.F. Lavin, M.D. Person, T.T. Paull (2010) ATM activation by oxidative stress. *Science.* 330:517–521.

[87] Dhillon, A.S., S. Hagan, O. Rath, W. Kolch (2007) MAP kinase signalling pathways in cancer. *Oncogene.* 26(22):3279–3290.

[88] She, Q.B., A.M. Bode, W.Y. Ma, N.Y. Chen, Z.G. Dong (2001) Resveratrol-induced activation of p53 and apoptosis is mediated by extracellular-signal-regulated protein kinases and p38 kinase. *Cancer Res.* 61:1604–1610.

[89] Shih, A., F.B. Davis, H.Y. Lin, P.J. Davis (2002) Resveratrol induces apoptosis in thyroid cancer cell lines via a MAPK- and p53-dependent mechanism. *J Clin Endocrinol Metab.* 87:1223–1232.

[90] Aggarwal, B.B., S. Shishodia (2006) Molecular targets of dietary agents for prevention and therapy of cancer. *Biochem Pharmacol.* 71:1397–1421.

[91] Kim, Y.H., D.H. Lee, J.H. Jeong, Z.S. Guo, Y.J. Lee (2008) Quercetin augments TRAIL induced apoptotic death: involvement of the ERK signal transduction pathway. *Biochem Pharmacol.* 75:1946–1958.

[92] Cagnol, S., J.C. Chambard (2010) ERK and cell death: mechanisms of ERK-induced cell death—apoptosis, autophagy and senescence. *FEBS J.* 277:2–21.

[93] Kong, E.H., Y.J. Kim, H.J. Cho, S.N. Yu, K.Y. Kim, J.H. Chang, S.C. Ahn (2008) Piplartine induces caspase-mediated apoptosis in PC-3 human prostate cancer cells. *Oncol Rep.* 20:785–792.

[94] Raj, L., T. Ide, A.U. Gurkar, M. Foley, M. Schenone, X. Li, N.J. Tolliday, T.R. Golub, S.A. Carr, A.F. Shamji, A.M. Stern, A. Mandinova, S.L. Schreiber, S.W. Lee (2011) Selective

killing of cancer cells by a small molecule targeting the stress response to ROS. *Nature.* 475:231–234.

[95]   Cadenas, E. (2004) Mitochondrial free radical production and cell signaling. *Mol Aspects Med.* 25(1–2):17–26.

[96]   Storz, P. (2007) Mitochondrial ROS—radical detoxification, mediated by protein kinase D. *Trends Cell Biol.* 17(1):13–8.

[97]   You, H., K. Yamamoto, T.W. Mak (2006) Regulation of transactivation-independent proapoptotic activity of p53 by FOXO3a. *Proc Natl Acad Sci USA.* 103(24):9051–6.

[98]   Janssen-Heininger, Y.M., M.E. Poynter, P.A. Baeuerle (2000) Recent advances towards understanding redox mechanisms in the activation of nuclear factor kappaB. *Free Radic Biol Med.* 28(9):1317–27.

[99]   Chen, G.G., J.F.Y. Lee, S.H. Wang, U.P.F. Chan, C Ip Ping, W.Y. Lau (2002) Apoptosis induced by activation of peroxisome-proliferator activated receptor-gamma is associated with Bcl-2 and Nf-κB in human colon cancer. *Life Sci.* 70(22):2631–2646.

[100]   Santandreu, F.M., A. Valle, J. Oliver, P. Roca (2011) Resveratrol potentiates the cytotoxic oxidative stress induced by chemotherapy in human colon cancer cells. *Cell Physiol Biochem.* 28(2):219–28.

[101]   Radhakrishnan, S., L. Reddivari, R. Sclafani, U.N. Das, J. Vanamala (2011) Resveratrol potentiates grape seed extract induced human colon cancer cell apoptosis. *Front Biosci.* 3:1509–1523.

[102]   Zhang, C., G. Lin, W. Wan, X. Li, B. Zeng, B. Yang, C. Huang (2012) Resveratrol, a polyphenol phytoalexin, protects cardiomyocytes against anoxia/reoxygenation injury via the TLR4/NF-κB signaling pathway. *Int J Mol Med.* 29(4):557–563.

[103]   Connors, T.A., R. Duncan, R.J. Knox (1995) The chemotherapy of colon cancer. *Eur J Cancer.* 31(7–8):1373–1378.

[104]   Chan, A.T., E.L. Giovannucci (2010) Primary prevention of colorectal cancer. *Gastroenterology.* 138(6):2029–2043.

[105]   Datsis, A., A. Tsoga, V. Langouretos (2010) The role of functional foods in the prevention of colorectal cancer. *Hell J Surg.* 82(4):224–232.

[106]   Boursi, B., N. Arber (2007) Current and future clinical strategies in colon cancer prevention and the emerging role of chemoprevention. *Curr Pharm Des.* 13(22):2274–2282.

[107]   Derry, M.M., R. Komal, A. Chapla, A. Rajesh (2013) Identifying molecular targets of lifestyle modifications in colon cancer prevention. *Front Oncol.* 3:119.

[108]   Farlex Partner Medical Dictionary. (2012) Retrieved January 26, 2016 from http://medicaldictionary.thefreedictionary.com/chemoprevention

[109] Castillo-Pichardo, L., S.F. Dharmawardhane (2012) Grape polyphenols inhibit Akt/ mammalian target of rapamycin signaling and potentiate the effects of gefitinib in breast cancer. *Nutr Cancer.* 64(7):1058–1069.

[110] Mahyar-Roemer, M., H. Köhler, K. Roemer (2002) Role of Bax in resveratrol-induced apoptosis of colorectal carcinoma cells. *BMC Cancer.* 2:27.

[111] Cal, C., H. Garban, A. Jazirehi, C. Yeh, Y. Mizutani, B. Bonavida (2003) Resveratrol and cancer: chemoprevention, apoptosis, and chemoimmunosensitizing activities. *Curr Med Chem Anti-Cancer Agents.* 3:77–93.

[112] Nicastro, H.L., E.B. Trujillo, J.A. Milner (2012) Nutrigenomics and cancer prevention. *Curr Nutr Rep.* 1(1):37–43.

[113] Banerjee, S., Y. Li, Z. Wang, F.H. Sarkar (2008) Multi-targeted therapy of cancer by genistein. *Cancer Lett.* 269(2):226–242.

[114] Nakamura, Y., S. Yogosawa, Y. Izutani, H. Watanabe, E. Otsuji, T. Sakai (2009) A combination of indole-3-carbinol and genistein synergistically induces apoptosis in human colon cancer HT-29 cells by inhibiting AKT phosphorylation and progression of autophagy. *Mol Cancer.* 8:100–115.

[115] Sanchez-Gonzalez, P.D., F. Lopez-Hernandez, F.P. Barriocanal, A.I. Morales, J.M.L. Novoa (2011) Quercetin reduces cisplatin nephrotoxicity in rats without compromising its anti-tumour activity. *Nephrol Dial Transplant.* 26:3484–3495.

[116] Shan, B.E., M.X. Wang, R.Q. Li (2009) Quercetin inhibit human SW480 colon cancer growth in association with inhibition of cyclin D1 and survivin expression through Wnt/beta-catenin signaling pathway. *Cancer Investig.* 27(6):604–12.

[117] Kawamori, T., R. Lubet, V.E. Steele, G.J. Kelloff, R.B. Kaskey, C.V. Rao, B.S. Reddy (1999) Chemopreventive effect of curcumin, a naturally occurring anti-inflammatory agent, during the promotion/progression stages of colon cancer. *Cancer Res.* 59:597–601.

[118] Johnson, I.T., E.K. Lund (2007) Nutrition, obesity and colorectal cancer. *Aliment Pharmacol Ther.* 26(2):161–181.

[119] Shao, H., K. Jing, E. Mahmoud, H. Huang, X. Fang, C. Yu (2013) Apigenin sensitizes colon cancer cells to antitumor activity of ABT-263. *Mol Cancer Ther.* 12(12):2640–50.

[120] Singh, B.N., S. Shankar, R.K. Srivastava (2011) Green tea catechin, epigallocatechin-3-gallate (EGCG): mechanisms, perspectives and clinical applications. *Biochem Pharmacol.* 82(12):1807–1821.

[121] Grabacka, M.M., M. Gawin, M. Pierzchalska (2014) Phytochemical modulators of mitochondria: the search for chemopreventive agents and supportive therapeutics. *Pharmaceuticals (Basel).* 7(9):913–42.

[122] Zeng, H., O.N. Trujillo, M.P. Moyer, J.H. Botnen (2011) Prolonged sulforaphane treatment activates survival signaling in nontumorigenic NCM460 colon cells but apoptotic signaling in tumorigenic HCT116 colon cells. *Nutr Cancer.* 63(2):248–55.

[123] Tang, F.Y., C.J. Shih, L.H. Cheng, H.J. Ho, H.J. Chen (2008) Lycopene inhibits growth of human colon cancer cells via suppression of the Akt signaling pathway. *Mol Nutr Food Res.* 52(6):646–54.

[124] Lin, M.C., F.Y. Wang, Y.H. Kuo, F.Y. Tang (2011) Cancer chemopreventive effects of lycopene: suppression of MMP-7 expression and cell invasion in human colon cancer cells. *J Agric Food Chem.* 59(20):11304–18.

[125] Bonnesen, C., I.M. Eggleston, J.D. Hayes (2001) Dietary indoles and isothiocyanates that are generated from cruciferous vegetables can both stimulate apoptosis and confer protection against DNA damage in human colon cell lines. *Cancer Res.* 61(16):6120–30.

[126] Zheng, Q., Y. Hirose, N. Yoshimi, A. Murakami, K. Koshimizu, H. Ohigashi, K. Sakata, Y. Matsumoto, Y. Sayama, H. Mori (2002) Further investigation of the modifying effect of various chemopreventive agents on apoptosis and cell proliferation in human colon cancer cells. *J Cancer Res Clin Oncol.* 128(10):539–46.

[127] Kaur, M., B. Velmurugan, A. Tyagi, C. Agarwal, R.P. Singh, R. Agarwal (2010) Silibinin suppresses growth of human colorectal carcinoma SW480 cells in culture and xenograft through down-regulation of beta-catenin-dependent signaling. *Neoplasia.* 12(5):415–424.

[128] Kauntz, H., S. Bousserouel, F. Gosse, J. Marescaux, F. Raul (2012) Silibinin, a natural flavonoid, modulates the early expression of chemoprevention biomarkers in a preclinical model of colon carcinogenesis. *Int J Oncol.* 41(3):849–54.

[129] Lee, E.R., Y.J. Kang, H.J. Kim, H.Y. Choi, G.H. Kang, J.H. Kim, B.W. Kim, H.S. Jeong, Y.S. Park, S.G. Cho (2008) Regulation of apoptosis by modified naringenin derivatives in human colorectal carcinoma RKO cells. *J Cell Biochem.* 104(1):259–73.

[130] Akpinar-Bayizit, A., T. Ozcan, L. Yilmaz-Ersan (2012) The therapeutic potential of pomegranate and its products for prevention of cancer. In *"Cancer Prevention—From Mechanisms to Translational Benefits"*, 331–373, InTech, Croatia, *Alexandros Georgakilas Ed.*, ISBN 978-953-51-0547-3.

[131] Adhami, V.M., N. Khan, H. Mukhtar (2009) Cancer chemoprevention by pomegranate: laboratory and clinical evidence. *Nutr Cancer.* 61(6):811–815.

[132] Jaganathan, S.K., M.V. Vellayappan, G. Narasimhan, E. Supriyanto (2014) Role of pomegranate and citrus fruit juices in colon cancer prevention. *World J Gastroenterol.* 20(16):4618–4625.

[133] Temraz, S., D. Mukherji, A. Shamseddine (2013) Potential targets for colorectal cancer prevention. *Int J Mol Sci.* 14:17279–17303.

[134] Rupnarain, C., Z. Dlamini, S. Naicker, K. Bhoola (2005) Colon cancer: genomics and apoptotic events. *Biol Chem.* 385(6):449–464.

[135] Galluzzi, L., O. Kepp, C. Trojel-Hansen, G. Kroemer (2012) Non-apoptotic functions of apoptosis-regulatory proteins. *EMBO Rep.* 13:322–330.

[136] Velmurugan, B., S.C. Gangar, M. Kaur, A. Tyagi, G. Deep, R. Agarwal (2010) Silibinin exerts sustained growth suppressive effect against human colon carcinoma SW480 xenograft by targeting multiple signaling molecules. *Pharm Res.* 27(10):2085–2097.

[137] Panaro, M.A., V. Carofiglio, A. Acquafredda, P. Cavallo, A. Cianciulli (2012) Anti-inflammatory effects of resveratrol occur via inhibition of lipopolysaccharide-induced NF-κB activation in Caco-2 and SW480 human colon cancer cells. *Br J Nutr.* 108:1623–1632.

[138] Kauntz, H., S. Bousserouel, F. Gosse, F. Raul (2012) The flavonolignan silibinin potentiates TRAIL-induced apoptosis in human colon adenocarcinoma and in derived TRAIL-resistant metastatic cells. *Apoptosis.* 17(8):797–809.

[139] Raina, K., C. Agarwal, R. Agarwal (2013) Effect of silibinin in human colorectal cancer cells: targeting the activation of NF-κB signaling. *Mol Carcinog.* 52:195–206.

[140] Hoh, C., D. Boocock, T. Marczylo, R. Singh, D.P. Berry, A.R. Dennison, A.J. Gescher (2006) Pilot study of oral silibinin, a putative chemopreventive agent, in colorectal cancer patients: Silibinin levels in plasma, colorectum, and liver and their pharmaco-dynamic consequences. *Clin Cancer Res.* 12(9):2944–2950.

[141] Yogosawa, S., Y. Yamada, S. Yasuda, Q. Sun, K. Takizawa, T. Sakai (2012) Dehydro-zingerone, a structural analogue of curcumin, induces cell-cycle arrest at the G2/M phase and accumulates intracellular ROS in HT-29 human colon cancer cells. *J Nat Prod.* 75(12):2088–2093.

[142] Tu, S.P., H. Jin, J.D. Shi, L.M. Zhu, Y. Suo, G. Lu, A. Liu, T.C. Wang, C.S. Yang (2012) Curcumin induces the differentiation of myeloid-derived suppressor cells and inhibits their interaction with cancer cells and related tumor growth. *Cancer Prev Res.* 5(2):205–215.

[143] Camacho-Barquero, L., I. Villegas, J.M. Sánchez-Calvo, E. Talero, S. Sánchez-Fidalgo, V. Motilva, C. Alarcón de la Lastra (2007) Curcumin, a Curcuma longa constituent, acts on MAPK p38 pathway modulating COX-2 and iNOS expression in chronic experimental colitis. *Int Immunopharmacol.* 7(3):333–342.

[144] Chen, C., Y. Liu, Y. Chen, J. Xu (2011) C086, a novel analog of curcumin, induces growth inhibition and down-regulation of NFκB in colon cancer cells and xenograft tumors. C086, a novel analog of curcumin, induces growth inhibition and down-regulation of NFκB in colon cancer cells and xenograft tumors. *Cancer Biol Ther.* 12(9):797–807.

[145] Patel, B.B., D. Gupta, A.A. Elliott, V. Sengupta, Y. Yu, A.P.N. Majumdar (2010) Curcumin targets FOLFOX-surviving colon cancer cells via inhibition of EGFRs and IGF-1R. *Anticancer Res.* 30(2):319–325.

[146] He, Z.Y., C.B. Shi, H. Wen, F.L. Li, B.L. Wang, J. Wang (2011) Upregulation of p53 expression in patients with colorectal cancer by administration of curcumin. *Cancer Investig.* 29:208–213.

[147] Li, Y.H., Y.B. Niu, Y. Sun, F. Zhang, C.X. Liu, L. Fan, Q.B. Mei (2015) Role of phytochemicals in colorectal cancer prevention. *World J Gastroenterol.* 21(31):9262–9272.

[148] Khan, N., H. Mukhtar (2008) Multitargeted therapy of cancer by green tea polyphenols. *Cancer Lett.* 269(2):269–280.

[149] Larsen, C.A., R.H. Dashwood (2010) (-)-Epigallocatechin-3-gallate inhibits Met signaling, proliferation, and invasiveness in human colon cancer cells. *Arch Biochem Biophys.* 501(1):52–57.

[150] Thakur, V.S., A.R. Ruhul Amin, R.K. Paul, K. Gupta, K. Hastak, M.K. Agarwal, M.W. Jackson, D.N. Wald, H. Mukhtar, M.L. Agarwal (2010) P53-Dependent p21-mediated growth arrest pre-empts and protects HCT116 cells from PUMA-mediated apoptosis induced by EGCG. *Cancer Lett.* 296(2):225–232.

[151] Steinmann, J., J. Buer, T. Pietschmann, E. Steinmann (2013) Anti-infective properties of epigallocatechin-3-gallate (EGCG), a component of green tea. *Br J Pharmacol.* 168(5): 1059–1073.

[152] Yang, C.S., H. Wang, G.X. Li, Z. Yang, F. Guan, H. Jin (2011) Cancer prevention by tea: evidence from laboratory studies. *Pharmacol Res.* 64(2):113–122.

[153] Yang, H., K. Landis-Piwowar, T.H. Chan, Q.P. Dou (2011) Green tea polyphenols as proteasome inhibitors: implication in chemoprevention. *Curr Cancer Drug Targets.* 11(3):296–306.

[154] Carrasco-Pozo, C., M.L. Mizgier, H. Speisky, M. Gotteland (2012) Differential protective effects of quercetin, resveratrol, rutin and epigallocatechin gallate against mitochondrial dysfunction induced by indomethacin in Caco-2 cells. *Chemico-Biol. Interact.* 195:199–205.

[155] Min, K., T.K. Kwon (2014) Anticancer effects and molecular mechanisms of epigallocatechin-3-gallate. *Integr Med Res.* 3(1):16–24.

[156] Adachi, S., T. Nagao, H.I. Ingolfsson F.R. Maxfield, O.S. Andersen, L. Kopelovich, I.B. Weinstein (2007) The inhibitory effect of (-)-epigallocatechin gallate on activation of the epidermal growth factor receptor is associated with altered lipid order in HT29 colon cancer cells. *Cancer Res.* 67(13):6493–6501.

[157] Park, S.Y., Y.J. Jeong, S.H. Kim, J.Y. Jung, W.J. Kim (2013) Epigallocatechin gallate protects against nitric oxide-induced apoptosis via scavenging ROS and modulating the Bcl-2 family in human dental pulp cells. *J Toxicol Sci.* 38(3):371–8.

[158] Adams, L.S., N.P. Seeram, B.B. Aggarwal, Y. Takada, D. Sand, D. Heber (2006) Pomegranate juice, total pomegranate ellagitannins, and punicalagin suppress inflammatory cell signaling in colon cancer cells. *J Agric Food.* 54(3):980–985.

[159] Kasimsetty, S.G., D. Blalonska, M.K. Reddy, G. Ma, S.I. Khan, D. Ferreira (2010) Colon cancer chemopreventive activities of pomegranate ellagitannins and urolithins. *J Agric Food Chem.* 58:2180–2187.

[160] Larrosa, M., F.A. Tomás-Barberán, J.C. Espín (2006) The dietary hydrolysable tannin punicalagin releases ellagic acid that induces apoptosis in human colon adenocarcinoma Caco-2 cells by using the mitochondrial pathway. *J Nutr Biochem.* 17:611–625.

[161] Patil, J.R., G.K. Jayaprakasha, K.N. Chidambara Murthy, S.E. Tichy, M.B. Chetti, B.S. Patil (2009) Apoptosis-mediated proliferation inhibition of human colon cancer cells by volatile principles of Citrus aurantifolia. *Food Chem.* 114(4):1351–1358.

[162] Pan, M.H., W.J. Chen, S.Y. Lin-Shiau, C.T. Ho, J.K. Lin (2002) Tangeretin induces cell-cycle G1 arrest through inhibiting cyclin-dependent kinases 2 and 4 activities as well as elevating Cdk inhibitors p21 and p27 in human colorectal carcinoma cells. *Carcinogenesis.* 23:1677–1684.

[163] Totta, P., F. Acconcia, S. Leone, I. Cardillo, M. Marino (2004) Mechanisms of naringenin-induced apoptotic cascade in cancer cells: involvement of estrogen receptor alpha and beta signalling. *IUBMB Life.* 56(8):491–9.

[164] Fridrich, D., N. Teller, M. Esselen, G. Pahlke, D. Marko (2008) Comparison of delphinidin, quercetin and (-)-epigallocatechin-3-gallate as inhibitors of the EGFR and the ErbB2 receptor phosphorylation. *Mol Nutr Food Res.* 52:815–822.

[165] Li, M., Z. Zhang, D.L. Hill, X. Chen, H. Wang, R. Zhang (2005) Genistein, a dietary isoflavone, down-regulates the mdm2 oncogene at both transcriptional and posttranslational levels. *Cancer Res.* 65(18):8200–8.

[166] Liu, B., Z. Zhou, W. Zhou, J. Liu, Q. Zhang, J. Xia, J. Liu, N. Chen, M. Li, R. Zhu (2014) Resveratrol inhibits proliferation in human colorectal carcinoma cells by inducing G1/S-phase cell cycle arrest and apoptosis through caspase/cyclin-CDK pathways. *Mol Med Rep.* 10:1697–1702.

[167] Fouad, M.A., A.M. Agha, M.M. Merzabani, S.A. Shouman (2013) Resveratrol inhibits proliferation, angiogenesis and induces apoptosis in colon cancer cells: calorie restriction is the force to the cytotoxicity. *Hum Exp Toxicol.* 32:1067–1080.

[168] Turktekin, M., E. Konac, H.I. Onen, E. Alp, A. Yilmaz, S. Menevse (2011) Evaluation of the effects of the flavonoid apigenin on apoptotic pathway gene expression on the colon cancer cell line (HT29). *J Med Food.* 14(10):1107–17.

[169] Cho, H., H. Jung, H. Lee, H.C. Yi, H.K. Kwak, K.T. Hwang (2015) Chemopreventive activity of ellagitannins and their derivatives from black raspberry seeds on HT-29 colon cancer cells. *Food Funct.* 6(5):1675–83.

[170] Umesalma, S., P. Nagendraprabhu, G. Sudhandiran (2015) Ellagic acid inhibits proliferation and induced apoptosis via the Akt signaling pathway in HCT-15 colon adenocarcinoma cells. *Mol Cell Biochem.* 399(1–2):303–13.

[171] Huang, R.F., Y.J. Wei, B.S. Inbaraj, B.H. Chen (2015) Inhibition of colon cancer cell growth by nanoemulsion carrying gold nanoparticles and lycopene. *Int J Nanomed.* 10:2823–46.

[172] Trejo-Solís, C., J. Pedraza-Chaverrí, M. Torres-Ramos, D. Jiménez-Farfán, A. Cruz Salgado, N. Serrano-García, L. Osorio-Rico, J. Sotelo (2013) Multiple molecular and cellular mechanisms of action of lycopene in cancer inhibition. *Evid Based Complementary and Alternative Medicine* (2013) Article ID 705121, 17 p., http://dx.doi.org/ 10.1155/2013/705121.

[173] Stefanska, B., H. Karlic, F. Varga, K. Fabianowska-Majewska, A.G. Haslberger (2012) Epigenetic mechanisms in anti-cancer actions of bioactive food components—the implications in cancer prevention. *Br J Pharmacol.* 167:279–297.

[174] Choi, K., M.G. Jung, Y.H. Lee, J.C. Yoon, S.H. Kwon, H.B. Kang, M.J. Kim, J.H. Cha, Y.J. Kim, W.J. Jun, J.M. Lee, H.G. Yoon (2009) Epigallocatechin-3-gallate, a histone acetyltransferase inhibitor, inhibits EBV-induced B lymphocyte transformation via suppression of RelA acetylation. *Cancer Res.* 69(2):583–92.

[175] Eberhart, C.E., R.J. Coffey, A. Radhika, F.M. Giardiello, S. Ferrenbach, R.N. DuBois (1994) Up-regulation of cyclooxygenase-2 gene-expression in human colorectal adenomas and adenocarcinomas. *Gastroenterology.* 107:1183–8.

[176] Saldanha, S.N., R. Kala, T.O. Tollefsbol (2014) Molecular mechanisms for inhibition of colon cancer cells by combined epigenetic-modulating epigallocatechin gallate and sodium butyrate. *Exp Cell Res.* 324(1):40–53.

[177] Ho, E., J.D. Clarke, R.H. Dashwood (2009) Dietary sulforaphane, a histone deacetylase inhibitor for cancer prevention. *J Nutr.* 139:2393–2396.

[178] Myzak, M.C., W.M. Dashwood, G.A. Orner, E. Ho, R.H. Dashwood (2006) Sulforaphane inhibits histone deacetylase in vivo and suppresses tumorigenesis in Apc-minus mice. *FASEB J.* 20(3):506–508.

[179] Traka, M., A. Gasper, J. Smith, C. Hawkey, Y. Bao, R. Mithen (2005) Transcriptome analysis of human colon Caco-2 cells exposed to sulforaphane. *J Nutr.* 135:1865–1872.

[180] Slaby, O., M. Sachlova, V. Brezkova, R. Hezova, A. Kovarikova, S. Bischofová, S. Sevcikova, J. Bienertova-Vasku, A. Vasku, M. Svoboda, R. Vyzula (2013) Identification of microRNAs regulated by isothiocyanates and association of polymorphisms inside their target sites with risk of sporadic colorectal cancer. *Nutr Cancer.* 65:247–254.

[181] Kaeberlein, M., T. McDonagh, B. Heltweg, J. Hixon, E.A. Westman, S.D. Caldwell, A. Napper, R. Curtis, P.S. DiStefano, S. Fields, A. Bedalov, B.K. Kennedy (2005) Substrate-specific activation of sirtuins by resveratrol. *J Biol Chem.* 280(17):17038–45.

[182] Tili, E, J.J. Michaille, H. Alder, S. Volinia, D. Delmas, N. Latruffe, C.M. Croce (2010) Resveratrol modulates the levels of microRNAs targeting genes encoding tumor-suppressors and effectors of TGF-beta signaling pathway in sw480 cells. *Biochem Pharmacol.* 80:2057–2065.

[183] Kumazaki, M., S. Noguchi, Y. Yasui, J. Iwasaki, H. Shinohara, N. Yamada, et al. (2013) Anti-cancer effects of naturally occurring compounds through modulation of signal transduction and miRNA expression in human colon cancer cells. *J Nutr Biochem.* 24:1849–1858.

[184] Del Follo-Martinez, A., N. Banerjee, X. Li, S. Safe, S. Mertens-Talcott (2013) Resveratrol and quercetin in combination have anticancer activity in colon cancer cells and repress oncogenic microRNA-27a. *Nutr Cancer.* 65:494–504.

[185] Knop, C., J. Putnik, M. Scheuermann, M. Schmitz (2010) Cutting Edge Technologies: Cell Analysis/2010, B. Ziebolz, ed., Springer Medizin, Springer Verlag, Heidelberg, Germany, 4–13, 58–68, 137–141.

[186] Hotnog, D., M. Mihaila, A. Botezatu, G.G. Matei, C. Hotnog, G. Anton, M. Bostan, L.I. Brasoveanu (2013) Genistein potentiates the apoptotic effect of 5-fluorouracyl in colon cancer cell lines. *Rom Biotechnol Lett.* 18(6):8751–8760.

[187] Hotnog, D., M. Mihaila, I.V. Iancu, G.G. Matei, C. Hotnog, G. Anton, M. Bostan, L.I. Brasoveanu (2013) Resveratrol modulates apoptosis in 5-fluorouracyl treated colon cancer cell lines. *Roum Arch Microbiol Immunol.* 72(4):255–264.

[188] Ivanov, K., N. Kolev, I. Shterev, A. Tonev, V. Ignatov, V. Bojkov, T. Kirilova (2014) Adjuvant treatment in colorectal cancer. *"Colorectal Cancer—Surgery, Diagnostics and Treatment"*, 305–328, InTech, Croatia, Jim S. Khan Ed., ISBN 978-953-51-1231-0.

[189] Nita, M.E., H. Nagawa, O. Tominaga, N. Tsuno, S. Fujii, S. Sasaki, C.G. Fu, T. Takenoue, T. Tsuruo, T. Muto (1998) 5-fluorouracil induces apoptosis in human colon cancer cell lines with modulation of Bcl-2 family proteins. *Br J Cancer.* 78(8):986–992.

[190] Wolmark, N., H. Rockette, B. Fisher, D.L. Wickerham, C. Redmond, E.R. Fisher, J. Jones, E.P. Mamounas, L. Ore, N.J. Petrelli, et al. (1993) The benefit of leucovorin-modulated fluorouracil as postoperative adjuvant therapy for primary colon cancer: results from National Surgical Adjuvant Breast and Bowel Project protocol C-03. *J Clin Oncol.* 11(10): 1879–87.

[191] Lowe, S.W., H.E. Ruley, T. Jacks, D.E. Housman (1993) p53-dependent apoptosis modulates the cytotoxicity of anticancer agents. *Cell.* 74(6):957–67.

[192] Piazza, G.A., A.K. Rahm, T.S. Finn, B.H. Fryer, H. Li, A.L. Stoumen, R. Pamukcu, D.J. Ahnen (1997) Apoptosis primarily accounts for the growth-inhibitory properties of

sulindac metabolites and involves a mechanism that is independent of cyclooxygenase inhibition, cell cycle arrest, and p53 induction. *Cancer Res.* 57:2452–59.

[193] Violette, S., L. Poulain, E. Dussaulx, D. Pepin, A.M. Faussat, J. Chambaz, J.M. Lacorte, C. Staedel, T. Lesuffleur (2002) Resistance of colon cancer cells to long-term 5-fluorouracil exposure is correlated to the relative level of Bcl-2 and Bcl-XL in addition to Bax and p53 status. *Int J Cancer.* 98(4):498–504.

[194] Zhang, N., Y. Yin, S.J. Xu, W.S. Chen (2008) 5-Fluorouracil: mechanisms of resistance and reversal strategies. *Molecules.* 13(8):1551–1569.

[195] Tomé-Carneiro, J., M. Larrosa, A. González-Sarrías, F.A. Tomás-Barberán, M.T. García-Conesa, J.C. Espín (2013) Resveratrol and clinical trials: the crossroad from in vitro studies to human evidence. *Curr Pharm Des.* 19(34):6064–6093.

Permissions

The contributors of this book come from diverse backgrounds, making this book a truly international effort. This book will bring forth new frontiers with its revolutionizing research information and detailed analysis of the nascent developments around the world.

We would like to thank all the contributing authors for lending their expertise to make the book truly unique. They have played a crucial role in the development of this book. Without their invaluable contributions this book wouldn't have been possible. They have made vital efforts to compile up to date information on the varied aspects of this subject to make this book a valuable addition to the collection of many professionals and students.

This book was conceptualized with the vision of imparting up-to-date information and advanced data in this field. To ensure the same, a matchless editorial board was set up. Every individual on the board went through rigorous rounds of assessment to prove their worth. After which they invested a large part of their time researching and compiling the most relevant data for our readers.

The editorial board has been involved in producing this book since its inception. They have spent rigorous hours researching and exploring the diverse topics which have resulted in the successful publishing of this book. They have passed on their knowledge of decades through this book. To expedite this challenging task, the publisher supported the team at every step. A small team of assistant editors was also appointed to further simplify the editing procedure and attain best results for the readers.

Apart from the editorial board, the designing team has also invested a significant amount of their time in understanding the subject and creating the most relevant covers. They scrutinized every image to scout for the most suitable representation of the subject and create an appropriate cover for the book.

The publishing team has been an ardent support to the editorial, designing and production team. Their endless efforts to recruit the best for this project, has resulted in the accomplishment of this book. They are a veteran in the field of academics and their pool of knowledge is as vast as their experience in printing. Their expertise and guidance has proved useful at every step. Their uncompromising quality standards have made this book an exceptional effort. Their encouragement from time to time has been an inspiration for everyone.

The publisher and the editorial board hope that this book will prove to be a valuable piece of knowledge for researchers, students, practitioners and scholars across the globe.

List of Contributors

Monica Ortenzi, Giovanni Lezoche, Roberto Ghiselli and Mario Guerrieri
Polytechnic University of Marche, Surgical Clinic, United Hospitals, Ancona, Italy

Paul Mitrut, Anca Oana Docea, Adina Maria Kamal, Radu Mitrut, Daniela Calina, Eliza Go ita, Vlad Padureanu, Corina Gruia and Liliana Streba
University of Medicine and Pharmacy of Craiova, Craiova, Romania

Yumi Z. H-Y. Hashim and Phirdaous Abbas
Department of Biotechnology Engineering, Kulliyyah of Engineering, International Islamic University Malaysia, Kuala Lumpur, Malaysia

Cheryl Latimer, Nigel Ternan and Chris I. R. Gill
School of Biomedical Sciences, Ulster University, Northern Ireland, United Kingdom

Valentin Ignatov, Anton Tonev, Nikola Kolev, Aleksandar Zlatarov, Shteryu Shterev, Dilyan Petrov, Tanya Kirilova and Krasimir Ivanov
Department of General and Operative Surgery, Medical University of Varna, Varna, Bulgaria

Zodwa Dlamini, Thandeka Khoza, Rodney Hull, Mpho Choene and Zilungile Mkhize-Kwitshana
Research, Innovation & Engagements Portfolio, Mangosuthu University of Technology, Durban, South Africa

Sandra Ríos-Arrabal and Francisco Artacho-Cordón
Department of Radiology and Physical Medicine, University of Granada, Granada, Spain,
Biosanitary Research Institute, Granada, Spain

José Antonio Muñoz-Gámez, Sergio Manuel Jiménez-Ruíz and Jorge Casado-Ruíz
Clinical Management Unit of Digestive Disease and Research Support Unit, San Cecilio
University Hospital Granada, Spain;
Biosanitary Research Institute Granada, Spain

Josefa León-López
Clinical Management Unit of Digestive Disease and Research Support Unit, San Cecilio
University Hospital Granada, Spain;
Biosanitary Research Institute Granada, Spain;
Ciber of Hepatic and Digestive Diseases (CIBERehd), Madrid, Spain

Serife Koc
Karamanoglu Mehmetbey University, Karaman School of Health, Karaman, Turkey

Melek Nihal Esin and Aysun Ardic
Istanbul University, Florence Nightingale Faculty of Nursing, Istanbul, Turkey

Gabriel Mak, Michele Moschetta and Hendrik-Tobias Arkenau
Sarah Cannon Research Institute, London, UK

Hendrik-Tobias Arkenau
University College London, London, UK

Valentin Ignatov, Anton Tonev, Nikola Kolev, Aleksandar Zlatarov, Shteryu Shterev, Tanya Kirilova and Krasimir Ivanov
Department of General and Operative Surgery, Medical University Varna, Bulgaria

Marinela Bostan, Mirela Mihaila, Camelia Hotnog, Viviana Roman and Lorelei Irina Brasoveanu
Center of Immunology Dept., "Stefan S. Nicolau" Institute of Virology, Bucharest, Romania

Coralia Bleotu
Cellular and Molecular Pathology Dept., "Stefan S. Nicolau" Institute of Virology, Bucharest, Romania

Gabriela Anton
Molecular Virology Dept., "Stefan S. Nicolau" Institute of Virology, Bucharest, Romania

Index